Clarence W. Donnelly, R.T.

PRINCIPLES OF

RADIOGRAPHIC EXPOSURE

AND

PROCESSING

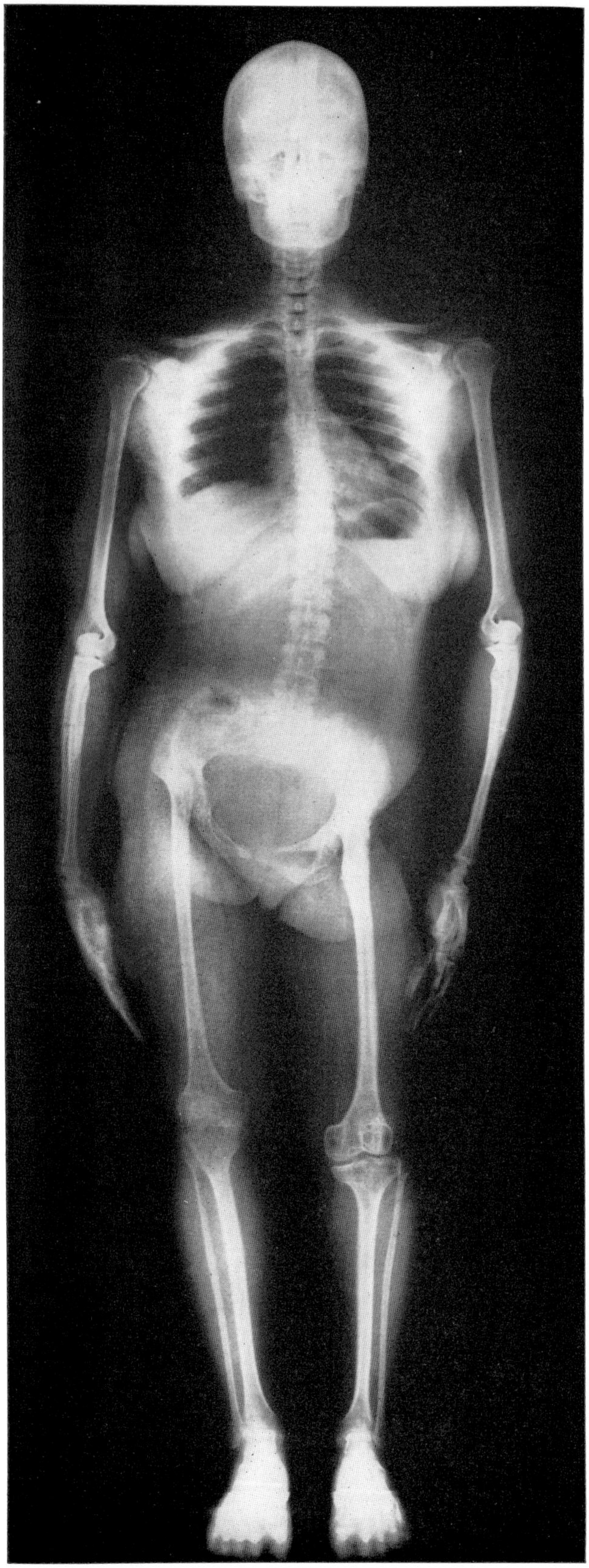

Figure 1. *Frontispiece.* X-ray film has been prepared in many sizes for medical work. The largest film (32 by 72 inches) used was for entire body radiography of a woman, aged thirty-three, exhibiting hip pathology. The radiograph was made with a one-second exposure, 75 KvP, 150 Ma., 12 feet focus-film distance, fast screens, and tissue compensating filtration.

(Second Edition, Eleventh Printing)

PRINCIPLES OF

RADIOGRAPHIC EXPOSURE AND PROCESSING

By

ARTHUR W. FUCHS

CHARLES C THOMAS • PUBLISHER
Springfield • Illinois • U.S.A.

Published and Distributed Throughout the World by
CHARLES C THOMAS • PUBLISHER
BANNERSTONE HOUSE
301-327 East Lawrence Avenue, Springfield, Illinois, U.S.A.

ISBN 0-398-00627-X

Library of Congress Catalog Card Number: 57-10431

First Edition, United States Printing Office, 1955
Second Edition, First Printing, Charles C Thomas, Publisher, 1958, 5000 copies
Second Edition, Second Printing, 1964, 2500 copies
Second Edition, Third Printing, 1966, 2500 copies
Second Edition, Fourth Printing, 1967, 2500 copies
Second Edition, Fifth Printing, 1968, 2500 copies
Second Edition, Sixth Printing, 1969, 2500 copies
Second Edition, Seventh Printing, 1970, 2500 copies
Second Edition, Eighth Printing, 1971, 2500 copies
Second Edition, Ninth Printing, 1972, 2500 copies
Second Edition, Tenth Printing, 1973, 5000 copies
Second Edition, Eleventh Printing, 1974, 5000 copies

With THOMAS BOOKS *careful attention is given to all details of manufacturing and design. It is the Publisher's desire to present books that are satisfactory as to their physical qualities and artistic possibilities and appropriate for their particular use.* THOMAS BOOKS *will be true to those laws of quality that assure a good name and good will.*

Printed in the United States of America
P-4

TO

WOLFRAM CONRAD FUCHS

Roentgen Pioneer

1865-1907

Preface

Principles of Radiographic Exposure and Processing is an outgrowth of the need for training x-ray technicians at an accelerated rate during World War II at the School for Medical Department Technicians, U. S. Army, Washington, D. C. Since that time, the methods, as taught, have crystallized as a result of presenting the subject matter in the form of refresher courses at a number of medical schools, hospitals, and the X-ray Branch of the Army Service School, Fort Sam Houston, Texas and before various radiological groups.

The approach employed in teaching the subject of x-ray exposure may be considered unorthodox, for it aims to make the theory and application of x-ray exposure factors singularly practical. Complex subject matter is treated in a thoroughly uncomplicated manner and only a small amount of mathematics is employed to solve a few problems. The original version of this text is currently contained in two U. S. Army training manuals, *X-ray Film Processing* and *Principles of Radiographic Exposure*. It was at the invitation of the late Lt. Col. Burt N. Coers, MC, and the encouragement of Col. C. G. Gruber, MSC, that these manuals were prepared.

For the many helpful suggestions, as a result of reading the text, my thanks and appreciation are sincerely extended to Rex B. Wilsey, formerly of the Kodak Research Laboratories and the late Aubrey O. Hampton, M.D. To the many radiologists and x-ray technicians who have stimulated me in the production of this book, I am grateful.

The purpose of any x-ray examination is to assist in the solution of a medical or surgical problem, i.e., to procure diagnostic information. The radiograph constitutes the record and it must satisfy one prime requisite—that of depicting all anatomical details of the body part being examined in such a way as to make possible a diagnosis. It is not an anatomical snapshot taken at random. To obtain this record, the examination is begun with x-ray film and ends with film. The x-ray apparatus exposes the film and the processing solutions transforms the exposed x-ray film into the radiograph. The making of a radiograph is essentially a photographic process. The exposure of the x-ray film, and the resulting physical and chemical activity leading to the formation of the latent image and the processing of the film to produce a visible silver image, is a very complex process. Fortunately, standardization of the several operations in the production of the image greatly simplifies the entire procedure.

Radiography should entail the use of standardized apparatus and projection technics so that all operations will consume a minimum of time. The excellent quality of x-ray film and processing solutions, today, aids materially when standardized exposures are employed to yield radiographs of the best quality. The training of x-ray technicians should include comprehensive and detailed instruction in the fundamentals of radiographic exposure and processing so that satisfactory radiography can be performed irrespective of assignment. The purpose of this text, therefore, is to describe the principles of radiographic exposure and x-ray film processing by means of theory, experiment, and application.

Radiographic results, whether good or poor, usually are unintelligible to the student technician. For that reason he must be made acquainted early with the kind of radiograph that is most useful to the radiologist—one that possesses correct diagnostic quality. The student cannot acquire that knowledge except by actually making radiographs under guidance and then, during a film clinic, have demonstrated to him *why* the quality is or is not satisfactory. This type of instruction instills immeasurable self-confidence in the student.

To facilitate this sort of training, a simple though exact exposure system is described which is based upon proved fundamental theories and practices. Wherever possible, the exposure factors have been reduced to constants, thereby eliminating many sources of possible error. This system permits the student to quickly become acquainted with better-than-average quality radiographs that can be produced during the course of his instruction.

The operations necessary to the correct handling and chemical treatment of exposed x-ray film to convert it to a radiograph are discussed in detail. The text serves as a guide for the x-ray technician and radiologist to the accepted procedures for the production of good quality radiographs from properly exposed x-ray film. Correct processing is an important function in radiography, for the procurement of uniformity in result is dependent not only upon the exposure technic employed but also upon the care with which the film is processed.

If this text assists the x-ray technician in the production of better radiographs of sick people, it has accomplished its mission.

A. W. F.

Rochester 19, New York

Contents

PART II

X-RAY FILM PROCESSING

PRINCIPLES OF

RADIOGRAPHIC EXPOSURE

AND

PROCESSING

Part I

Radiographic Exposure

Chapter 1

X-Rays

A SATISFACTORY UNDERSTANDING of exposure and processing terms requires at least a limited knowledge of x-rays and their characteristics. X-rays are a form of invisible radiant energy and were discovered by Wilhelm Conrad Röntgen on November 8, 1895. They are quite similar to light in their general properties since they travel at the same speed and obey many of the same laws. A distinguishing feature of x-rays, however, is their extremely short wave length—only about one ten-thousandth the wave length of *visible* light. It is this property that is responsible for the x-rays' ability to penetrate materials that ordinarily would absorb or reflect light.

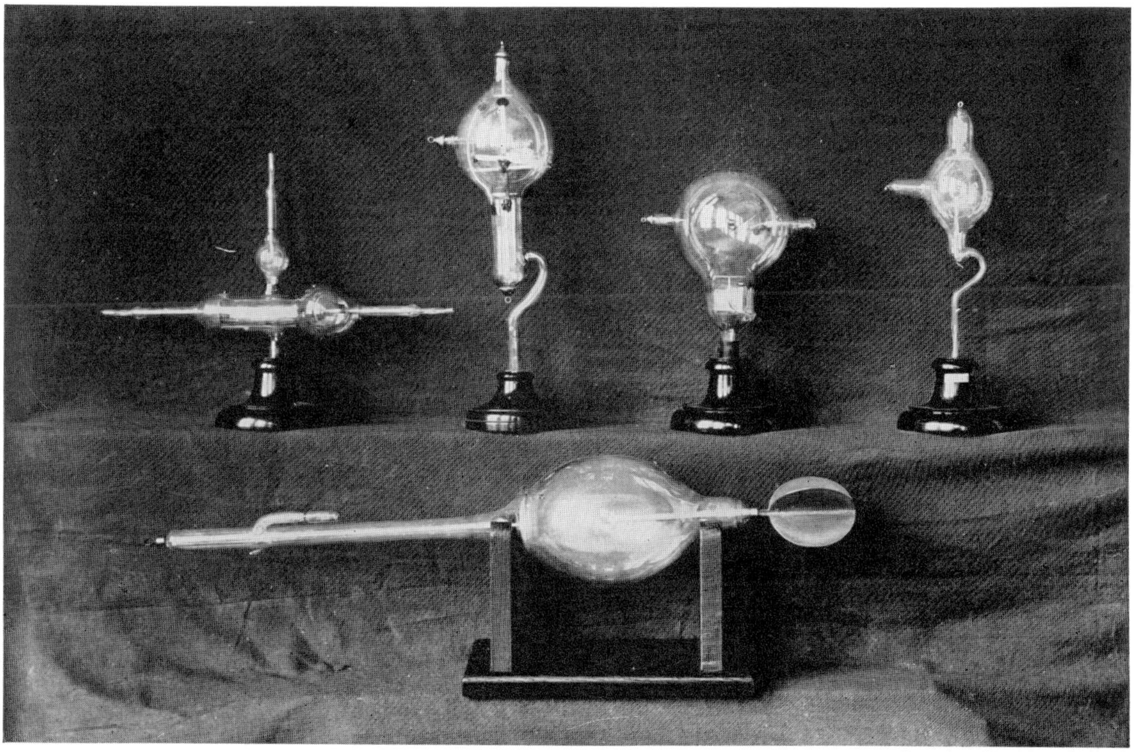

Deutches Museum—Munich

Figure 2. Photograph of the gas discharge tubes employed by Röntgen in his experiments that led to his discovery of the x-rays.

GENERATION OF X-RAYS

The generation of x-rays is a complex process. Fortunately, a knowledge of only a few of the principles is necessary. The essential feature of x-ray production is the striking of matter by high speed electrons; this may occur within or outside a vacuum. Basically, the device in which x-rays are generated is the x-ray tube.

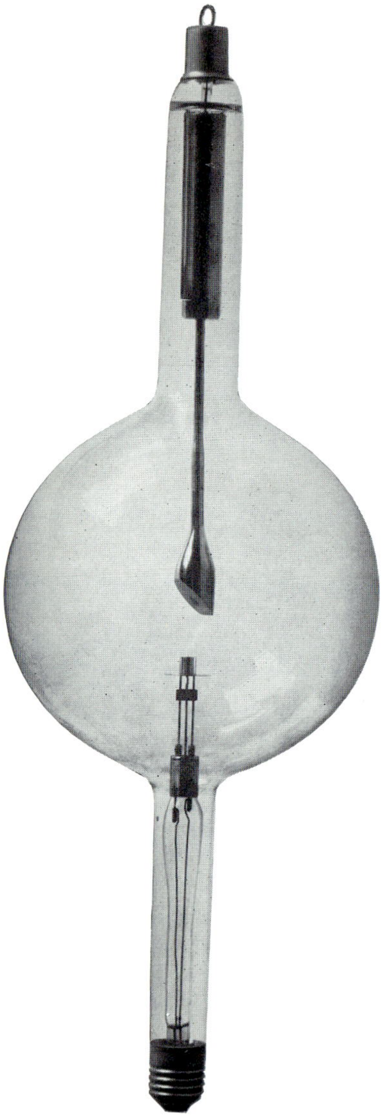

Figure 3. Photograph of an early Coolidge stationary anode tube in which the electrons originate in a heated tungsten filament.

X-rays are produced in an x-ray tube when electrons, traveling at great speed in a high vacuum, under stress of high voltage, collide with a metallic target of high molecular weight such as tungsten. The efficiency of production of x-rays is very small, for only about one part in a thousand of electron energy at average kilovoltages is converted into x-rays that are penetrating enough to make a radiograph; the balance of energy is dissipated as heat.

The x-ray tubes employed by the early workers contained gas under low pressure. These tubes were known as Crookes or Hittorf tubes. Röntgen's early tubes (Figure 2) were of the Crookes type which consisted of a pear-shaped glass tube filled with air under reduced pressure. An aluminum cathode was installed in the small end of the tube and, through a stem of glass on the side of the tube was inserted an aluminum anode.

When a high voltage current was passed between the cathode and anode, the residual gas in the tube became ionized and a stream of electrons was repelled by the cathode. Many of these electrons were attracted to the anode because of its location in the tube, but the majority of the electrons were bombarded against the glass at the end of the tube. The sudden stoppage of the electrons against the glass produced x-rays.

When the Jackson *focus* tube was made, the electron stream was focused on to a metal anode inclined at an angle so that a larger amount of radiation could be concentrated on a particular area.

Maintenance of a constant pressure in the early gas tubes was almost impossible for the pressure would vary with each use of the tube. These early tubes were quite erratic. The advent of the Coolidge hot cathode x-ray tube made possible the generation of a constant source of x-rays that could be easily duplicated at will. This tube was invented by Dr. W. D. Coolidge of the General Electric Company and announced December 27, 1913 (Figure 3).

X-RAY TUBE

The modern x-ray tube consists of a highly evacuated glass bulb into which are sealed two electrodes — the cathode, or *negative* electrode (the source of electrons), and the anode, or *positive* electrode (the source of x-rays). The degree of vacuum of the x-ray tube and the arrangement of the electrodes are such that no electrical discharge between the cathode and the anode is possible until the filament in the cathode is heated (Figure 4).

Electron Emission

Employing the principle that all *hot* bodies emit electrons, a spiral, incandescent filament of tungsten wire is incorporated in the cathode of the usual form of x-ray tube. This filament is heated by a current of low amperage from a low voltage step-down transformer. The temperature of the filament, as governed by the amount of current that passes through it, controls the number of electrons emitted—the higher the filament temperature, the greater the electron emission. Because of its small mass an electron rapidly develops greater speed in an electric field. Surrounding the filament is a shield that serves to focus the electron stream from the heated filament to the *focal spot* on the tungsten target located at the end of the anode. The stream of electrons from cathode to anode constitutes the tube current and is measured in milliamperes. The electron stream is propelled by high-voltage electricity impressed on the tube electrodes by a high-voltage transformer. This voltage, which may be varied at will, regulates the *speed* with which the electrons cross the gap between the cathode and the anode. Thousands of volts (kilovolts) are normally used for this purpose. The stream of electrons forms a conducting path for the high voltage current to reach the anode. Upon impact with the focal spot of the tube, the electrons produce a stream of x-rays which are emitted over a 180° angle from the focal spot of the target.

X-ray Wave Length

Despite the enormous energy in the electron stream, only a small portion is converted to x-rays; the bulk is dissipated as heat at the anode. The greater the force of impact of the electrons on the focal spot, the shorter is the wave length of the x-rays produced and the more readily do they penetrate the object being examined. In other words, the higher the voltage, the

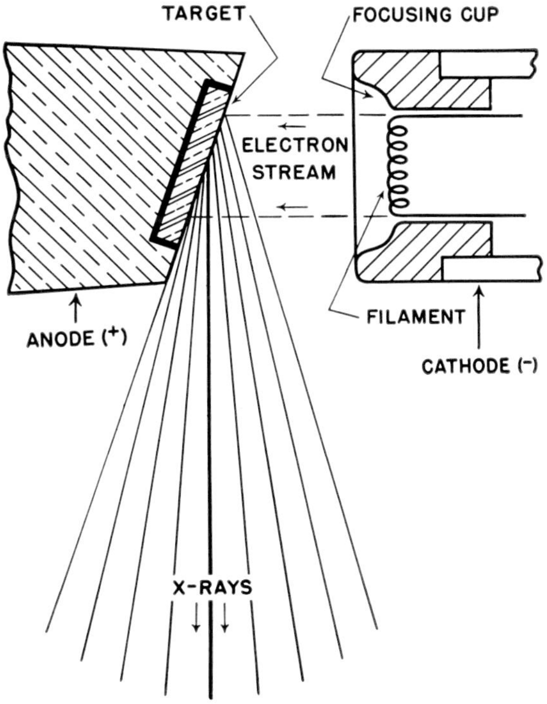

Figure 4. Diagram of the essential elements of a modern x-ray tube wherein electrons generated by a heated filament in the cathode are bombarded against a tungsten target in the anode, resulting in x-ray production.

greater is the speed of the electrons striking the focal spot. The result is a decrease in wave length of the x-rays emitted and an increase in both their intensity and penetrating power. Wave lengths are measured in *ångstrom (Å) units;* an ångstrom unit is equal to 10^{-8} centimeter. The useful range of wave lengths for medical radiography is approximately 0.50 to 0.100 *ångstrom units.*

The Roentgen

Defined and adopted in 1937, the *roentgen* is the international unit of quantity for both x-rays and gamma rays. It is designated by the symbol *r*.

PROPERTIES OF X-RAYS

Although x-rays exhibit all of the properties of visible light, and many similarities between light and x-rays may be readily noted, the effects produced are so different that it is preferable to consider the properties of x-rays separately from other types of radiation. For example, light is refracted by glass and, consequently, is capable of being focused by a lens in such instruments as cameras, microscopes, etc. X-rays can also be refracted, but to such a very slight degree that it requires the most refined apparatus to detect this phenomenon. Hence, the use of any kind of lens is quite out of the question.

An outstanding characteristic of the x-rays is their ability to penetrate matter of any kind. They are also able to expose photographic film, which makes radiography possible. When lengthy exposures are employed, x-rays have the power to change the color of many chemicals. Another important characteristic is the ability of x-rays to excite fluorescence in many substances, such as barium platino-cyanide, zinc sulfide, calcium tungstate, and many others. This fact makes possible the use of fluoroscopic and intensifying screens made with these substances for fluoroscopy, or for reducing the x-ray exposure in radiography. X-rays are a powerful agent in the treatment of cancer and other diseases. Air can be ionized by x-rays—a principle employed in the *r*-meter or ionization chamber used for measuring various kinds of x-radiation.

THE X-RAY BEAM

The x-ray beam may be likened to the *reflected* light from an object that passes through the lens of a camera to expose a photographic film. The x-ray beam, however, *passes through* the human body or object to expose the x-ray film.

The x-ray beam (Figure 5) may be divided into two parts, the *primary* beam and the *remnant* beam.

Primary Radiation

The primary radiation (PR) is confined to the portion of the x-ray beam emitted from the focal spot (FS) of the x-ray tube. It is not materially altered in its quality nor in its intensity as it passes toward the object (OB) being examined despite the fact that it usually passes through an aluminum filter that absorbs some of the longer wave lengths of radiation which are not needed in medical radiography. This filter is employed as a safety measure for the patient.

Remnant Radiation

The remnant radiation (RR) is that portion of the primary radiation that emerges from the body tissues to expose the x-ray

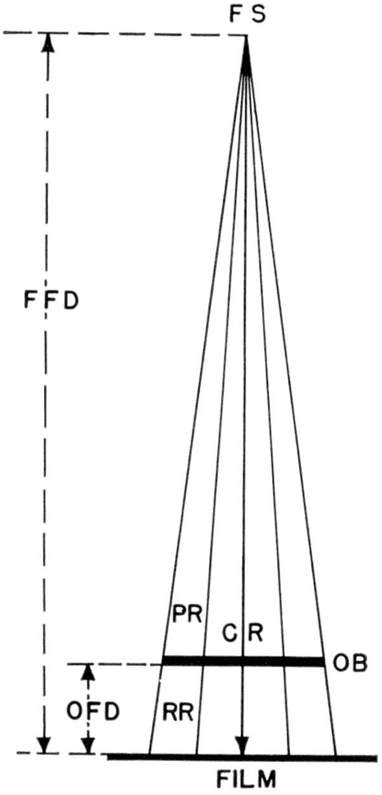

Figure 5. Diagram illustrating the various components of an x-ray beam with relation to an object and an x-ray film.

film and record the radiographic image. Actually, the remnant radiation is primary radiation that has been selectively diminished in intensity by reason of absorption as it passed through the body tissues. It is the *image-forming* radiation. The remnant radiation also contains secondary radiation emitted by the tissues, the amount depending upon its wave length and the manner in which it is controlled.

The Central Ray

The central ray (CR) is the center of the x-ray beam. The term is employed in describing the direction of the x-rays in a given projection. The course of the central ray may be considered to extend from the focal spot of the x-ray tube to the x-ray film. The entire distance traversed by the central ray is known as the focus-film distance (FFD). The distance from the object or body part of the x-ray film measured along the course of the central ray is known as the object-film distance (OFD).

Secondary Radiation

When x-rays strike any form of matter (Figure 6), such as body tissue, apparatus, etc., secondary x-rays (SR) are produced that possess the same and longer wave lengths than the primary radiation. Since secondary radiation is unfocused and may come from any direction, its action on the film is such that it may cover the entire image with a veil of fog unless it is well controlled by certain accessories employed during the exposure. Radiographically, fog tends to destroy contrast, hence makes the

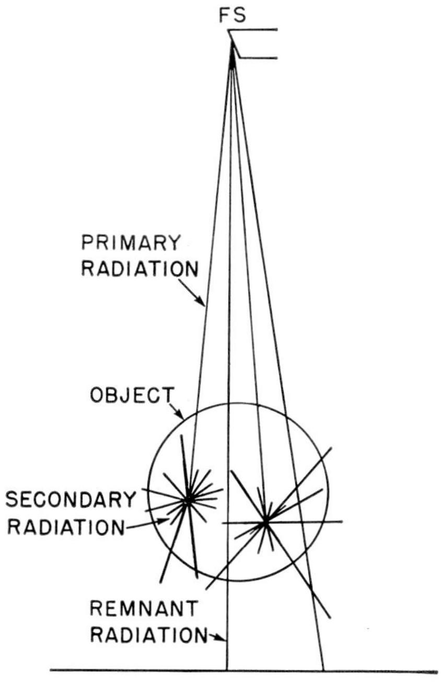

Figure 6. Diagram illustrating manner in which secondary radiation is generated when x-rays strike any form of matter.

visualization of image details more difficult.

Filtered Radiation

When any material such as a sheet of aluminum is placed in the x-ray beam at the x-ray portal of the x-ray tube, the quality of the emergent radiation is altered. Since sheet aluminum is a common type of filtering material in radiography, the longer wave lengths tend to be absorbed by the filter. As the thickness of the filter increases, more and more of the long wave lengths are filtered out and only the shorter wave lengths emerge.

Filtered radiation tends to reduce the dosage of the more damaging long wave length radiation to the patient. Under no circumstances should radiography be performed without a filter at the x-ray tube portal. The degree of x-ray absorption when employing one millimeter of aluminum as a filter has no discernible radiographic effect, but the filter is a highly valuable protective element to the patient.

Chapter 2

Radiographic Terms

THE NOMENCLATURE of x-ray exposure comprises electrical and sundry terms that are commonly employed under the general designation of *radiographic factors.* Each of the factors listed below influences the character of the radiographic image. The terms employed in this text, together with their respective symbols, should be thoroughly memorized.

Term	*Symbol*
1. Central ray	CR
2. Focal spot	FS
3. Focus-film distance	FFD
4. Kilovolts peak	KvP
5. Milliamperes	Ma
6. Milliampere-seconds	MaS
7. Object-film distance	OFD
8. Primary radiation	PR
9. Remnant radiation	RR
10. Secondary radiation	SR
11. Time of exposure in seconds	S

There are several items of apparatus that, when used, have a definite influence on the radiographic image. Through usage, these accessories are usually considered together with the actual exposure factors.

Screens. X-ray intensifying screens in cassettes are employed to augment the exposure effect of the x-rays. (See Chapter 14.)

Cone. The cone is a device that limits the size of the x-ray beam irradiating the body part and should be employed for all projections.

Stationary Grid. The stationary grid is a device used to prevent secondary radiation generated in the body from reaching the x-ray film.

Potter-Bucky Diaphragm. The Potter-Bucky (P-B) diaphragm is a device similar to the stationary grid, but it is mechanized so that it will move during the exposure. Its function also is to absorb secondary radiation.

ELECTRICAL TERMS

There are various electrical terms employed in radiography which should be known. Electricity, like water, is capable of flowing through a conductor, and this flow or *current* is measured in *amperes.* However, the ampere is too large a unit to employ in radiography and the *milliampere* ($1/1000$ ampere) is used instead. For electricity to flow, it must be under pressure; the unit of pressure is the *volt.* Thousands of volts are required when making exposures and the term usually employed is the *kilovolt* (1000 volts). The number of amperes or volts respectively does not indicate the amount of power in a circuit; however, when volts and amperes are multiplied, the product is the unit of power called the *watt.* Thousands of watts are used by x-ray apparatus, therefore, the term *kilowatt* (1000 *watts*) is more commonly employed. The term *milliampere-seconds* (MaS) is the product of the milliamperage (Ma) and time of exposure in seconds (S).

PHOTOGRAPHIC TERMS

To describe the various characteristics of the finished radiograph, a few terms of photographic origin are in common use. These terms and their definitions are as follows:

RADIOGRAPHIC DENSITY

Radiographic density is the resultant deposit of black metallic silver on the x-ray film after x-ray exposure and processing. Details of the elements of tissue examined are rendered as deposits of black metallic silver of various concentrations.

TONE VALUE

The degree of silver concentration determines the brightness or *tone* value of each radiographic density as viewed on a standard x-ray illuminator.

RADIOGRAPHIC CONTRAST

Radiographic contrast is the condition under which two or more densities (tones) can be compared in the image when viewed on a standard x-ray illuminator. There are two general types of contrast seen in medical radiography:

1. Short-scale Contrast

When the range of image densities is short and each density exhibits a large tonal difference from its neighbor, short-scale contrast exists. It is not often useful in medical radiography.

2. Long-scale Contrast

When the range of image densities is wide and great in number, and each density exhibits relatively small difference from its neighbor, long-scale contrast prevails. This scale of contrast is ideal for medical radiography.

Chapter 3

X-Ray Film

Radiography is photography.* The only dissimilarity between them is the means employed for exposing the film and producing a latent image. In photography, visible light is employed; and, in radiography, invisible light. It is then a matter of wave length. The longer wave lengths, of course, occur in visible light, and the very short wave lengths in x-rays, gamma radiation, etc. But the manner in which an x-ray film is exposed is fundamentally the same in photography as in radiography, i.e., by means of radiant energy.

> Of especial interest in many ways is the fact that photographic dry plates show themselves susceptible to x-rays. We are thus in a position to corroborate many phenomena in which mistakes are easy, and I have, whenever possible, controlled each important ocular observation in fluorescence by means of photography.

Thus, Röntgen's original communication indicated the importance of the photographic plate as a means of *recording* the x-ray image and opened the way to a new science — radiography. He demonstrated this point by showing the first radiograph, one of Mrs. Röntgen's hand, and also the first one taken through metal, which showed a compass card and needle enclosed in a metal case.

In radiography, one starts with x-ray film and ends with x-ray film. The apparatus, the positioning, etc., are agents in the production of the radiographic image. The technician's job is to take x-ray film and put the maximum amount of diagnostic information on it—that is what the radiologist is interested in. Also, one should not produce an image that is only partially informative. What must be accomplished is the production of an image of a given body part that includes all of the anatomy required for the diagnosis. It is most important, therefore, that the x-ray film to be used should be one that will help to achieve this objective.

Since radiography made use of photographic emulsions as recording media, the history of x-ray film actually reaches back into the beginning of photography itself when it was observed that certain salts of silver responded to the action of light.

* Photography is the art or process of obtaining images on sensitized surfaces by the action of light or other radiant energy. (*Encyclopedia Americana*, 1955.)

BEGINNINGS OF PHOTOGRAPHY

In the early 18th century it became known that some silver compounds blackened when exposed to light; thus began the art of photography. In 1727, a German chemist, John H. Schultz, discovered that a paste of silver carbonate or chloride mixed with chalk became dark when it was exposed to light in a glass tube. After stencils of letters were placed on the tube and the material exposed to sunlight, black lettered images were seen when the stencils were removed. However, these images were only transient; since he knew of no way to make them permanent, the areas originally protected from light eventually darkened.

Further investigation of this phenomenon followed the direction of satisfying man's innate longing for pictures—a desire to capture the beauties of nature in its many existent forms, family life and all it entailed as a matter of sentiment, and as a matter of record. So it was that the fundamentals of photography were gradually, though energetically, pieced together that man might record the present in permanent form by his photographic handiwork.

In 1802, Thomas Wedgewood and Sir Humphrey Davy recorded silhouettes on glass by contact printing on paper coated with silver chloride. A crude camera was made in 1816 by Joseph N. Niepce from a jewel box in which a lens from a microscope was inserted. With this device, he secured an image. None of the images obtained could be made permanent. It was one thing to produce an image by exposing a silver salt to light. It was quite another to treat the image so that it would become permanent.

William Henry Fox Talbot, an Englishman, exposed silver chloride paper in a camera obscura to secure a visible image which was made permanent by treatment with sodium chloride. Talbot made an important discovery in 1840, when he found that he could develop a latent image after exposure of the silver layer. He obtained a negative image and by printing on sensitized paper was able to obtain positive images. Talbot became the inventor of the *negative-positive* method of photography. It is interesting to note that Sir John Herschel, an outstanding scientist of the period. wrote Talbot under the date of February 28, 1839, using the coined word "photography"—drawing with light—in referring to Talbot's work. He also coined the term *negative* and *positive* in reference to photographic images. The word "photography" then was acquired by the vocabulary of all languages.

In 1819, Herschel discovered the solvent action of hypo (sodium thiosulfate) on silver chloride. However, the Rev. J. B. Reade was the first (1937) to use sodium thiosulfate to dissolve the unexposed silver salts remaining in the photograph. This treatment prevented the possibility of the image darkening upon further exposure to light.

The Frenchman, Louis J. J. Daguerre, recorded images (1839) on plates covered with a silver salt that had been fumed with iodine to form a layer of silver iodide. Long exposures of these plates in a camera produced faint, unsatisfactory visual images. One day he placed one of the exposed plates in his cupboard. Upon removing the plate at a later date, he found that there was a well-defined positive image on the plate. Some mercury had been spilled in the cabinet and its fumes had "developed" the image completely. The unexposed silver iodide was removed by a solution of sodium chloride. Daguerre thereby discovered the phenomenon of development.

Paper negatives were used up to this time, but the grainy paper structure was reproduced on the prints. To overcome this condition, C. F. A. Niepce de St. Victor in 1847 coated glass with an albumen emulsion containing silver iodide. Gallic acid was used for developing and resulted in a good image of fine grain.

Frederick Scott-Archer, in 1851, published the details of a process wherein wet collodion was used as a binder for the silver salts and coated on glass. The exposure was made before the collodion dried. It soon superseded all other processes. However, the method was laborious and inconvenient. Many variations of the collodion process was tried but none was too satisfactory. Hence, various attempts were made to find a method of coating a plate that could be dried and perhaps stored until used.

The invention of the gelatin silver bromide *dry* plate (September 8, 1871), by Richard L. Maddox of England served as the basis for modern photography. These plates were slow and the salts often crystallized in the emulsion, since he did not realize the need for washing away the excess of silver salts. In 1873, J. Burgess manufactured the first practical dry plate with a washed emulsion. Also, in 1873, H. W. Vogel discovered that such plates normally sensitive to blue and violet light could be made sensitive to all colors by the addition of certain dyes.

Dry plates were found to be several times faster than the wet plate and soon were manufactured in several countries. At first, dry plates were coated by hand. The first mechanically coated glass plates were made in 1879 by George Eastman who had invented a plate-coating machine. Another product called *American Film* was introduced by Eastman in 1885. This was a stripping film which used paper as a temporary support for the emulsion. After exposure and processing, the paper was stripped away leaving a thin transparent "film" from which prints could be made. At this time also, Eastman began the manufacture of paper sensitized with an emulsion for use in cameras and called Eastman *Negative Paper.* After exposure and development, the paper was made transparent for printing by chemical treatment. In 1889, this firm introduced a flexible transparent base of nitrocellulose coated with a sensitive silver halide emulsion. This product served to advance photography greatly. Thenceforth, photosensitive materials became progressively more efficient as more knowledge concerning the science of photography accrued. Thus, the stage was set for one of man's most important discoveries wherein the photographic emulsion was to play a dominant role.

BIRTH OF RADIOGRAPHY

On November 8, 1895, Wilhelm Conrad Röntgen proved the existence of x-rays by exposing and processing a dry plate, thus opening to the world a vast new field of endeavor—radiography.

The moment of the actual discovery of the x-rays proved it to be the beginning of a new era. The very nature of the x-rays was such that the whole scientific and lay world would become absorbed in it, not alone by its very spectacular nature but also by the possibility that these new rays would open the door of knowledge to the ultimate nature of matter—something that had perplexed the best scientific minds. It was the dawn of the atomic age.

After the first few months of wild exaggeration and rumor, the discovery was stripped of its sensationalism and left to the conservative experimenter who rejoiced in the possibilities of this new discovery, for it opened to him a new field in which the reward of virgin labors could be obtained. These efforts he later found were based upon the sensitive dry plate which not alone proved the presence of the x-rays but also became the biggest factor in the ultimate development of the science of radiology.

EARLY PLATES

At first the dry plate was used to record x-ray images but the exposures required were exceedingly long. Soon, manufacturers made plates that were more sensitive to the exposure effect of the x-rays—but they were still exceedingly slow and lacked the qualities now found in modern x-ray film. Another disadvantage of the dry plate used in those early days was that the glass of which they were made was easily broken. The development of an x-ray intensifying screen by Thomas Edison, which was composed of calcium tungstate fluorescent crystals, and its first use by Professor Michael Pupin of Columbia University, in 1896, served to augment the exposure effect of the x-rays when using glass plates, thereby extending the usefulness of the radiographic method in medicine. Until 1917, however, radiography was largely performed with fast photographic plates that were specially designed for x-ray work.

EARLY X-RAY FILM

During World War I, x-ray film was produced, but the sensitive emulsion coated only on one side of a sheet of cellulose nitrate caused excessive curl. It was also highly inflammable. The objectionable curl was shortly eliminated by coating the emulsion on *both* sides of the cellulose support. This treatment of the film gave it greater speed, and *two* x-ray intensifying screens could then be employed to further reduce the time of exposure. The quality of the film was also improved. In 1924, *safety* x-ray film was introduced. The film base upon which was coated the silver emulsion was made of cellulose acetate, a material that has the same slow-burning properties of a like quantity of newsprint. Since that time, the quality and uniformity of film has been greatly enhanced. It is a far cry from the days of 1896 when a radiograph of a hand required an x-ray exposure of over an hour to the present time when only a fraction of a second is required.

COMPOSITION OF X-RAY FILM

X-ray film is manufactured today with a remarkable consistency as to uniformity and quality so that its exposure and processing may be standardized. If you ever go through a film manufacturing plant, notice the utmost cleanliness and fine housekeeping that exists wherever film is made, handled and inspected. X-ray film consists of an *emulsion* of finely precipitated silver bromide crystals suspended in gelatin that is coated on *both* sides of a transparent blue-tinted cellulose support called the *base*. The base furnishes support for the emulsion and provides the correct degree of stiffness for handling. The principal components of an x-ray film are: (1) the film base, and (2) emulsion. In general, the making of an x-ray film comprises the steps of procedure shown in Figure 7.

FILM BASE

The film *base* for the emulsion is made by dissolving wood or cotton in acetic anhydride in the presence of sulfuric acid. The cellulose combines with the acetic anhydride to form a thick solution. It is then washed in water and the cellulose acetate separates out of the solution. After further washing, it is dried and shredded into small particles that are dissolved in a special solvent containing a blue dye. The resulting solution is carefully spread over the surfaces of huge, heated and highly polished slowly moving drums. The solvent evaporates from the cellulose acetate which solidifies to a transparent sheet with a thickness of about eight thousandths of an inch. It is finally passed over other heated drums for thorough drying.

Blue Tint of Base

At various times attempts were made to improve the over-all quality of film by tinting the film. The purpose was to emphasize contrast and thus make it easier to visualize the densities present in the image. The colors used or locally applied were various shades of green, pink, orange, or blue.

The first commercialized (patented) method to be applied to x-ray film in America was described in 1933 by George A. Scanlan and Charles Holzwarth of Parlin, New Jersey who introduced a blue tint in x-ray film. The idea became popular with

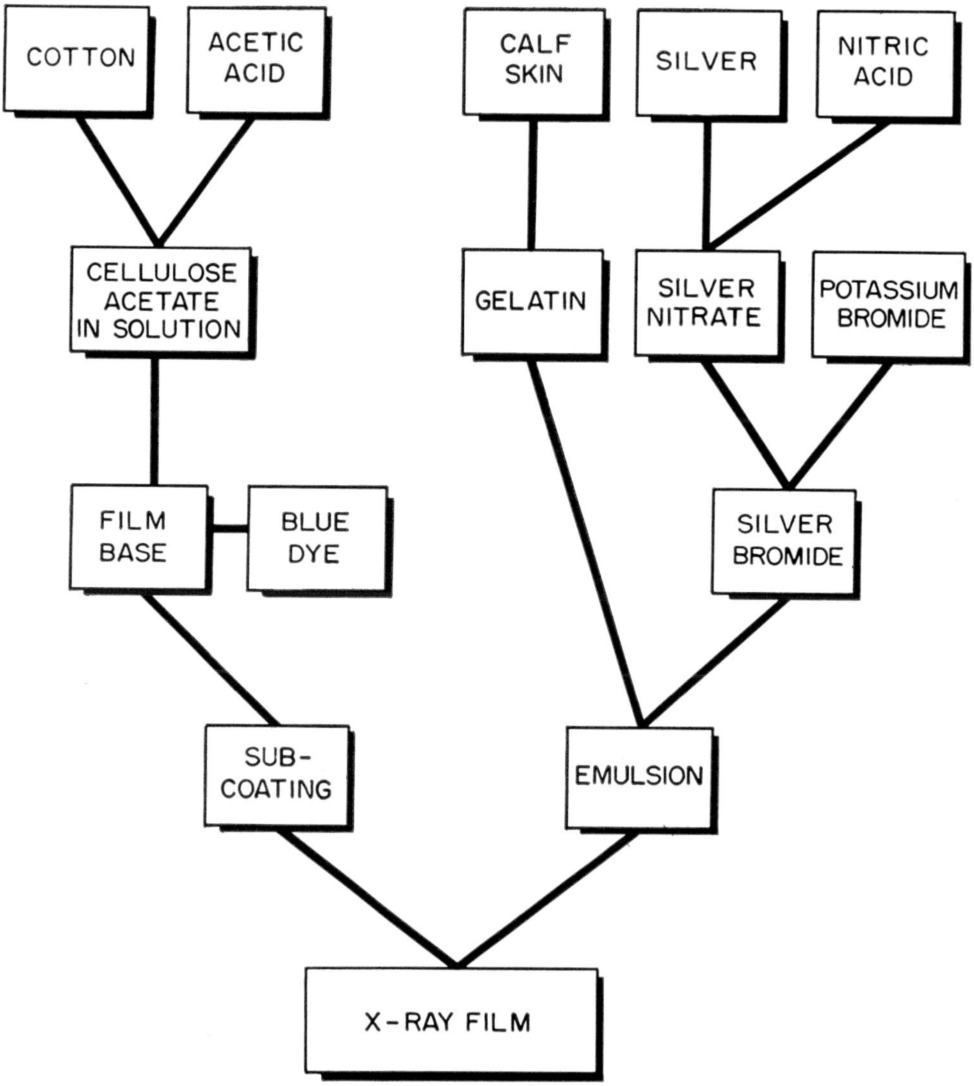

Figure 7. Steps in the procedure for manufacturing x-ray film.

radiologists because they found that the presence of the blue tint slightly emphasized contrast differences. Modern x-ray film is blue tinted.

Subcoating

After the base is made, it is covered on both sides with a thin adhesive-type material so that the sensitive emulsion will adhere to the base. This is called the *subcoating* and prepares the base for emulsion coating.

EMULSION

The *emulsion* itself starts with gelatin. Next, virgin silver is dissolved in nitric acid to form silver nitrate; then the silver nitrate solution is mixed with potassium bromide and gelatin to produce an emulsion of silver bromide crystals. It is then coated on both sides of the film base. After drying, the surfaces of the emulsion coatings are specially treated to prevent surface abrasion.

The purpose of the silver emulsion is to *absorb* radiation during an x-ray exposure and produce a latent image. The degree of exposure depends upon the intensity of the radiation *emerging* from the object that is interposed between the focal spot of the x-ray tube and the film, to reach the film.

Since gelatin is a most important constituent of the emulsion, some details regarding its source and characteristics are of interest.

Gelatin

Gelatin is a necessary constituent of the x-ray film emulsion and its properties should be familiar to all technicians. A most important discovery in the manufacture of photographic sensitive materials occurred many years ago as previously mentioned when gelatin was found to be an ideal medium for suspension of silver salts. Its ability to withstand action of the developer and fixer solutions at the processing temperatures normally employed without affecting the distribution of the silver crystals within it was most important. The fact that it assisted in the sensitization of the emulsion came as an after development.

Gelatin for photographic purposes is extracted from calf or cattle skins. In the early days of photography some gelatin was found to be good and some not. A study of this fact revealed that cattle grazing on pasturage containing mustard plants retained microscopic traces of sulfur in their hides, which in turn was carried in the gelatin obtained from them. Moreover, the silver bromide crystals suspended in this kind of gelatin were much more sensitive to the action of x-rays or light than crystals obtained in gelatin having no trace of sulfur. Film manufacturers obviously cannot depend upon the vagaries of bovine grazing habits when making film, but the problem was solved by adding the proper amount of natural synthetic mustard oil and now, other chemicals, to the emulsion formula.

Chemically, gelatin is a colloid and a very complex substance. Without special treatment, gelatin becomes soft and flexible when soaked in water because it absorbs an amount several times its bulk. An important physical property of gelatin is that in both liquid and solid forms it is clear and transparent so that no optical impairment of the image occurs when it is used in film manufacture. Gelatin immersed in hot water will dissolve to a liquid but it will not dissolve in cold water. This is an advantage for two reasons: (1) the liquid state is necessary for emulsion mixing and coating, and (2) the gelatin should not dissolve at the temperatures employed in processing the x-ray film. In the manufacture of the emulsion the gelatin can be given additional hardness without seriously impairing its porosity or clarity. Another favorable characteristic is the fact that when incorporated in the emulsion, it can swell considerably in a cool solution without dissolving thereby permitting action of the processing chemicals on the silver crystals without altering their places in the emulsion; afterwards the gelatin can be shrunk and hardened in the fixing bath so that the radiograph can be washed and dried. The influence of gelatin on sensitivity varies with different gelatins; therefore the gelatin must be carefully selected. Increased sensitivity can be given to the emulsion by adding certain substances to the gelatin during manufacture.

Silver Salts

In the preparation of the emulsion, a solution of potassium bromide is made with water. Pure silver nitrate is made by dissolving virgin silver in nitric acid. The solutions of potassium bromide and silver nitrate are slowly added to the gelatin solution in total darkness. The potassium bromide and silver nitrate solutions combine to form a precipitate of silver bromide in gelatin. This results in a thick, creamy emulsion. The chemical reaction is as follows:

$$KBr + AgNo_3 \longrightarrow AgBr \downarrow + KNO_3$$

KBr	AgNo₃	AgBr	KNO₃
Potassium Bromide	Silver Nitrate	Silver Bromide	Potassium Nitrate

The silver bromide emulsion is now heated to temperatures that vary from 50-80° C. This process is known as digestion and tends to increase the sensitivity of the emulsion. It is next cooled to a thick jelly and cut up into fine shreds which are washed in water for several hours to remove the potassium nitrate and other soluble salts. The washed emulsion is again heated and mixed with additional gelatin. In this state it is ready to be coated on the film base.

When examined under the microscope, the emulsion is seen to be made up of countless tiny crystals of silver bromide embedded in the gelatin (Figure 8, Left). Upon exposure and development, these crystals are changed into irregular clumps and strands of black metallic silver that in the aggregate compose the image, Right.

EMULSION COATING

In the coating operation, the film base is passed at high speed through a trough containing the sensitive emulsion where it acquires a coating of uniform thickness. The coated film next passes into a chamber of cold air where the emulsion is chilled to a jelly. It then traverses other chambers where it is dried and a nonabrasive coating is applied. It is then tested and spooled into a huge roll. The finished film is finally cut to the various sizes required by the radiologist. Each emulsion layer is about one-thousandth of an inch in thickness. Since x-rays pass readily through x-ray film —and also through x-ray intensifying screens when used—an emulsion layer is coated on *both* sides of the film base, providing thereby a greater effect upon exposure to x-rays than would be possible with an emulsion coated only on one side.

This completes the x-ray film. That, in brief, is the way x-ray film is made. It seems very simple—actually, it is tremendously complicated. Even after years of research in the manufacture of x-ray film, there are still things to be learned about the emulsion. Experience over the years has proved that certain methods of manufacture will produce a given uniform result. As time goes on and more is known regarding the physical and chemical characteristics of the emulsion, even better x-ray film should be produced than is manufactured today.

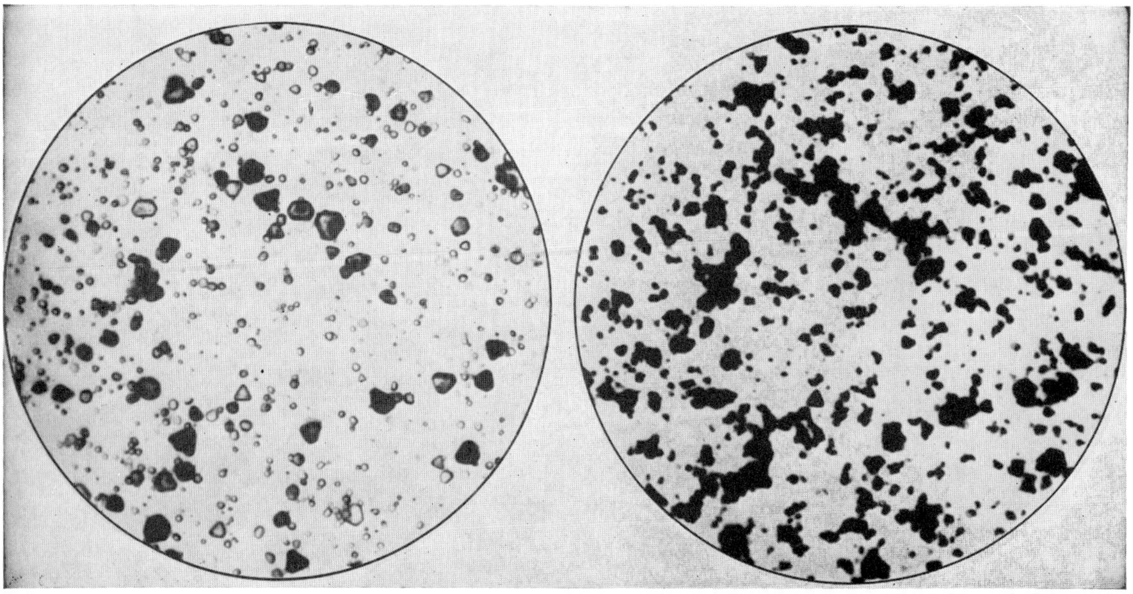

Kodak Research Laboratories

Figure 8. Photomicrograph (2500 X) of silver emulsion. (*Left*) before exposure, the emulsion is seen to be made up of countless tiny crystals of silver bromide isolated from one another by gelatin. (*Right*) after exposure and development, the original crystals have been broken down to form clumps or strands of black metallic silver.

TYPES OF MEDICAL X-RAY FILM

While an image may be formed on film by light, gamma rays, or other forms of radiation including x-rays, the properties of the latter in producing a radiographic image are of a distinct character. For this reason, x-ray film must be distinctly different from that used in photography. It has not been possible to manufacture a film that is solely sensitive to the action of x-rays and not to light. In fact, modern radiography depends greatly upon the use of the visible fluorescent light emitted by x-ray intensifying screens to augment the x-ray action on the film. Two general types of x-ray film are employed in medical radiography, *screen-type* film and *direct-exposure* film.

SCREEN-TYPE

Film that is particularly sensitive to the *fluorescent* light of x-ray intensifying screens is known as screen-type x-ray film. The visible fluorescent light from screens amplifies the direct action of the x-rays. When used with intensifying screens, screen-type film is much faster than the direct-exposure type. When screen-type film is used without intensifying screens, however, it is slower than the direct-exposure type. However, it is frequently exposed without screens. In radiography of the smaller thicknesses of the body such as the hand, ankle, etc., screen-type film provides a wider range of densities than when it is employed with screens. Because of its lower sensitivity to direct action of the x-rays, the background density of the processed radiograph is usually less than that of the direct-exposure type.

DIRECT-EXPOSURE TYPE

Direct-exposure film (no-screen film) is especially sensitive to the *direct* action of the x-rays. It is used only for the thinner body parts. Its silver content is greater and the film has a higher inherent contrast than the screen-type film when directly exposed. It is about three times faster than screen-type film under these conditions and the development time is longer. This film cannot be used with x-ray intensifying screens, for it is largely insensitive to their fluorescent light.

DENTAL X-RAY FILM

Dental x-ray film is individually wrapped in moisture-proof packets for use in dental radiography. These films are modifications of the medical x-ray films and are available in different speeds and sizes. They are classified as:

Periapical

Periapical dental x-ray film is packed in lighttight moisture-proof paper packets for examining the roots of teeth. The emulsions are usually classified as slow, average, and fast as to their sensitivity or speed.

Interproximal

Interproximal (bite-wing) film in the form of packets is used for locating cavities between the teeth.

Occlusal

Occlusal film is larger than the periapical film and is employed for examining larger dental areas than can be covered with the periapical film. It, too, is supplied in packet form.

PHOTORADIOGRAPHIC FILM

Photoradiographic film is single coated and employed for photography of the fluorescent screen by a camera in mass health examinations, particularly of the chest. The films vary in speed and are used either in 4 x 10-inch sheet or 50-100-foot rolls in the 35mm and 70mm widths. One type is more sensitive to the *blue* fluorescence of one kind of fluorescent screen; the other is most sensitive to the *green* fluorescence of another kind of screen.

FILM SPEED

The shortest exposure required in making a good quality radiograph, the faster the film is said to be. To know the speed of the film you are using is important when building an exposure chart. All films are fast enough for radiography, but the important things to remember are: the uniformity of the film speed as used from year to year; the film's response to time-temperature development; and, a constant radiographic quality when correct exposure and processing procedures are employed. Extreme speed in an x-ray film is attained only at the expense of some of the qualities that make a good radiograph. Actually, with the proper use of kilovoltage, the sensitivity of modern x-ray film will satisfy all the demands of medical radiography.

Chapter 4

Silver Image Formation

ELECTRONIC ENERGY and its many uses are of fascinating interest, for this is an electronic age. Electronic energy is not a strange new thing. The movement of electrons has been harnessed in may ways to accomplish useful purposes. The flow of electrons through a copper wire becomes the flow of electric current; the flow at high speed of electrons from an incandescent wire to a tungsten button in an evacuated x-ray tube produces x-rays; an x-ray film emulsion in its small way is also a veritable electronic powerhouse.

All matter, in the course of existence, is dependent upon the flow of electrons. The movement of electrons causes chemical reactions or the emissions of light and x-rays. The manufacture, exposure, and processing of an x-ray film is dependent at one time or another upon electron flow to produce the radiograph. Matter consists of atoms. Each atom is an aggregation of electrons, carrying negative charges of electricity; and protons, carrying positive charges. This is the normal state of all matter whether it is air, rock or water.

PHOTOGRAPH VS. RADIOGRAPH

The production of a radiograph is in a sense similar to the making of a photograph. Both radiography and photography use various wave lengths of light to expose the film and in each instance, after processing, the image is made up of various degrees of concentration of silver deposits. When making a *photograph,* the various deposits of black metallic silver and their distribution over the film are dependent upon the amount and kind of visible light *reflected* from the object being photographed, as gathered by the lens of a camera and focused on the film. Since different areas of the object being photographed *absorb* more light than others, the *intensity* of the light reflected to the camera is variable. Hence the resulting silver deposits vary in concentration after the film is exposed and processed, to produce the photographic image. This situation is analogous to the mechanics of production of an image by x-rays—another form of light—when making a *radiograph,* with this difference. As an x-ray beam passes *through* a part of the human body, its intensity is decreased by selective absorption of the various tissues it penetrates. The resulting variation in intensity within the beam as it emerges from the body causes differences in the amount of exposure given to the x-ray film. When the film is developed, these exposure differences are manifested by silver deposits that vary in their concentration to compose the radiographic image.

The outstanding difference in the mechanics of image production between the photograph and the radiograph is that, in radiography, the variations in intensity of the x-rays reaching the film are dependent upon the difference in *absorption* of the x-rays as they pass through body tissues, whereas in photography the image is formed by the variation in intensity of the light *reflected* from the subject.

The creation of any photographic or radiographic image is based upon the performance of the gelatin emulsion containing the silver bromide crystals. The absorption of x-rays, light or any other external stimulus by the molecules of silver bromide in the emulsion initiates a chain of atomic activities which results in the formation of the *latent image*. The silver bromide crystals have the ability to store energy from these sources and the resultant effect on the crystal is increased manyfold by chemical treatment. The production of a silver image (radiograph), therefore, is dependent upon two phases of activity: latent image formation and development.

The nature of the latent image and the development process are closely allied and their understanding is dependent upon some knowledge regarding the atomic structure and reactions of the silver bromide emulsion upon exposure and development.

THE ATOM

The *atom* is a kind of building block that when added to others, becomes the structure of matter. Atoms vary in structure depending upon the substance or chemical they are destined to comprise. All matter in the universe is composed of nearly one hundred varieties of atoms. The atom is the smallest particle of matter or *element*, such as silver, oxygen, hydrogen, etc., that is capable of entering into a chemical reaction. It is too small to be visible to the eye.

All atoms have a similar pattern consisting of a central positively charged *nucleus* about which whirls at speeds in excess of millions of times per second, negatively charged *electrons* in orbits that are at definite distances many thousand times greater than the diameter of the nucleus. The relationship between the nucleus and the electron is similar to that the planets exercise in their relation to the sun. The nucleus of a stable atom consists of equal numbers of *protons* that carry a positive charge and *neutrons* that are electrically neutral. It contains the bulk of the weight of the atom. The nucleus is surrounded by an equal number of electrons that are *negatively* charged. The positive charge on the nucleus is always equal to that of the aggregate of negative charges carried by the electrons. This makes the atom electrically neutral. The number and arrangements of the electrons determines the identity of the atom—whether it is hydrogen, iron, or some other element. The simplest atom (hydrogen) consists of a nucleus and one electron. The number of the electrons in the atom determines the chemical nature of the element it represents. The number of protons in the nucleus of a given atom is equal to the number of electrons and is known as the *atomic number*. This number serves to identify the element. For example, an atom containing 47 electrons is the element silver.

The structure of a simple atom of a given element may vary slightly as one or more neutrons are added to the nucleus. The element then assumes a relatively unstable form and is called an *isotope* (of the element). For example, when a neutron is added to a hydrogen atom, it becomes deuterium—an isotope of hydrogen

IONIZATION

Electricity is made up of positive (+) and negative (−) charges. Charges of *like* sign (a plus charge and a plus charge or a negative charge and a negative charge) repel each other. Charges of *unlike* sign (a positive charge and a negative charge) attract each other and when they meet, each is neutralized. A positive ion (*cation*) carries a positive charge of electricity and a negative ion (*anion*) carries a negative charge. When matter is partially or wholly converted into *ions*, a state of ionization exists. This means that the components of a molecule can be changed, in a sense, to positive and negative charges of electricity. For example, when sodium chloride is dissolved in water, the sodium chloride separates into sodium ions that are positively charged and chlorine ions that are negatively charged. The chemical reaction may be written as follows:

$NaCl \longrightarrow$	Na^+	+	Cl^-
Sodium Chloride	Sodium ion		Chlorine ion

This fact is quite important in the exposure and development of the silver bromide crystal for these phenomena are dependent upon ionization.

Chemical changes of substances also cause a redistribution of electrons in the atoms involved in the chemical reaction. Normally, electrons are packed in an orderly fashion in an atom. Yet depending upon their position in the atom, an electron can free itself and pass to another atom that is deficient in electrons. These electrons are known as *valence electrons.* If an atom loses an electron, it will have an excess of positive charge. On the other hand, if one or more electrons are added, it will have a negative charge.

To explain how two separate elements will produce a separate and distinct compound when joined together, silver and bromine may be employed as an example. In solution, atoms of silver are able to lose electrons to atoms of bromine when mixed together for the elements become ionized. A typical example may be cited. A solution of silver nitrate is mixed with a solution of potassium bromide in the correct proportions and since the chemicals become ionized when in solution, the positively charged silver ions join the negatively charged bromine ions; one charge neutralizes the other and solid crystals of silver bromide are formed as a precipitate in a solution of potassium nitrate.

$Ag^+\ NO_3^-$	+	$K^+\ Br^- \longrightarrow$	$Ag\ Br \downarrow$	$K\ NO_3$
Silver Nitrate		Potassium Bromide	Silver Bromide	Potassium Nitrate

When an x-ray film emulsion is made, the silver bromide crystals have been prepared in such a manner that they will be readily susceptible to the x-ray stimulus that starts them on the way to becoming a radiographic image. A crystal is a package of atoms. It is the way of nature to put a large amount of a single substance in a pure form. Chemists take advantage of this fact to make large quantities of a chemical by separating it from other substances by crystallization.

LATENT IMAGE FORMATION

Exposure of an x-ray film occurs when x-rays strike the silver bromide crystals in the emulsion; they can only absorb a very small amount of x-ray energy to convert them into a latent image. The crystals ionize into positively charged silver ions and negatively charged bromine ions—the degree of ionization within the crystal depends upon the amount of exposure received. When this situation is created, a *latent image* is produced. The ionic equation can be written as follows:

AgBr	+	X-rays $\longrightarrow$	Ag^+	+	Br^-
Silver Bromide Crystal			Silver ion		Bromine ion

The latent image cannot be seen or detected by any ordinary physical means. It is contained in the emulsion of the x-ray film from the time of exposure until it is changed into a visible silver image by chemical processing. Many theories have been advanced as to the nature of the changes occurring in the production of the latent image. However, a general pattern of the process can be described.

It was early assumed that the latent image was composed of metallic silver. On that supposition, the manner in which the silver of the latent image was formed and its distribution among the crystals, formed the basis for exhaustive research to prove the theory. This work was also extended to include the nature of the development process whereby the presence of a minute amount of metallic silver on or in the crystal (development center) makes development of exposed silver bromide possible.

SENSITIZATION SPECKS

During manufacture, the emulsion is treated with certain chemicals that produce what are known as sensitization specks on the crystal surfaces. They provide the future sites for the beginning of the development phenomenon leading to the production of the visible image. In the study of the latent image, it was found that these specks were tiny particles of atomic silver and silver sulfide on the surfaces of the silver bromide crystals after they were mixed with the right kind of gelatin to form an emulsion. These particles or specks of silver can only be seen with the electron microscope. Development only can be continued by the *growth* in size of these specks, and *not* by the continual formation of new specks all over the crystals. Crystals that did not possess the specks cannot develop. In other words, these specks constituted nuclei for future development.

It has been fairly well established that the formation of the latent image is a process wherein the energy of the light or x-rays is absorbed by the crystal with resultant ionization. The general aspects of this activity is diagrammatically shown in Figure 9. In this diagram of a silver bromide crystal, a few sensitization specks are shown on the surface of the crystal (A). Let us see what happens to one of these specks when the crystal is exposed to x-rays (B). As soon as x-rays are absorbed by the crystal, (C), it becomes a weak conductor for electrons are released by the atoms in the crystal and they, as well as the slower moving positive ions begin to move within it. This electronic activity, as stimulated by exposure, causes the crystal to become *ionized.* The hitherto neutral sensitization speck now acquires a negative charge (D) because the electrons have been trapped by it and the slower moving positive silver ions are attracted to it (E). As the silver ions reach the negatively charged speck, both are neutralized with the result that tiny particles of atomic silver are deposited at the speck (F). Obviously, the amount of atomic silver that is deposited depends upon the amount of exposure. When sufficient silver has been accumulated at the speck, it acts as a development center making the crystal potentially developable (G). In other words, a latent image has been produced. When the crystal is attacked by the developing solution, it is changed from silver bromide to a clump of filamentous black metallic silver merely by oxidation. These silver

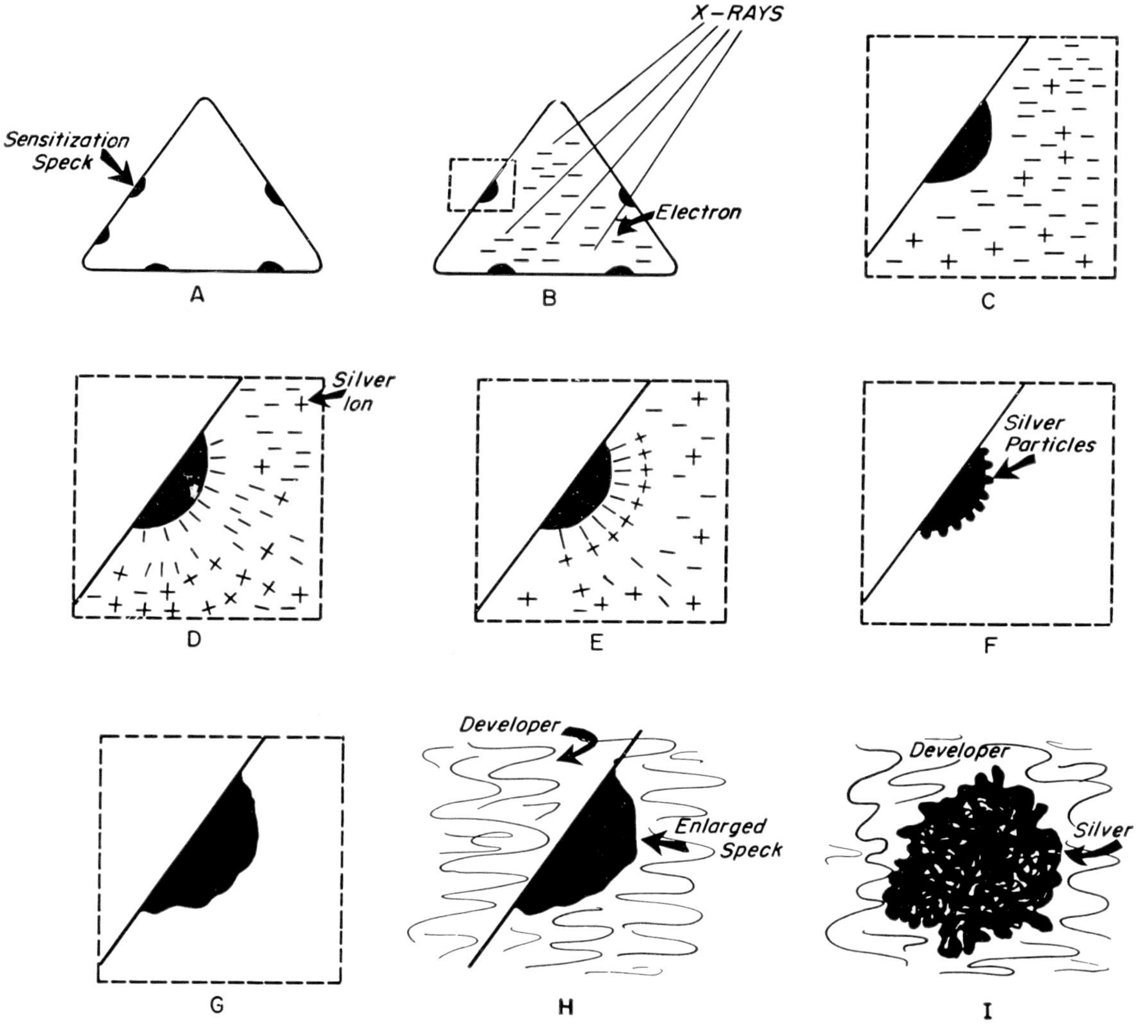

Figure 9. Changes occurring within the silver bromide crystal upon exposure to x-rays and development.

deposits (I) in the aggregate compose the image. If the quantity of x-rays that strikes a crystal happens to be insufficient, the sensitization speck will not grow to the point where it can break down the entire crystal upon development. The fully exposed crystal will usually develop and be reduced to black metallic silver within the normal time of development at a given temperature.

PRODUCTION OF SILVER IMAGE

The process of converting the latent image to a metallic silver image comprises two important chemical reactions—development and fixation.

DEVELOPMENT

The purpose of development is to make the latent image visible. The chief function of a developing solution is to reduce progressively the exposed silver bromide crystal to black metallic silver. The silver nuclei on the silver bromide crystals that are formed by the action of an external stimulus such as x-rays serve as the starting points for this reaction. This transition involves two chemical reactions—reduction and oxidation—wherein electrons play an important role. Certain chemicals have the ability to liberate elements from their compounds. These are known as *reducers* and are materials that can be *oxidized.* When development occurs, reduction of the silver bromide takes place and the developing agents become oxidized.

Oxidation

Reduction actually is chemical oxidation. The term "oxidation" does not necessarily mean a chemical reaction involving oxygen for it may occur with or without oxygen. If an electron is *removed* from an atom of silver, it may be considered as oxidized. Since the electron is negatively charged, a positively charged silver *ion* is left behind. In chemical symbols this reaction of *oxidation* is written as follows:

$$\underset{\text{Silver atom}}{Ag} \longrightarrow \underset{\text{Silver ion}}{Ag^{+}} + \text{electron}^{-}$$

When an electron is *removed* from a bromine ion, *oxidation* takes place and an *atom* of bromine is formed. The reaction is written as follows:

$$\underset{\text{Bromide ion}}{Br^{-}} \longrightarrow \underset{\text{Bromide atom}}{Br} + \text{electron}^{-}$$

Reduction

When an electron is *added* to a silver ion, the reaction is one of *reduction* with the formation of an atom of silver. This reaction is as follows:

$$\underset{\text{Silver ion}}{Ag^{+}} + \text{electron}^{-} \longrightarrow \underset{\text{Silver atom}}{Ag}$$

Silver is a metal that can liberate electrons but it cannot easily acquire any. On the other hand, bromine acquires electrons readily and thereby is easily reduced. When an electron is *added* to an atom of bromine, reduction takes place and the reaction may be written as follows:

$$\underset{\text{Bromine atom}}{Br} + \text{electron}^{-} \longrightarrow \underset{\text{Bromine ion}}{Br^{-}}$$

Reduction of Exposed Emulsion

A reducing agent cannot be a photographic developer unless it reacts more rapidly with *exposed* silver bromide crystals than those that are unexposed. Hence, an x-ray exposure must be of sufficient degree that a sufficient quantity of exposed crystals can be reduced in a given developmental period to form a satisfactory image. In a properly exposed radiograph, this action is usually completed upon full development and *before* the unexposed crystals have an opportunity to develop to any perceptible degree.

When the exposed x-ray film is placed in the developer, the gelatin in the emulsion becomes swollen and porous due to the presence of water and the activity of the alkali in the developer solution. The exposed silver bromide crystals being ionized, the reducing agents can attack them. As previously mentioned, the x-ray exposure causes the sensitization specks to acquire atomic silver to the point where they act as nuclei for the deposition of more silver as the crystals break down by the action of the developer (Figure 9 I). As development progresses, more and more metallic silver accumulates on the specks until the silver ions from the disintegrating silver bromide crystals are exhausted. The bromine ions are freed from the emulsion and react with the potassium ions from other chemicals in the developer solution to form potassium bromide. Upon completion of development, the *exposed* silver bromide crystals are reduced to black metallic silver to constitute the image. The unexposed silver bromide is unaffected by this treatment during the development period.

FIXATION

After the silver image has been produced on the film, the unexposed and undeveloped silver bromide crystals must be dissolved away from the emulsion by the action of a fixing bath so that the silver image may become permanent.

RESUME OF IMAGE PRODUCTION

When the exposed emulsion is considered as a whole rather than as its constituent silver bromide crystals, the various stages in the production of the silver image can be diagrammatically illustrated as in Figure 10. Let us assume that an object (A) in the form of an aluminum step wedge is correctly exposed using an x-ray film (B) as the recording medium. When the film is represented in enlarged cross section, a latent image of the object is produced upon exposure in the silver bromide emulsion (C). The latent image is represented by the dotted area and consists of representations of the six portions of the wedge. The radiation reaching the film is of varying intensity after its passage through the various thicknesses of the wedge and the relative absorption of each thickness is represented. The radiation passing through step number 1 of the object (A) is only partially absorbed, hence more silver bromide is exposed than that portion of the film under steps No. 4 or No. 6 wherein greater absorption takes place. Hence, upon development, the quantity of silver deposited in these areas is *less* than under step number 1. In other words, each step is recorded as a deposit of silver that is proportionate to the intensity of the emergent radiation reaching the film. Upon development (D), the latent image silver bromide is reduced to metallic silver and the unexposed silver bromide (thin diagonal lines) is not affected. (Mixed with the metallic silver deposits are unexposed and undeveloped silver bromide crystals.) After the film has been treated as in fixation (E), all the unexposed and undeveloped silver bromide is dissolved from the emulsion and the metallic silver remains on the film to constitute the radiographic image of the step wedge shown in (A). When the radiographic image (F) is later viewed on an x-ray illuminator, all the various deposits of silver representing the steps of the wedge are seen in their proper silver concentration with various degrees of translucency to the transmission of light from the illuminator.

SUMMARY

The initial effect of exposure on the silver bromide crystal is to ionize the crystal and produce free electrons and, the subsequent formation of tiny particles of atomic silver at the sensitization speck. The amount of silver on the speck is in proportion to the amount of exposure it received. The aggregate of specks containing silver in all the silver bromide crystals constitutes what is known as the *latent*

→

Figure 10. Stages of exposure of a step wedge (A), and development of x-ray film (B). Creation of latent image (C) as a result of exposure; latent image changed to silver image (D) as a result of development; unexposed and undeveloped silver bromide emulsion removed from silver image (E) by process of fixation; image as seen on the x-ray illuminator (F).

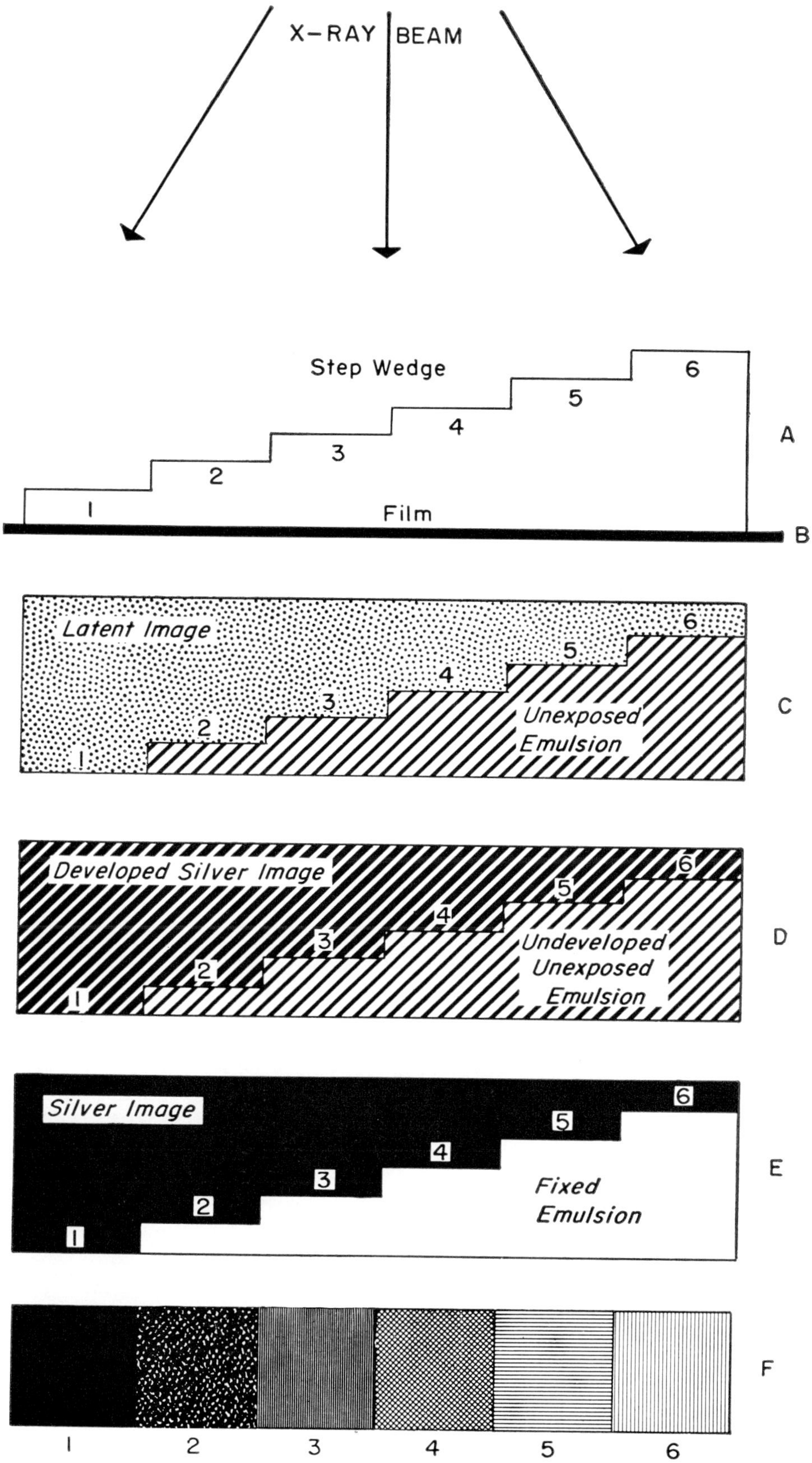
X-RAY BEAM
Step Wedge
1
2
3
4
5
6
Film
A
B
Latent Image
Unexposed Emulsion
C
Developed Silver Image
Undeveloped Unexposed Emulsion
D
Silver Image
Fixed Emulsion
E
F

image. The specks provide the future sites for the beginning of development that results in the production of a visible silver image. The latent image for all practical purposes is permanent. It should be realized that only the radiation *absorbed* by the silver bromide crystals causes ionization of the crystal and silver growth on the speck making it subject to development. This is the basic response of any photographic or x-ray emulsion when it is exposed to light, x-rays or a situation wherein external energy is absorbed by the crystals from other causes. When an exposed x-ray film is developed, the reducing agents in the developer attack the exposed crystals reducing the silver bromide to black metallic silver. The fixing bath then removes all the unexposed and undeveloped silver bromide from the film. Upon completion of the processing procedure a black metallic silver image is contained on the base. A radiograph is produced.

Chapter 5

Image Characteristics

THE RADIOGRAPHIC IMAGE is composed of many deposits of black metallic silver distributed over both surfaces of the radiograph. These deposits constitute radiographic *details* that blend into an image to represent the anatomical structures in the part of the body examined. There are two major characteristics of the image that directly influence the diagnostic quality of the radiograph. They are radiographic *density* and *contrast*.

RADIOGRAPHIC DENSITY

When an x-ray film is directly exposed by primary x-radiation and then processed, a uniform deposit of black metallic silver appears on both sides of the film, Figure 11, *Left*. This silver deposit is a *radiographic density* and is a measure of

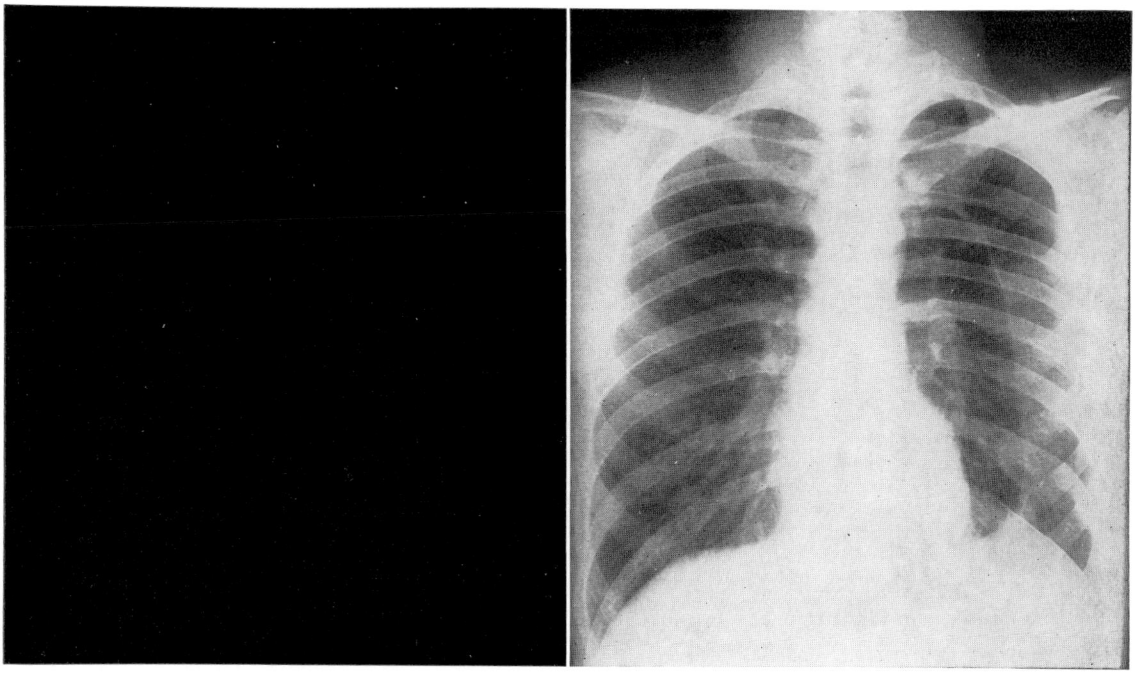

Figure 11. Radiographs illustrating: (*Left*) A single radiographic density; (*Right*) Many radiographic densities. The latter radiograph exhibits radiographic contrast; the former does not.

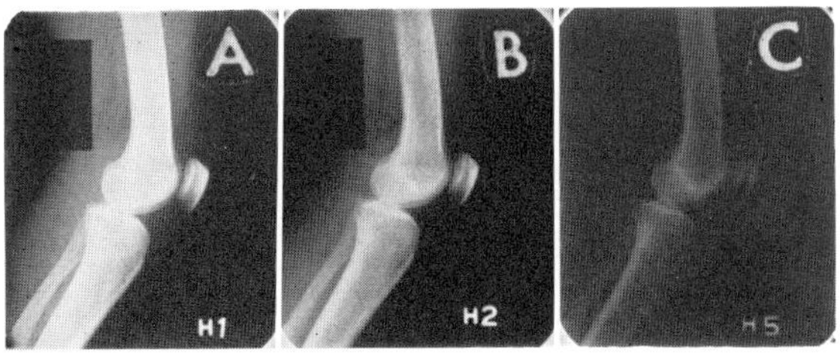

Figure 12. Series of radiographs demonstrating results of underexposure (A); correct exposure (B); overexposure (C). Note opaque silver deposits in (C) and absence of some silver deposits in (A), indicating loss in detail visualization.

the quantity of radiation absorbed by the film.

TONE VALUE

During their passage through a body part, the x-rays are absorbed selectively by various tissue components. This absorption results in the production of a number of *different* silver deposits on the radiograph. Each deposit has a certain degree of translucency or *tone value* when the radiograph is viewed on an x-ray illuminator.* The greater the silver concentration in a density, the less light from the illuminator that can pass through it and vice versa. For example, a heavy deposit of silver in the image transmits very little light; a modest deposit of silver permits a greater amount of light to pass through it. The former appears very dark to the eye—it has little brightness—whereas the latter appears very bright. As a consequence, it is easy to differentiate one from the other. Each density possesses tone value by virtue of the intensity of the light transmitted.

Radiographic images are made up of a large number of densities that have different tone values. The visibility of image details, therefore, depends upon the tone value. If the object is fairly complex in structure and the exposure factors employed are correct, the tone of each image density is radiographic evidence of a structural detail. Obviously, the greater the number of tones present (correct tone rendition), the greater the number of structural details that can be visualized in the image. Assuming that the radiograph is processed by a standardized method, *opaque* deposits are known as *overexposures;* areas of the image possessing little silver deposit are almost totally transparent and are known as *highlights* or *underexposures*. Under standard conditions of illumination, highlights possessing little silver, and, therefore, of detail, are diagnostically worthless. Also, areas of overexposure may be considered diagnostically useless since the opaqueness of the silver deposit obscures image details when the radiograph is viewed before the light from a standard x-ray illuminator (see Figure 12). The range of tones in an image is photographically known as the "gray scale," and it is intimately associated with radiographic contrast.

* Modern x-ray illuminators emit light of standard intensity and color usually provided by two 15-watt daylight, fluorescent lamps.

RADIOGRAPHIC CONTRAST

In the visualization of radiographic detail, it is the *tonal* relationship between one density and another that enables image details to become visible. This constitutes *radiographic contrast.* Radiographic contrast comprises the differences in light-transmitting properties (translucence) between the various radiographic densities that compose the image. Stated in another way, radiographic contrast is the observable differences in optical density that occur in the image. Generally speaking, visualization of details depends upon the degree of contrast and sharpness with which they are rendered. Practically, if the radiographic densities differ enough in tone value that anatomical details are readily discernible, the radiographic objective has been attained (Figure 11, *Right*).

CONTRAST SCALE

The scale of contrast in a radiographic image is determined by the number and tone value of the various densities. Radiographic contrast may vary widely or within some acceptable *average* range depending upon the nature of the part being examined. A good radiograph is one that possesses a correct balance of densities (gradation) over the entire contrast scale. The contrast should be such that, with prevailing exposure technics, good differentiation is shown between tissue details portrayed over the whole area of diagnostic interest, without loss of detail in the lighter or darker areas of the radiographic image.

The scale of densities that determines the contrast and the visibility of details is directly influenced by the x-ray wave length which, in turn, is regulated by the factor of kilovoltage. This fact may be demonstrated by two diagrams, Figures 13 and 14. An aluminum step-wedge is shown being irradiated by x-rays; the exposed x-ray film in enlarged cross section is shown beneath the step-wedge; and the resulting radiographic image as it appears when viewed on the illuminator is depicted below the film cross section in both illustrations.

Short-Scale Contrast

In the diagram (Figure 13) it is assumed that long wave length radiation is directed toward a step-wedge. The radiation easily penetrates step No. 1 and the remnant radiation strongly affects the silver emulsion. Upon development, a radiographic density representing step No. 1 is produced. This density appears opaque when viewed on the illuminator. Step No. 2 is also easily penetrated and although the intensity of the remnant radiation is somewhat reduced by absorption, another opaque density is produced. The radiation is greatly absorbed by step No. 3 resulting in remnant radiation of such low intensity that a translucent density with a gray tone is produced. The x-rays traversing step No. 4 are largely absorbed and the remnant radiation has just sufficient intensity to produce a density with a light gray tone. The radiation passing to steps Nos. 5 and 6 is almost totally absorbed and the film covered by this area is not exposed because there is too little remnant radiation. Differentiation between densities Nos. 1 and 2 representing the thin portion of the wedge cannot be made when the image is viewed on the illuminator. The film area that should contain details of steps Nos. 5 and 6 is devoid of silver, hence, there is no image. Steps Nos. 3 and 4 are represented by two densities of different tone value. A representative image of the entire wedge was not recorded because of an inadequacy of remnant radiation. Note that the differences between densities are wide and few in number and that the number of densities are insufficient to portray a complete image of the subject.

This diagram illustrates the fact that radiographic details of an object cannot be seen in the image unless there are discernible differences in tone value between densities and that there must be a silver deposit on the film if a detail within the object is to be demonstrated. The above situation is typical for *short-scale* contrast. Photographically, the image may be likened so that in Figure 13 *Left,* wherein a large number of details in the image are absent.

When an image of a body part is rendered with densities that are either ex-

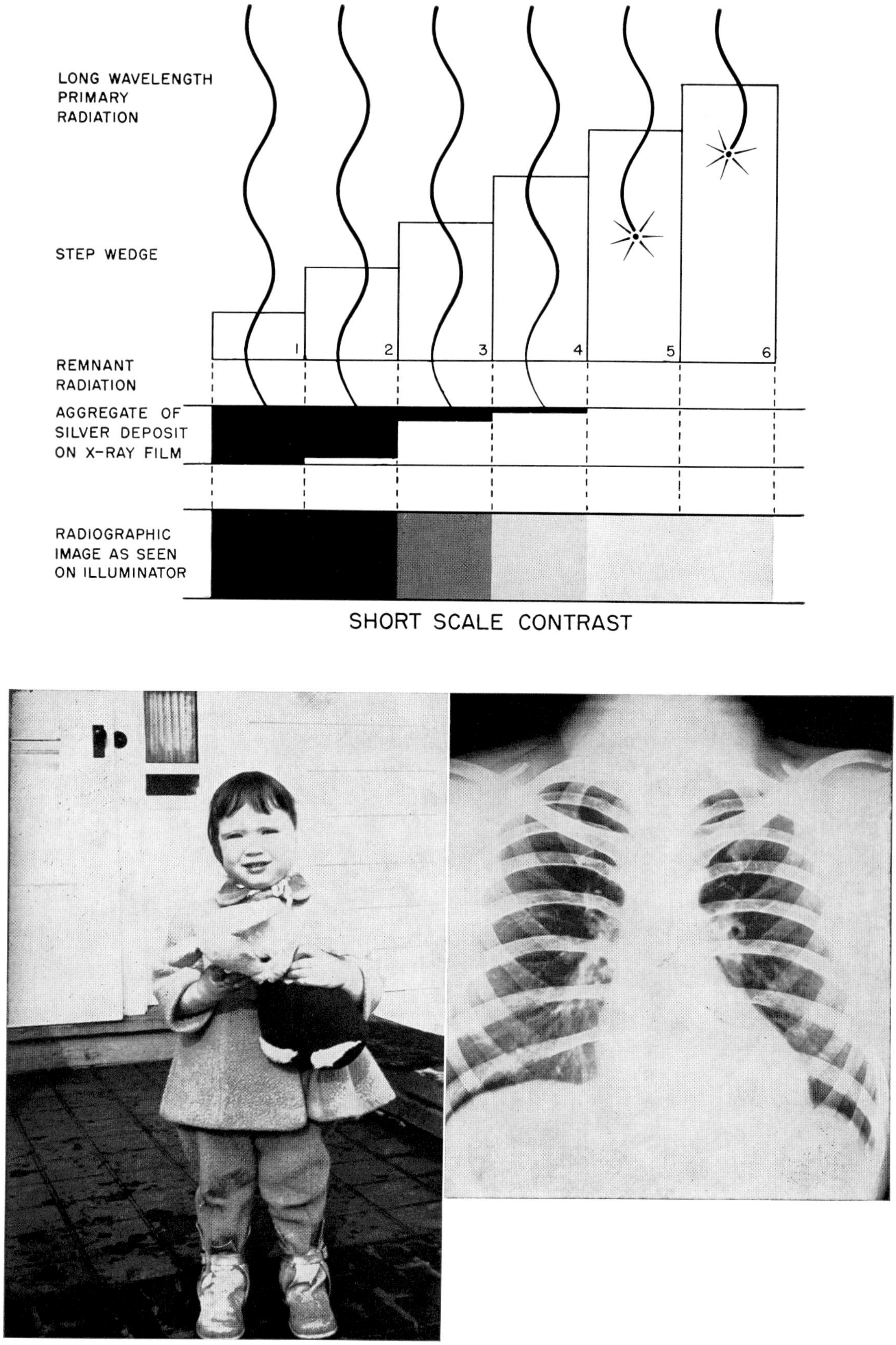

Figure 13. Diagram (*Top*), photograph (*Left*), and radiograph (*Right*), illustrating *short-scale* **contrast.**

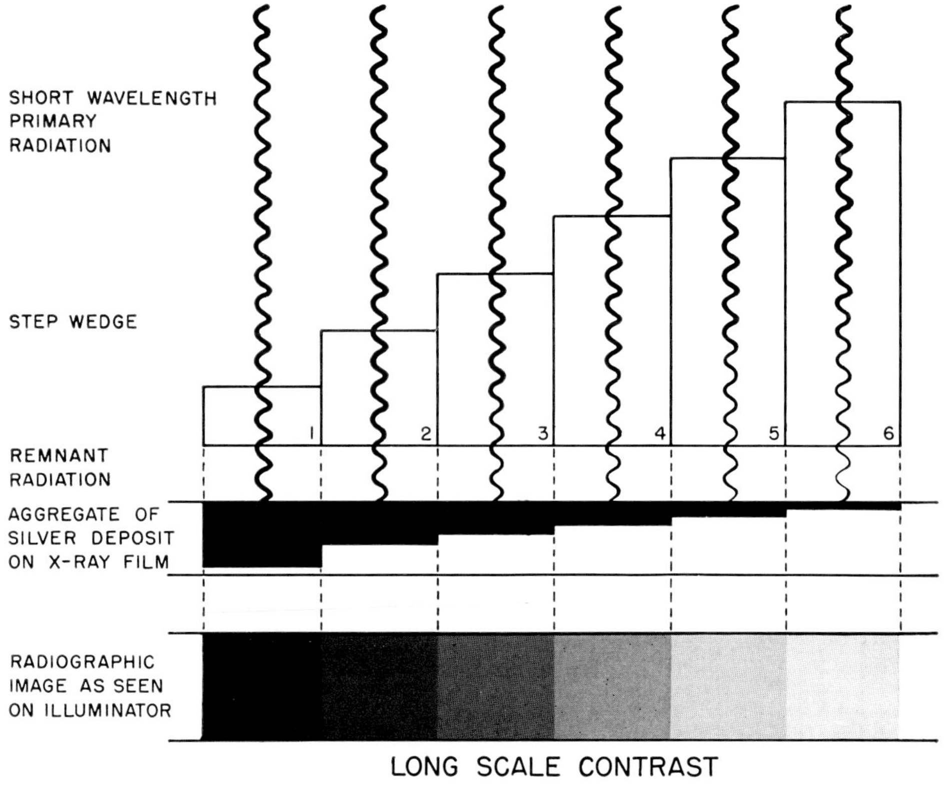

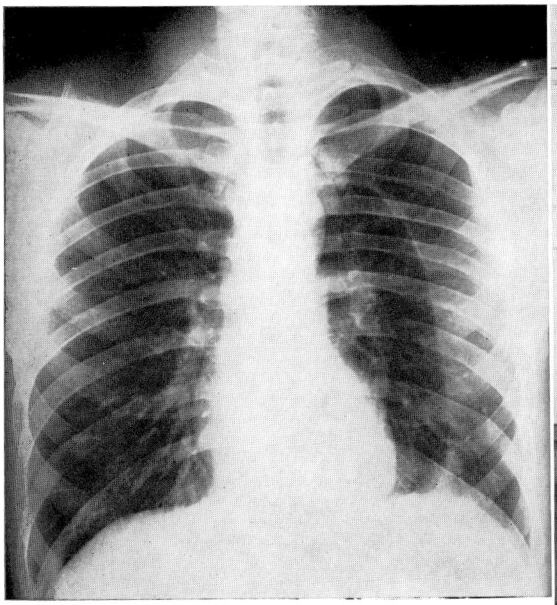

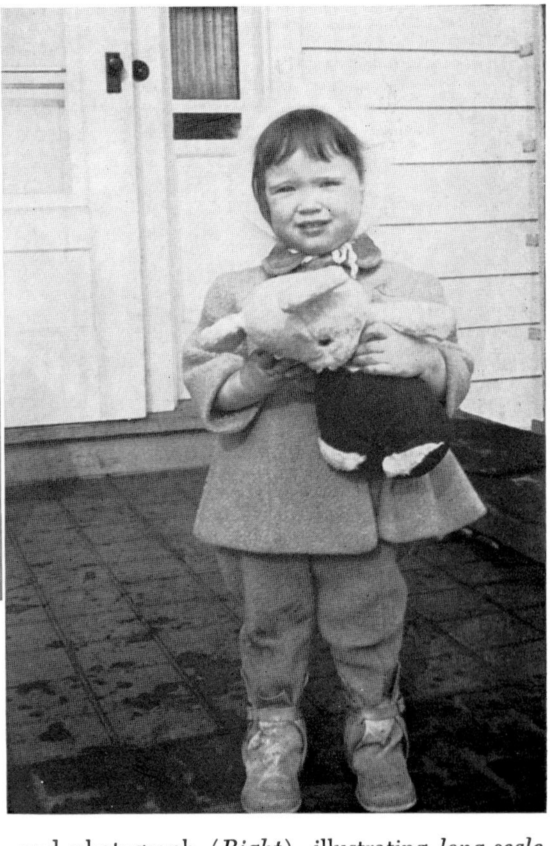

Figure 14. Diagram (*Top*), radiograph (*Left*), and photograph (*Right*), illustrating *long-scale* **contrast.**

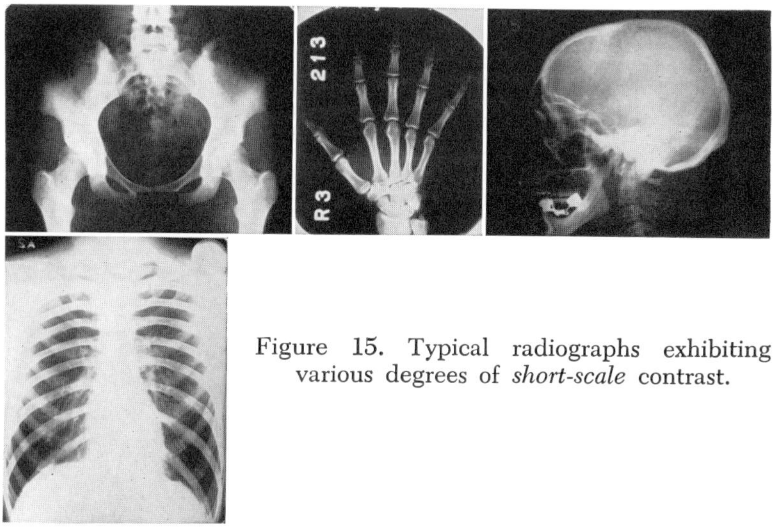

Figure 15. Typical radiographs exhibiting various degrees of *short-scale* contrast.

cessive or virtually nonexistent with a short range of widely different intermediate translucent densities, short-scale contrast exists. Such radiographs are pictorially pleasing to look at, for they possess instant eye appeal but they have little diagnostic worth and are economically wasteful, Figure 13 *Right.*

When low kilovoltage is used for thin tissue parts such as the hand, elbow, etc., greater contrast occurs between the bones and the flesh. In fact, a point may be reached in which the thinner portions such as the skin and subcutaneous tissues and even some muscle detail are obliterated by opaque silver deposits; and, some bone detail may also be lost because the denser bone tissue absorbs so much radiation that little remnant radiation reaches the film. Even when exposures are increased to impractical limits by the MaS factor in order to obtain satisfactory bone detail, opaque silver deposits will still obscure details of the less dense fleshy areas.

On the other hand, when the exposure is decreased to exhibit flesh details satisfactorily, then osseous details are lost. In other words, as kilovoltage is decreased, the number of intermediate tones diminishes and over-all detail diminishes in the same ratio. So only those details in the image produced by exposure factors that happen to be optimum for the area are rendered with maximum visibility and the remainder of the image becomes diagnostically useless.

There are occasions when it seems advisable to shorten the scale of contrast in a specific area but when this is done, there is always that danger of losing detail visibility in other adjacent areas. On the whole, the entire image exhibiting short-scale contrast is invariably incomplete, for details that represent the thinner and thicker portions of the body part are not always shown. Short-scale contrast has its place only as a special procedure in more adequately visualizing details of *small* tissue areas and then only after preliminary survey radiographs have been made. Typical examples of short-scale contrast are shown in Figure 15.

Long-Scale Contrast

Portraying the same situation as shown in Figure 13, but using *shorter wave length radiation,* the diagram, Figure 14, exhibits a different result. The radiation readily penetrates all portions of the wedge and the selective degree of absorption by each step has permitted remnant radiation to emerge with different intensities that are recorded as separate translucent densities. These densities of varying tone value represent the several steps in the wedge. The transition between tones is gradual and each tone is distinctive. The image is completely informative and is typical of long-scale contrast. Desirable long-scale contrast is produced when the kilovoltage is adjusted to delineate all normal structures satisfactorily. Absorption of radiation by the silver bromide crystals decreases as the kilovoltage increases and when exposures are correct there is little opportunity to produce excessive densities in the image.

In the case of human radiography, when the scale of densities representing a departure from the normal occurs, the image becomes open to pathologic or physiologic suspicion. In the final analysis, the criterion of good diagnostic contrast is whether one sees all one expects to see. Compare the photographs shown in Figures 13 and 14 and note that the long-scale contrast in the photograph, Figure 14, *Left,* exhibits a larger number of details than the short-scale contrast picture, Figure 13, *Left.*

Long-scale contrast is characterized by a large number of translucent densities of varying tone value, each of which represents some structural element of the part examined. The transition between tones is gradual. Long-scale contrast makes possible visualization of small units of image density. The short wave length radiation employed effects greater penetration of the tissues resulting in an abundance of remnant radiation of varying intensity that, in turn, produces a large number of translucent densities (Figure 14, *Right*). The contrast scale, however, should never be so long that differentiation between structures is difficult. If the maximum of diagnostic information is to be obtained in the survey film, a compromise must be made between the radiograph with short-scale contrast or that exhibiting the longer-scale contrast. Typical examples of long-scale contrast are shown in Figure 16.

OTHER CONTRAST FACTORS

There are a number of factors other than kilovoltage that influence radiographic contrast. They are: (a) developer contrast, (b) film contrast, and (c) tissue contrast. It is fortunate that these factors may be so regulated that they can in a measure be considered as constants and standardized. As will be explained later, the exposure factor of kilovoltage, then, can be used as the active variable in altering radiographic contrast.

Developer Contrast

Two types of x-ray film developers are in common use. The *regular* developer is usually a sodium carbonate developer that produces long-scale contrast in the radiographic image. The other type developer is one containing a more active alkali (kodalk) or sodium hydroxide which produces greater contrast in the image as compared to that produced by the regular developer. Each type of contrast is inherent to each developer and established by the manufacturer, and it should be treated as a constant.

Since the type of contrast rendered by the developer can be changed in some measure by the time and temperature of development, the maximum radiographic contrast from either type of developer will be obtained when *full* development is employed. Attempts to change contrast by alteration of the solutions or by use of a nonstandardized method of development invariably yields unsatisfactory results. Comparisons between the contrasts produced by the use of both types of developer may be made by reference to Figure

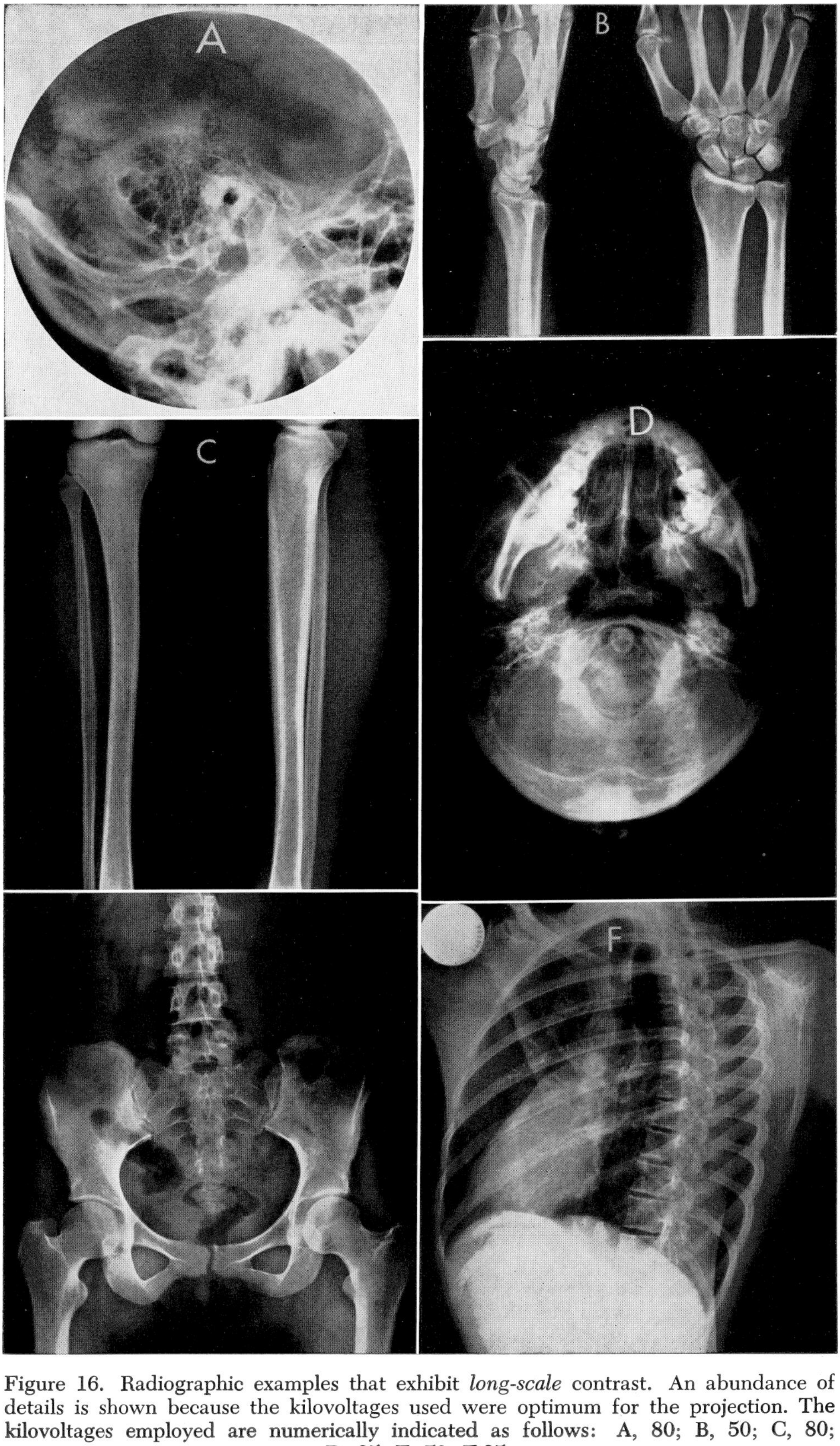

Figure 16. Radiographic examples that exhibit *long-scale* contrast. An abundance of details is shown because the kilovoltages used were optimum for the projection. The kilovoltages employed are numerically indicated as follows: A, 80; B, 50; C, 80; D, 85; E, 70; F,85.

149, Chapter 20, wherein the time of development at 68° F. in each case has been varied in 1-minute intervals.

Film Contrast

X-ray film is manufactured with inherent contrast characteristics that are most suitable for the type of radiograph it is designed to produce. It is axiomatic that different kinds of x-ray films made by one manufacturer or those made by another manufacturer yield different contrasts even though the same developer and processing procedures are employed. Two general types of medical x-ray film are normally employed that can yield any one of several kinds of radiographic contrast depending upon the manner in which the films are exposed. The use of either type is based primarily on the speed and image definition requirements for the various projections.

Screen-type film possesses an emulsion that is particularly sensitive to the blue-violet fluorescent light emitted by x-ray intensifying screens. It is less sensitive to the direct action of x-rays. The characteristics of this film are such that a relatively *higher* contrast is obtained when it is exposed with intensifying screens than when the same film is directly exposed to x-rays at the same kilovoltage.

When two posteroanterior radiographs at 50 KvP and 36″ FFD are made of a body part such as the hand (Figure 17), one with 1.5 MaS and intensifying screens (*Left*) and the other without them (*Right*) at 40 MaS, the images differ materially in contrast and sharpness of definition. In the case of the screen exposure, bone details exhibit greater contrast, but there is some loss in image sharpness. The soft tissues show higher density and in some areas details cannot be easily visualized because of some opaque densities. The radiograph made *without* screens, however, will show a lower contrast and greater detail sharpness, while the densities representative of *all* tissues are translucent. However, screens should always be employed in radiography of the heavier body parts and where shortness of exposure is necessary to stop movement.

The direct-exposure film has an emulsion that is predominantly sensitive to the *direct* action of x-rays rather than to screen-light. It should not be used with screens. This film has thick silver emulsion layers and provides relatively higher radiographic contrast than the screen-type film when direct exposures are employed using the same kilovoltage. It is about three times faster than screen-type film under these conditions. Upon direct exposure, using either film, most of the silver deposit will be found distributed *throughout* the emulsion. Because of the heavier silver emulsion of the direct-exposure film, more silver bromide crystals are present for exposure and heavier densities occur than are found on the screen-type film when the same kilovoltage is used. The higher contrast provided by direct-exposure film makes possible the use of higher kilovoltages to lengthen the contrast scale and utilize shorter exposures to greater advantage (Figure 18).

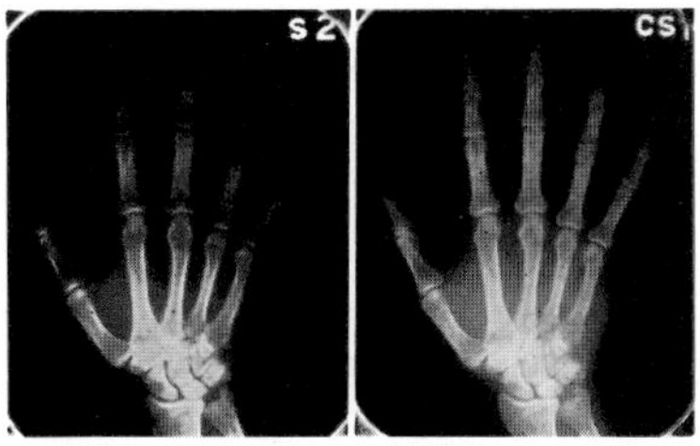

Figure 17. Two posteroanterior radiographs of a thin part (hand) of the body: (*Left*) made with intensifying screens; note shorter scale contrast. (*Right*) made without intensifying screens.

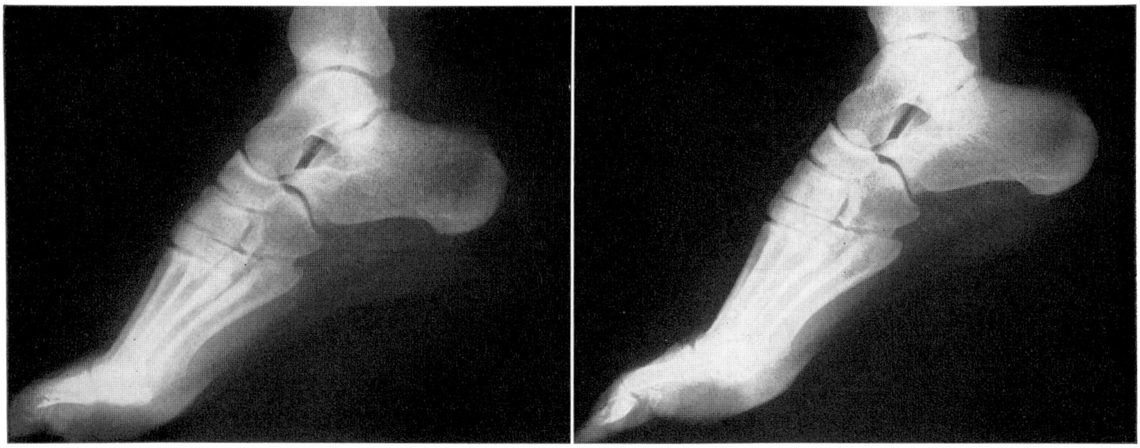

Figure 18. Radiographs of the foot employing the same kilovoltage and direct exposure: (*Left*) with screen-type film; (*Right*) with direct exposure film. Note longer contrast scale in image on screen-type film.

CONTRAST AND DIAGNOSIS

The radiologist knows that certain anatomical areas must be depicted in a particular manner when a given projection is used. All radiologists use the same basis for evaluating the diagnostic worth of the radiograph. The means by which these structures are presented to him in the image is photographic and comprises the visual appeal created by differences in concentration of the silver deposits which represent the various tissue components. In the main, these silver deposits (density differences) are all the eye has to work on. However, detail sharpness is also a factor in visualization. In general, the greater the range of densities within the image, the greater the ease with which a diagnosis can be made because details are more readily evident. The type of body part being examined has a decided bearing upon detail visualization and the wide range of available kilovoltages makes possible good detail representation of any part of the body. Since kilovoltage (Chapter 9) can alter the contrast within the image to reveal essential details, all body parts as they are presented by each projection should, therefore, be carefully evaluated. The image should be such that it can be interpreted by anyone with the necessary experience—there is no place for conjecture in diagnosis. There must be radiographic evidence.

Geometric Characteristics. The geometric character of the silver image is discussed in Chapter 13.

SUMMARY

RADIOGRAPHIC DENSITY

Radiographic density is the resultant deposit of black metallic silver on an x-ray film after it has been exposed and processed. Details of the tissue elements examined are rendered as radiographic densities of varying concentration.

RADOGRAPHIC DETAIL

Radiographic detail comprises all silver deposits on an x-ray film that in the aggregate compose the radiographic image.

TONE VALUE

The *tone value* of any radiographic density is influenced by the degree of silver concentration in the deposit. Tone value is considered to be the degree of light transmission (brightness) of the various densities when they are viewed in the aggregate as an image before an x-ray illuminator.

RADIOGRAPHIC CONTRAST

Radiographic contrast is that characteristic of the image that provides sufficient differentiation between translucent radiographic densities to reveal all possible anatomical details when viewed on an x-ray illuminator. Contrast cannot exist unless two or more radiographic densities are present. In other words, contrast facilitates the visualization of all important tissue structures irrespective of their type. Kilovoltage is the exposure factor that regulates radiographic contrast, hence visibility of details. There are two general types of contrast—

Short-scale contrast, wherein the range of image densities is short and small in number; each density exhibits a large tonal difference from its neighbor. This type of contrast is impractical in medical radiography.

Long-scale contrast, wherein the range of image densities is wide and great in number; each density exhibits only a relatively small tonal difference from its neighbor. This scale of contrast is ideal for medical radiography.

OTHER INFLUENCING CONTRASTS

The contrast inherent to the x-ray developer, the type of film, the x-ray intensifying screens and the type tissue contribute to the sum total of radiographic contrast.

X-RAY PENETRATION

Penetration of the tissues is determined by the x-ray wave length, which is directly influenced by the kilovoltage; it is also affected by the density of the tissues as well as their thickness.

Chapter 6

Radiographic Exposure

A STUDY OF radiographic exposure factors in relation to image characteristics demonstrates two important aspects: (1) photographic, and (2) geometric. The photographic aspect is related to the over-all *quantity* of silver deposited on the film (radiographic density) and its over-all *distribution* (radiographic contrast). The geometric aspect is related to the form and sharpness of definition of the image that will be discussed in Chapter 13. Radiographic exposure denotes the sensitizing action of the silver bromide crystals within the film emulsion by x-rays. The action is based upon the combined effects of: (1) the intensity of the x-rays reaching the film from a given focus-film distance; (2) the duration of the time that the x-rays act on the emulsion; and (3) the wave length of the x-rays. If the x-rays do not penetrate the object or body part and reach the film, there is no exposure; hence, no emulsion response.

X-RAY PENETRATION AND ABSORPTION

X-rays have wide variations in their ability to penetrate human tissues. The penetration of tissue is directly associated with the x-ray absorption properties exercised by the composition and thickness of the tissues irradiated. Penetration is a property of the applied x-ray wave length and the means for providing correct radiographic contrast. It should be realized that only a very small fraction of the original primary radiation emitted is effectively utilized in an exposure because the bulk of the x-rays is either absorbed by the tissues or converted into secondary radiation. For example, it has been estimated that in a posteroanterior projection of the chest only 5 per cent of the traversing radiation emerges to expose the film. An anteroposterior view of the abdomen uses about 0.1 per cent and a lateral abdominal projection about 0.01 per cent. It is evident, therefore, that a correct application of exposure factors depends upon an intelligent analysis of tissues thickness and composition if the most efficient use is to be made of the image-forming radiation.

As an x-ray beam leaves the x-ray tube, it is composed of radiation possessing many *different* wave lengths. Predominant are the wave lengths typical of the specific kilovoltage applied to the tube. These are the wave lengths required when making a radiograph of a particular part of the body. In every x-ray beam there are a number of long wave lengths that are largely absorbed by the tissues. There are also wave lengths that are shorter than those produced by a specific kilovoltage. Some of this radiation tends to augment in minor degree the exposure effect of the predominant wave lengths.

As the primary x-ray beam traverses the tissues, various portions of the beam are selectively absorbed in accordance with the composition and thickness of the tissues. In consequence, the intensity of the remnant beam is *not* uniform as it emerges from the body. The greater the tissue absorption, the less intense is the emergent radiation that can expose the film and record the image, and vice versa. Upon development of the exposed film, black metallic silver constituting the image is deposited in proportion to the varying intensities of radiation contained in the remnant beam. A relationship, therefore, exists between tissue absorption and penetration, and radiographic density. A correct radiographic exposure is based upon the penetration qualities of the radiation and its amount. In other words, the x-radiation must be both *qualitatively* and *quantitatively* adequate.

FACTOR OF X-RAY WAVE LENGTH

In routine radiography, satisfactory image densities result only when the radiation penetrates the entire part. Attempts to circumvent this fact invariably result in the use of prolonged impractical exposures that seldom yield satisfactory images. This type image cannot be diagnostically useful, for many of the denser and thicker tissues are not penetrated. In general, long wave length radiation, produces short-scale contrast in the image. Bone absorbs a large amount of radiation and few osseous details may be shown in a radiograph, yet soft tissue details are visible. The absorption properties between these two tissues under these circumstances are exceedingly wide and details of both tissues cannot be shown in a single image. As a measure of economy and diagnostic expediency, therefore, a single radiograph that records *both* classes of tissue is preferable.

An x-ray beam consisting of predominantly long wave lengths does contain some of the shorter wave lengths. These shorter wave length rays actually create most of the image when an impractically *long* exposure is employed since the longer wave lengths are largely absorbed. There are a number of practical objections to an exposure procedure of this kind and its use is not recommended for an exposure routine because the maximum safe dosage to the patient would soon be reached—it often is exceeded in one exposure; the patient may move during an impractically long exposure; the latitude of exposure would be such that no margin for error would be possible; and, most important, complete penetration would not be attained. When the wave length is shortened, the absorption properties of flesh and bone are brought closer together because of a more uniform penetration of the tissues. The manner in which the film responds to various wave lengths may be diagrammatically explained as follows.

Long Wave Length Exposure

Reference to Figure 19 will serve to explain theoretically the penetration and absorption of x-rays. In diagram (A), a small unit of an x-ray beam of long wave length is projected toward an object. The predominantly long wave length x-rays are shown to partially penetrate the object but none emerges to expose the film because they have been absorbed by the object. Actually, a limited number of the shorter wave lengths in this primary beam do penetrate the object and expose the film slightly as shown in (E). For practical radiographic use, however, their number is so small that they cannot be depended

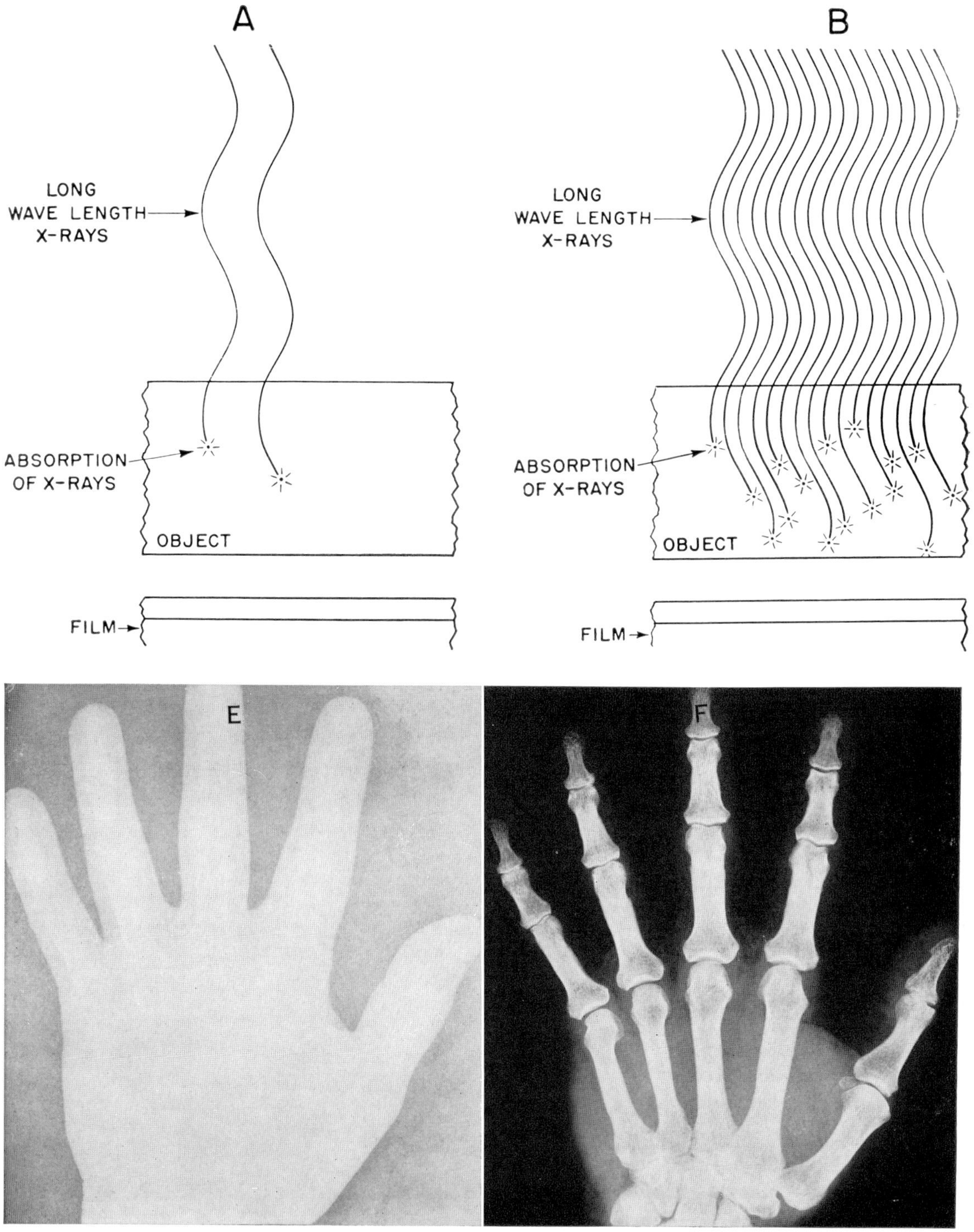

Figure 19. Illustrations demonstrating the penetration properties of the x-ray beam. (A) and (B) effects of long wavelength radiation; (C) and (D) effects of short wavelength radiation. Radiographs of the hand (E) to (H) that simulate the theoretical conditions shown above.

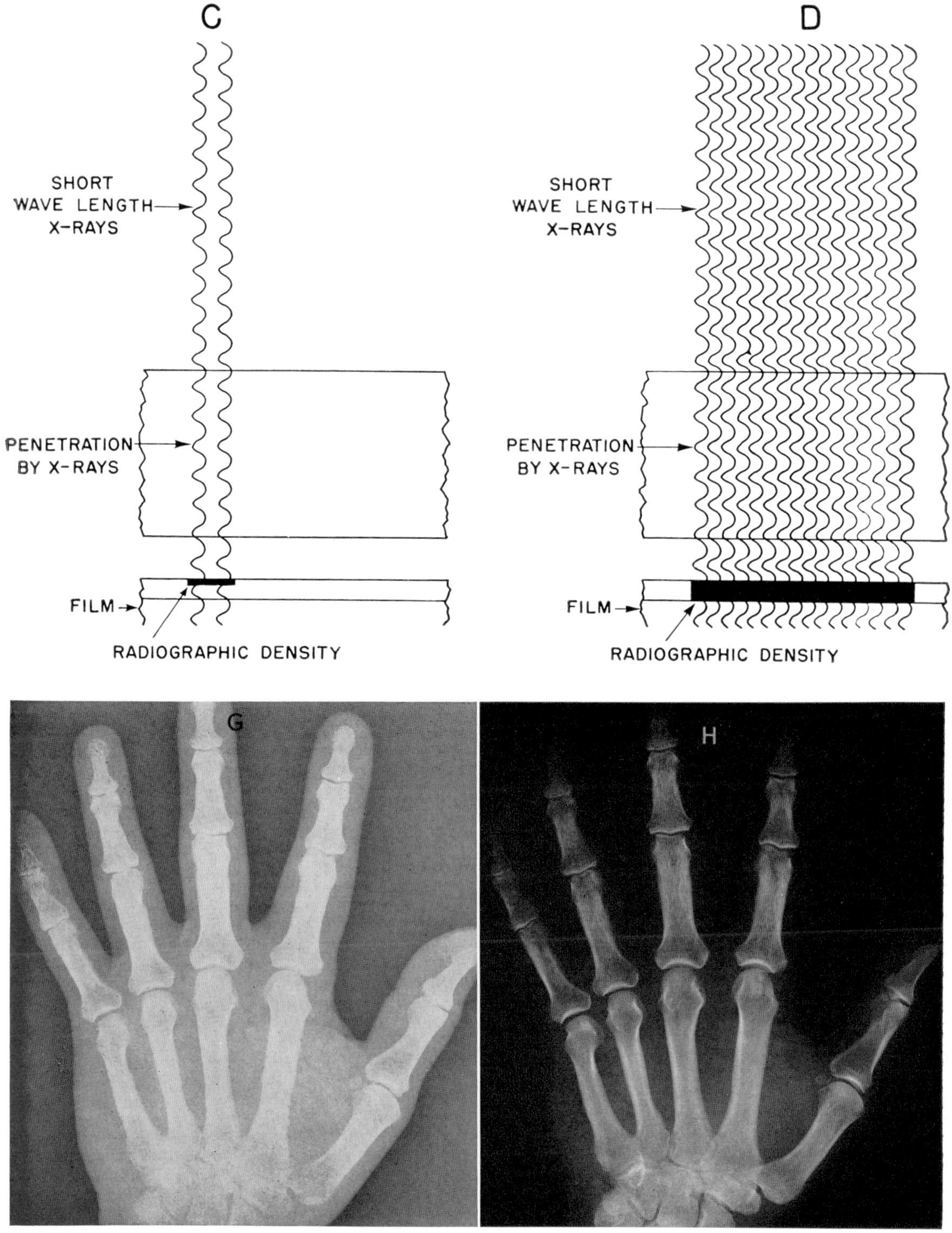

Figure 19. (*Continued. See legend on opposite page.*)

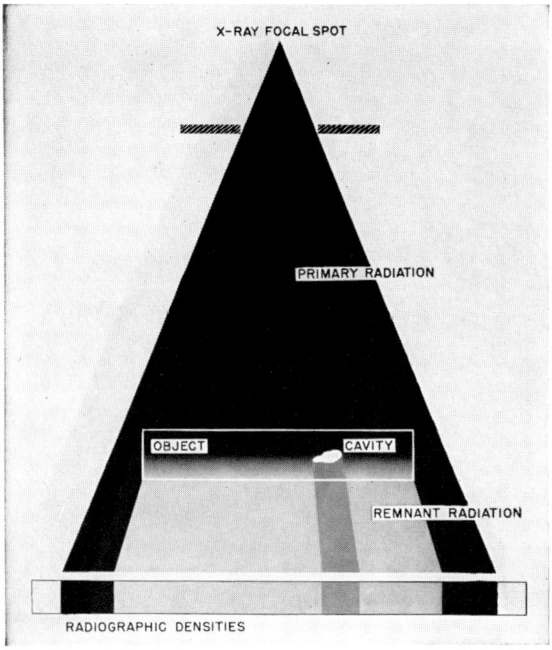

Figure 20. Diagram illustrating passage of x-rays through a homogeneous substance containing a cavity.

upon to produce a satisfactory image with a practical exposure time. When the *number* of long wave length x-rays is increased (B), they are also absorbed and fail to reach the film. The radiograph of the hand (F), was made employing the same wave length as in A but the exposure was very long and impractical. A satisfactory image was not obtained. Because the wave length was very long and insufficiently penetrating for the thicker portions of the hand, no appreciable gain in the amount of silver deposit occurred except in the image details representing the very thin tissues (fingers).

Short Wave Length Exposure

When the wave length is shortened (C), and a small unit of this x-ray beam is directed toward the object, penetration of the object easily takes place. The emergent x-rays (remnant radiation) sensitize a small unit of silver bromide emulsion in the x-ray film that upon development changes to a deposit of black metallic silver —a radiographic density. This is comparable to the image shown in (G), wherein weak radiographic densities in the image representing the *thicker* portions of the hand indicate that the radiation is sufficiently penetrating but it is inadequate in quantity. The radiation may now be considered *qualitatively* correct and penetration of the hand attained. However, the *number* of short wave length x-rays is still too small to expose the film sufficiently and produce a satisfactory image. With the same kilovoltage and an increase in exposure a satisfactory image is obtained (D) and (H).

ABSORPTION

Radiographically, absorption actually refers to the reduction in x-ray intensity that occurs as the x-ray beam traverses the body part. Absorption is influenced by the atomic weight (composition) of the tissue traversed as well as its thickness and the wave length of the radiation employed. Organic tissue offers no particular penetration problem but it necessitates control over the large amounts of secondary radiation that often are emitted. Inorganic tissue contains such a large quantity of mineral matter that extreme absorption of radiation may occasionally constitute a problem. High tissue density is often associated with large tissue thicknesses and special procedures are required to secure satisfactory radiographs.

ABSORPTION BY HOMOGENEOUS OBJECT

A homogeneous object is one in which

the material composing it is structurally uniform such as a block of aluminum.

Uniform Thickness

A diagrammatic representation of the passage of an x-ray beam through a homogeneous object such as an aluminum block of uniform thickness containing a cavity is shown in Figure 20. As the x-rays pass through the object in the area of the cavity, less substance capable of absorbing x-rays is present as compared to other portions of the object. The intensity of the remnant beam emerging from the area of the cavity is greater than that from the balance of the object. Consequently, the radiographic density in this portion of the image is greater. The difference in the density representing the major portion of the block and the cavity is due to the differences in intensity of the remnant radiation.

Unequal Thickness

To demonstrate the absorption character of an object of homogeneous consistency but unequal in thickness, an aluminum step-wedge (Figure 21) may be employed. X-ray absorption by an aluminum step-wedge is diagrammatically shown in Figure 22. The portion of the x-ray beam passing through the first step of the wedge is slightly absorbed and the remnant radiation produces a high density to represent this step. The absorption by the second step of the wedge is greater than that of the first step because it has twice the thickness; the intensity of the remnant radiation is thereby further reduced and a lesser density is produced; and, so on for the remainder of the steps. As the thickness of the object increases with each step of the wedge, the intensity of the primary beam is reduced so that less and less radiation emerges to expose the film. The image, therefore, consists of a graduated scale of densities with different tone values.

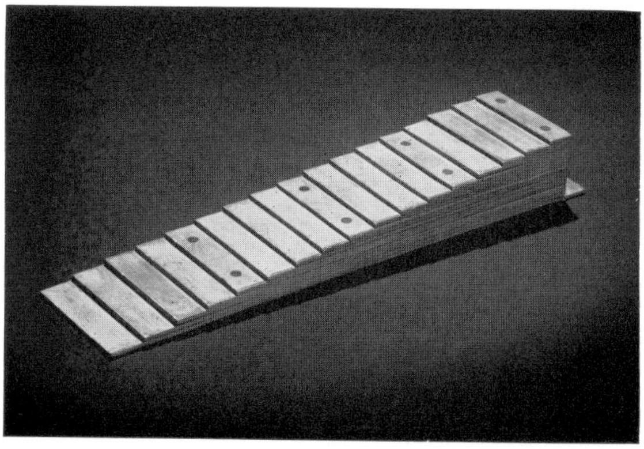

Figure 21. Photograph of typical aluminum step-wedge used for experimental purposes in radiography.

Absorption-Density Relation

It may be seen from the above that the difference in x-ray absorption of each step of aluminum had a direct relationship to its respective radiographic density. Since each step of the wedge was homogeneous

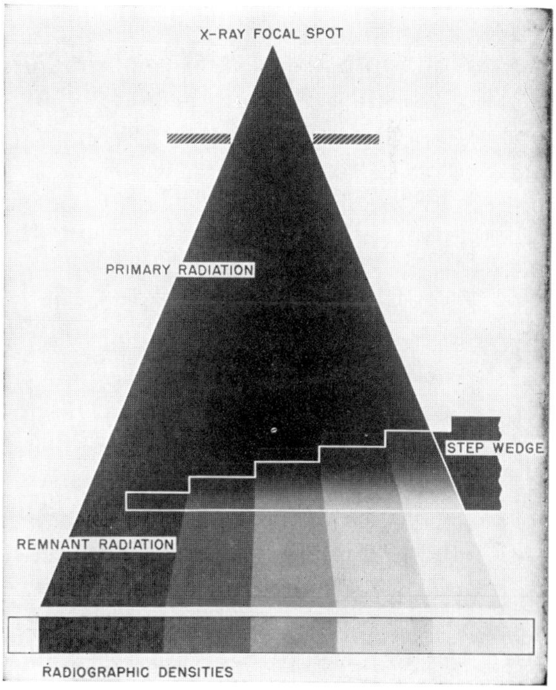

Figure 22. Diagram showing passage of x-rays through a homogeneous material (step-wedge) that varies in thickness.

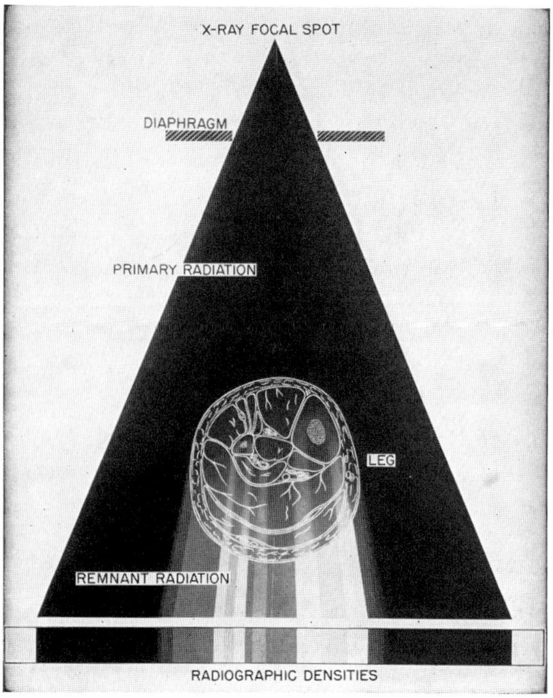

Figure 23. Diagram illustrating the penetration and absorption of an x-ray beam as it traverses a body part (leg) whose components absorb the x-rays in varying degree depending upon their thickness and tissue-density.

and uniform in its x-ray absorption, radiographic densities varying in tone value representative of each step resulted. The image density of each step was directly related to the intensity of the remnant radiation reaching the film.

ABSORPTION BY BODY PART

When x-rays pass through human tissue, each type of tissue absorbs its proportion of radiation according to its own tissue density and thickness. For example, as x-rays pass through one thickness of flesh, then through a thickness of bone and finally through another thickness of flesh, the total absorption is the sum of the various degrees of absorption exercised by the different tissues (Figure 23). Radiographic delineation of human tissues cannot be predicated upon their thicknesses alone. Their physical state (tissue density) is of the greatest importance from the standpoint of x-ray absorption. Absorption by various tissue components introduces the element of *tissue contrast* which is of major importance.

Tissue Contrast

Tissue contrast—sometimes called subject contrast—represents the differences in x-ray absorption occurring in an anatomical part. The greater the x-ray absorption of a tissue with relation to adjacent tissue, the greater the tissue contrast; the lower the tissue absorption, the lower the contrast. For example, greater tissue contrast is exhibited between bone and surrounding soft tissues than between kidney tissue and muscle. Also, the selective absorption of each tissue component within the leg causes different intensities within the remnant beam to produce variations in the image densities. As illustrated by the wedge (Figure 22), it was possible to differentiate between the various thicknesses of metal simply by comparing the tone value of one density with another. The same situation in a measure holds true with the leg, but, in addition, the composite absorption of x-rays by superimposed tissues of different types at different planes materially affects the image. Variation in thickness and composition is often evidenced as small differences in radiographic density. Since these differences are to be interpreted by the radiologist as anatomic details, they should be easily visible and translucent when viewed on the x-ray illuminator.

ABSORPTION VARIABLES

In radiography there are a number of unpredictable absorption variables in body tissues that are influenced by physiologic or pathologic changes and they may be disregarded in some measure if the exposure system provides enough latitude.

Generally, small deviations from the normal in tissue density or thickness can be ignored. Recognizable abnormal conditions, of course, may be easily compensated by adjustment of the variable exposure factor selected, usually the MaS.

Large Absorption Differences

When structural tissue details are widely different, each presents wide differences in absorbing power and wide differences in tone value will exist in the radiograph. Where a body part contains thick heavy bone surrounded by a large quantity of muscle and fat, as in the lumbar vertebral region, x-ray absorption differences become relatively wide (Figure 24). The image of a calcified body (Figure 25), outlined by the darker adjacent densities of its containing tissues also exhibits great tonal differences and provides easy visibility. As a rule, such parts provide little difficulty in recording even though large errors in exposure may be made.

Small Absorption Differences

At times, absorption differences between some tissues may be very small and differ-

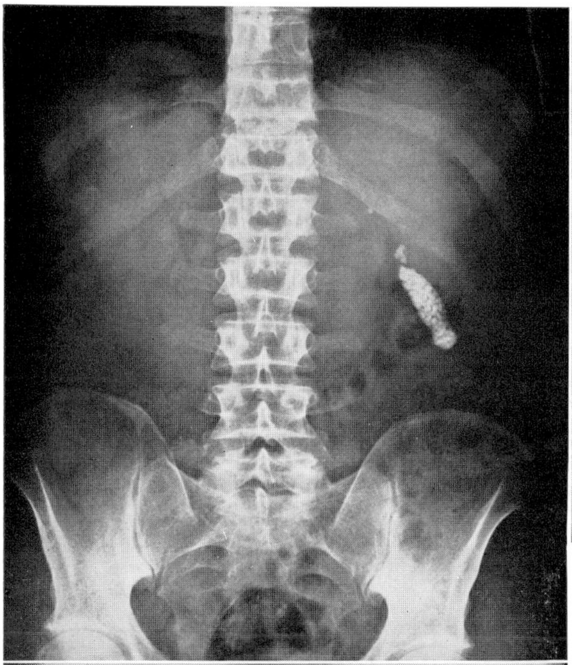

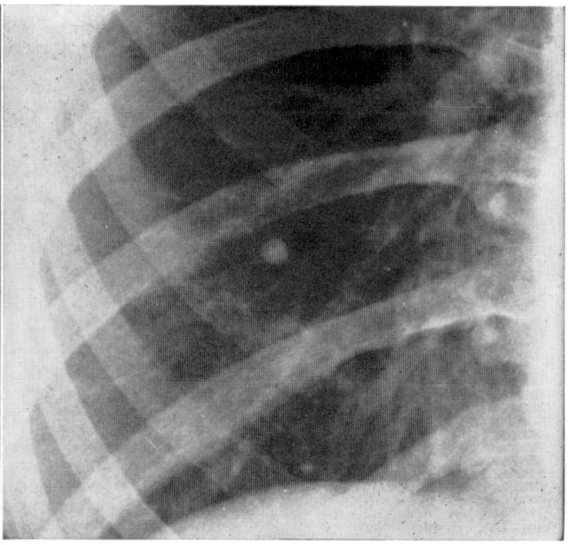

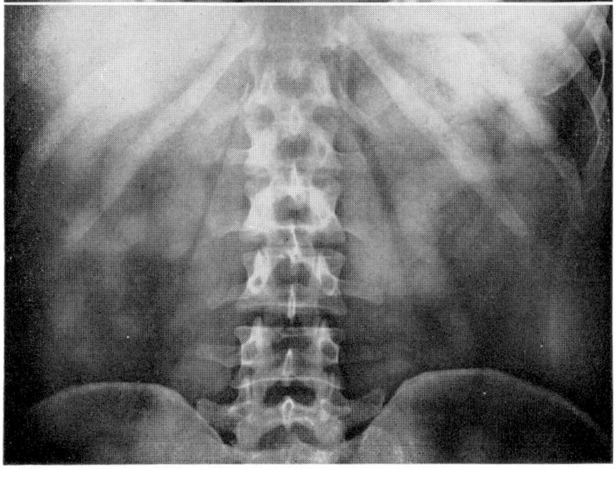

Figure 24 (*Left*). Anteroposterior screen-grid radiograph of the lumbar vertebrae. Wide absorption differences of the tissues produce a variety of radiographic densities in the image.

Figure 25 (*Above*). Portion of a posteroanterior chest screen-radiograph showing a calcification of high contrast against a low contrast background group of densities representing small differences in absorption by pulmonary tissues.

Figure 26 (*Left*). Anteroposterior screen-grid radiograph of the kidney region that exhibits small differences in density because the tissues penetrated are almost comparable in tissue density.

entiation becomes difficult. The kidney, gallbladder and liver areas are typical examples in which the x-ray absorbing power of the tissues is almost the same (Figure 26). The tonal differentiation of a small portion of lymphatic tissue within its surrounding tissues, also, cannot be as distinctive against its background density as could a calculus because of the small tissue absorption differences. A shorter scale of contrast in the image would therefore be helpful and perhaps necessary.

The use of exposure factors that produce favorable contrast patterns in the radiograph is based upon a knowledge of the relative tissue absorption properties of the anatomy. Where there is an appreciable density difference, as between bone and flesh, a compromise in detail rendition must be made in order to attain a satisfactory image of bone and flesh. However, in other areas, because of relatively small tissue absorption differences, the tonal differences between densities are exceedingly slight and may be lost if sufficient image contrast is not available. Such areas may be obliterated when an incorrect exposure is made.

The scale of radiographic contrast may best be well regulated if the type and nature of the anatomy being examined are properly evaluated. The differences in tissue absorption can be scaled to radiographic requirements by an appropriate selection of kilovoltage. For example, in the hand there are wide x-ray absorption differences between the flesh and the bones. The flesh is easily penetrated and has low x-ray absorption properties while the bones, although penetrable, absorb more x-radiation. In this situation it is necessary to use a *quality* of radiation that will record minor details within the flesh such as fingernails, muscle, or tendon details, as well as the osseous details. Shortening the scale of contrast increases the visibility of details within the soft tissues provided the exposure is correct but the thicker portions of the part may be either rendered as very weak opaque silver deposits, or not at all, due to the inadequacy of the kilovoltage employed. With prolonged exposure the flesh details may be obliterated by opaque silver deposits and the osseous details will be rendered with high contrast. Some osseous areas may be deficient in silver even under these exaggerated exposure conditions. On the other hand, when a correct exposure reveals details in both soft tissues and bone by the use of a compromise wave length, a diagnostic image is secured. When the wave length of the radiation is deemed to be optimum for a given projection, tissue contrast becomes a constant.

USE OF CONTRAST MEDIA

Contrast media are employed to render high tissue contrast in a viscus that normally has very low tissue contrast. These media comprise various nontoxic chemical preparations that have high x-ray absorption properties. They are either injected or ingested into the viscus before radiography is performed. Air is also very useful on occasions because of its very low x-ray absorption properties. The alimentary tract normally cannot be differentiated from surrounding tissues and it must be filled with a 'test meal' containing barium sulfate of high purity (A), Figure 27. For localization of abnormalities of the brain, air is often used to outline the ventricles (B). Study of the urinary tract function requires the absorption of a contrast medium by the body and upon excretion by the kidneys, details of the urinary tract can be radiographically delineated. This type of radiograph is called an intravenous pyelogram. Study of the urinary tract can also be accomplished by inserting radio-

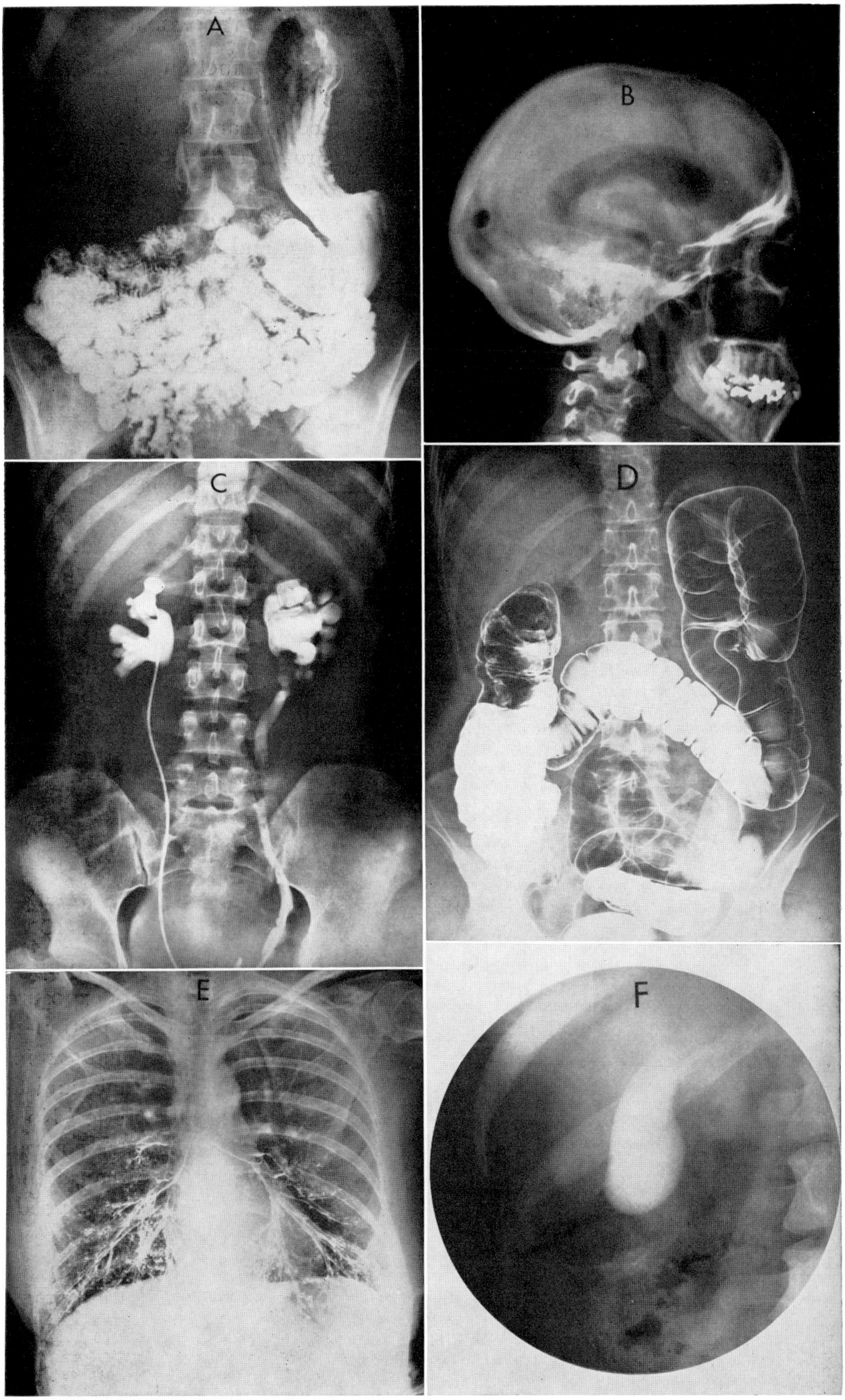

Figure 27. Radiographs in which contrast media have been employed to delineate anatomic structures. (A) Stomach and small intestine; (B) ventricles of the brain; (C) kidneys and ureters; (D) colon; (E) bronchi; (F) gall bladder.

paque catheters into the ureters and injecting a contrast medium into the pelvis of the kidney (C). This type of radiograph is known as a retrograde pyelogram. Air is often injected into the large intestine to augment the contrast properties of the barium sulfate meal or enema (D). The bronchi can be made visible by injecting an opaque substance into the lung (E). To study the function of the gallbladder, a harmless dye is injected into a vein. This substance is carried to the liver by the blood stream and is secreted with the bile into the gallbladder. Since the dye in the bile is opaque to x-rays, an image of the gallbladder and its contents can be visualized (F).

VALUE OF CONSTANTS

To understand the many factors that influence the radiographic image, the function of each factor in the exposure system must be thoroughly appreciated. The role of any factor must be determined by the use of the factor as a variable while all other factors remain constant. The influence of development on the radiographic image must also be known to appreciate the necessity for establishing as a constant the whole processing procedure; so that any variations in radiographic quality may then be attributed to exposure variations rather than to development. For example, if kilovoltage is to be studied to determine its radiographic influence in the exposure system, it should be employed as the variable and all other exposure and processing factors should be constant. The establishment of an exposure system should be based upon the employment as constants of those factors that have the *greatest* influence on the quality of the image and the selection of one factor that possesses only a single radiographic function as the variable.

METHOD STUDY

The principal radiographic functions of focus-film distance, kilovoltage, and milliampere-seconds are discussed separately in subsequent chapters in relation to radiographic density and contrast; for example, their photographic effects. The factors that exert geometric influence on the radiographic image are discussed in Chapter 13. The associated theory and arithmetic required to solve exposure problems will precede practical laboratory experiments that the student should perform, for they provide initial training in handling x-ray apparatus and its accessories, and exposure and processing practices. It is advised, however, that the experiments requiring exposures of the human body be postponed until the student has been instructed in body positioning.

ARITHMETICAL RELATIONS

Occasions arise in radiography wherein it is necessary to change an exposure factor to conform to a new projection requirement. Calculations for changes in focus-film distance, milliamperage, and time are matters of simple arithmetic. No reliable formula is available for compensating changes in kilovoltage because the radiographic image is greatly influenced by unpredictable absorption factors exercised by the human tissues in relation to the penetrating power of the radiation employed.

EXPOSURE EXPERIMENTS

To familiarize the student with the manipulation of x-ray apparatus and the use of exposure factors, simple experiments will be outlined. In performing these experiments, it is well to adjust the apparatus to produce the desired exposure factors before the object or the patient is positioned. Many radiographic exposures fail because insufficient care is taken in setting up the factors on the control panel of the x-ray apparatus. In setting up the exposure factors, the following procedure should be employed in sequence:

1. Select the milliamperage station that is to be employed.
2. Adjust the kilovoltage to the value desired.
3. Set the timer for the duration of exposure required.
4. Be sure the focus-film distance is correct.

Be sure exposure time, Ma or KvP values do not exceed the safey limits indicated by the capacity chart for the x-ray tube. When employing 1/60-second exposures, remember that this exposure time uses two impulses of current. If the timer is defective, an impulse may be lost and only one-half the exposure may be received by the film.

Lead Aperture Mask

A lead aperture mask is a very practical device for making the experiments. The resulting densities obtained after exposure may be easily compared. By placing lead numerals or letters in the apertures before exposure, an accurate record of the factors employed may be made. The mask (Figure 28) consists of a sheet of lead 1/16 x 8 x 10 inches, in which circular apertures 1.5 inches in diameter are cut. By using additional small sheets of lead as covering material, any single aperture or group of apertures may be selected through which exposures can be made.

Lead Figures and Letters

So that each experiment can be readily identified, suitable lead figures should be placed on the film before the exposure is made. Identifying exposure factors can then appear on each radiograph for reference.

VALUE OF PROTECTIVE FILTRATION

The radiographic effect of aluminum filtration is to screen out the long wave length radiation that is not needed for routine radiography and which may be hazardous to a patient. The primary effect of filtration is to alter the *quality* of the radiation and secondarily, the *quantity* of the radiation. As aluminum filtration is increased, some of the longer wave lengths of radiation are absorbed while the shorter wave lengths pass with the result that the contrast scale is lengthened in radiography of the thinner parts. However, the contrast scale is not influenced in radiography of heavy parts. In the interest of radiographic quality, there is a limit to the amount of aluminum filtration that should be used. It is most advisable, however, always to maintain at least 1 millimeter of external aluminum filtration in the filter channel. For reducing patient dosage, radiological authority now advocates 2 mm.

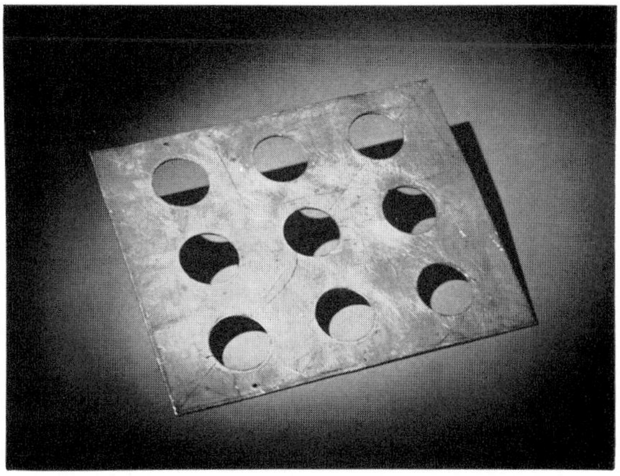

Figure 28. Lead aperture mask

Chapter 7

Body Tissues

The study of radiographs is actually an inquiry into living anatomy in its normal form or its deformation as a result of physiologic, pathologic, or structural change. The human body is a highly integrated chemical and structural entity with well-defined physiologic and mental processes. The relative differences in the composition and thickness of tissue components of a body part exert great influence on the radiation traversing it. This applies not alone to different parts of the same body, but also to the same parts of different bodies.

Absorption is intimately associated with the atomic number of the tissue elements being irradiated. Bone is less penetrable than the surrounding soft tissue. Body fluids possess about the same absorption characteristics as soft tissue. The pathologic and physiologic states of the tissues are also important when considering absorption differences. Selection and alteration of exposure factors must be made with these facts in mind. A good knowledge of human anatomy, therefore, helps in analyzing the various types of tissue combinations that are presented in routine radiography.

PHYSIQUE

Adequate study and analysis of the human body requires the conception for radiographic purposes of a geometric figure of bone and flesh. However, no two human physiques are identical. Not only do they differ in their general family and racial physical characteristics but individual parts vary widely in size, shape, and tissue density. Naturally, gradations between types of physiques do occur.

In radiography, therefore, any x-ray exposure system should encompass all of the body deviations with sufficient latitude so that radiographs of diagnostic utility can be produced with some measure of standardization.

BODY TYPES

The analysis of a living body for radiographic purposes requires its classification into one of three types, or more pertinently, somatotypes. Also, some discernment as to the physiology of the body should be made as well as an estimate as to the influence of disease or trauma on the tissues. There are three general types of physique classified under the term habitus —hypersthenic, sthenic, and asthenic. These types have been recently identified and renamed by Sheldon,* respectively,

* Sheldon, W. H.: *The Varieties of Human Physique.* New York, Harper and Brothers, 1940.

as endomorphic, mesomorphic and ectomorphic.

The characteristics of each type resolve into states wherein they can be generally separated almost as an entity from each other. It is not possible to strike much of an average in classification because the features of all body types are extensively interrelated. By study of the extremes of each type, however, a definite understanding of the variables in physique that must be met in radiography can be achieved and exposure compromises, usually of a low order, can be effected.

Hypersthenic

The hypersthenic type is characterized by softness and roundness throughout the various bodily regions. The tissues tend to be flabby with an excess of subcutaneous fat. The bones are small. Physically, however, this type often exhibits great strength. The torso is barrel-like. The digestive tract is large, and tends to dominate the individual, hence, the tendency to accumulate fat. The anteroposterior and lateral thicknesses are quite comparable in the head, neck, trunk, and limbs. Abdominal and thoracic volume is predominant as compared to the head and extremities. The well developed chest is relatively short and wide at the base. The shoulders are square and high with soft contours. The neck is short and thick and the waistline is high. Muscle relief is minimal. The head is almost spherical and the face is wide. The hands and feet are comparatively small. The vertebral column is relatively straight when viewed laterally and the back is usually well padded with fat. The skin is soft and smooth. The hard palate is wide and low. The heart is usually transverse.

This type tends to become obese and is often a victim of hypertension. Degenerative diseases of the heart, arteries and kidneys are common to the type.

Sthenic

The sthenic type is strong and active. Movements are relatively slow and awkward because of the heavy muscle development. The shoulders are fairly wide. The joints and bones are large. The abdominal wall is muscular and slightly prominent just beneath the umbilicus. The physique is heavy in muscle and bone and relatively rectangular in shape. The skin is thick with an abundance of underlying connective tissue. These persons are physically and emotionally well balanced.

The anteroposterior trunk thicknesses are less than those in the hypersthenic type. The lateral dimensions are usually large. Forearm thicknesses may equal the upper arm. The wrist and hand are large and heavy. The well developed chest is larger than the abdomen. The trunk is long and the pectoral area is wide; the waist is slender and low. The pelvis is sturdy with broad hips. The head varies widely in size and tends toward a cubical shape. The forehead is low. The neck is long, strong, and the transverse thickness is greater than the anteroposterior dimension. The clavicles are heavy and prominent. The face is long and broad.

Asthenic

The asthenic type exhibits a sense of fragility, linearity, and delicacy of body. The head varies widely in size but tends to be large. The lower jaw appears underdeveloped. The facial bones are delicate and lack prominence. The neck is long and slender and projects forward. Small bones and stringy muscles prevail. The thorax is long, flat and narrow. The ribs are thin and prominent and the shoulders are narrow without muscle relief. The shoulder girdle lacks muscular support and the scapulae tend to protrude posteriorly. The trunk is short and the limbs long. The abdomen is flat and shallow in depth; the lower abdomen is prominent. The abdominal viscera tend to be ptosed. The lumbar curve is flat and the thoracic curve is often prominent. The hard palate is narrow and high. Weakness of the thighs and upper arms is a typical feature of the asthenic type.

The type is physically weak, nervous, and prone to functional nervous disorders.

The foregoing physical characteristics are of course the extreme variants of the three somatotypes. As a matter of familial and hereditary characteristics, there is a blending of one type into another resulting in physiques of mixed components. In example, a dominant asthenic type may have some less dominant characteristics of the sthenic while a sthenic may have many characteristics of the other types. However, anatomical studies indicate that the external appearance of an individual presents a good indication of what is inside the body—anatomically and temperamentally. The body being an intermixture of all types may exhibit in a more or less dominant manner special characteristics of one or the other type. Knowing the general characteristics of the extremes makes the analysis of the patient a little easier for radiographic purposes.

Geographic Differences

The region of the country in which one is born seems to exercise definite influence on the kind of body one possesses by reason of original settlement by various European or American racial elements. The population at large is primarily a mixed group with little that can be designated as "pure" stock.

The larger heavy people seem to dwell largely in the states located west of the Mississippi River. These people in general are taller and heavier and possess relatively greater tissue density.

Those people that may be termed of "average" build live in Arkansas, Louisiana, Alabama, Mississippi, New York, New Jersey, Pennsylvania and New England.

The influx of Central and South American strains as well as French to the Southern United States is reflected in the smaller Latin physiques. The large interracial mixtures of whites and American Indians in Texas and Oklahoma have resulted in heavier strains, comparable to those found west of the Mississippi.

BODY COMPOSITION

The bony framework in all normal human beings has similarity of structure, and the distribution of soft tissue and bone in various parts of the body in a given body type is relatively proportional and may, for radiographic purposes, be considered a constant. The influence of disease, trauma, and physiologic disturbances does, of course, upset these normal relationships to some degree. There are three principal constituents of body composition other than bone—fat, lean tissue, and water. Of these, only fat widely varies independently of the others in a healthy, normal person. Therefore, the habitus of the body (physique) is an excellent guide to its relative tissue content.

BODY TISSUES

For radiographic purposes, body tissues may be divided roughly into two groups: those consisting largely of *organic* materials (soft tissue) and those containing organic materials impregnated with *inorganic* substances (bone).

ORGANIC TISSUE

Organic tissue generally constitutes the soft tissues or flesh and comprises skin, fat, muscle, cartilage, tendon, nerve trunks, brain, blood vessels, viscera, etc., which all contain a large amount of fluid when compared to inorganic tissues. Organic tissues are composed of carbon, hydrogen, nitrogen, and oxygen, and possess low x-ray absorption properties. Muscle tissue contains approximately 75 to 80 per cent fluid; fat stores little fluid—about 20 per cent. Pulmonary tissue contains a large quantity of moisture-laden air in the living state.

Soft Tissues

Radiographically, soft tissues may be generally grouped as follows: solid and hollow viscera; viscera surrounded by fat; intramuscular inclusions such as fat, air, or mineral salts; pools or body fluids, such as blood; musculature; and, fat. Soft tissues that are not demarcated by fat (or air), such as the stomach, cannot always be delineated, and it is then necessary to introduce a suitable contrast medium. The x-ray absorption properties of individual soft tissues vary; muscles, body fluids, connective tissue, and solid viscera have about the same degree of absorption as water whereas fat and air-laden pulmonary tissue offer considerably less absorption. The absorption differences between these two groups of soft tissues are not as great as that between soft tissues as a group, and bone. Circulatory vessels and nerves are slightly less penetrable than surrounding muscles. The difference is so small, however, that little or no distinction between them can usually be made.

Fat

Females and young children have more body fat than males. Alteration in the fat content is probably the most important single variable, other than disease, that determines the water content of the body at any specific period in its life. For example, a malignancy may cause a patient to lose weight. If the weight loss is principally fat, the water content remains unchanged. However, the body water may be expected to increase upon disappearance of the fat. Endocrine disturbances are often evidenced by fat accumulation. Aged obese persons exhibit a wide disproportion between muscle and fat, the latter predominating.

BONE

Organic tissues containing inorganic materials are largely confined to bone, dentine, calcified cartilage and dental enamel or to those tissues in which inorganic salts are normally deposited and, as a result of some repair or disease process. These tissues contain a much smaller percentage of fluid than organic tissues as a group. The normal adult bony and cartilaginous skeleton comprises approximately 20 per cent of the total body weight.

Living Bone

Living bone is a versatile tissue possessing an organic matrix (collagen) upon which mineral salts have been deposited. It furnishes the supporting framework of the body. It is soft in young persons and hard in the older. It bears most of the blood cells; it stores minerals and releases them to various parts of the body as they are needed. It is capable of repairing itself after injury and of growing like other tissues until the body reaches adulthood. Blood vessels penetrate the bony substance. The minerals in bone are calcium phosphate and calcium carbonate in a ratio of 2:1. It is the hardest tissue in the body and comprises approximately 30 per cent organic substances, 45 per cent inorganic materials, and 25 per cent fluid. Most interesting is the ability of the body to absorb calcium or release it into the blood to maintain a constant level. The fluid content is largely confined to the organic matrix of the bone substance. In developing bone, the fluid content may be as high as 60 per cent, while in senile cortical bone it may be as low as 10 per cent. Infants' bones are seldom as well delineated radiographically as those of an adult because their mineral content is less than that in the normal adult bone. Living bone acts as a reservoir of calcium salts, and accumulates or disposes of them in accordance with the physiologic requirements of the body as a whole. Certain bones react more quickly than others to this physiologic flux. Cancellous bone is more sensitive to calcium metabolic requirements than is cortical bone. The radiographic appearance of bone is directly related to its mineral content. Normal adult bone possesses high x-ray absorption characteristics.

Bone marrow is widely dispersed in the human body; its function is to form blood. The space within the bone is filled with blood-forming tissues. The total marrow space is greater in the adult male than the female and its average volume is about 168 cubic inches. The volume increases in elderly persons because of the aging process perhaps at the expense of cortical bone.

Bone is in a constant state of building up and tearing down a little at a time. In growth, bone is built by erosion (by osteoclasts) of the inside of the bone (medulla) thereby enlarging the medullary cavity while bone forming cells (osteoblasts) build up the bone externally. Bone fractures are repaired by the laying down of a soft fibrous tissue called callus that largely originates in the periosteum and joins the ends of the fractured segments. The callus is replaced gradually with hard, new bone due to the action of the osteoblasts. The jagged edges that might interfere with function are smoothed away by the osteoclasts; also, any excess bone produced during the repair process.

Growth in length of the bone is a bit different. In childhood each bone contains a disk of cartilage (epiphysis) at its ends. As growth takes place, the cartilage disk extends itself and the part nearest the bone absorbs calcium to make bone. When the bone reaches its normal length the cartilage is entirely replaced by bone.

More than 99 per cent of the calcium of the body is in the bones but calcium is also important to the other body tissues. It is necessary for the heart movements, the clotting of blood, contraction of skeletal muscles and the proper functioning of the nervous system. Calcium reaches all tissues by means of blood plasma and is regulated by the parathyroid glands.

BODY FLUIDS

Human body fluids comprise approximately 62 per cent of body weight distributed throughout all of the tissues. The range in males may be 55 to 70 per cent; in females, 46 to 60 per cent. Bodies of the lean muscular type may contain approximately 70 per cent fluids; whereas obese bodies may contain as little as 42 per cent fluid. Fluid content is a major factor in the generation of secondary radiation by the body tissues.

Fluids exist in localized quantities in the urinary, gastrointestinal, and biliary tracts, the circulatory vessels, joint spaces, glands, spinal cord, and intraventricular spaces of the brain. If body fluids are to be differentiated from the body structures, they must be surrounded by, or infused with, some medium that will provide the necessary differential contrast.

EVALUATION OF PATIENT

The technician must continually train his eyes and mind in evaluating the patient for radiographic purposes. He should try to view the body as a physiologic or pathologic entity; each part is pulsating with blood or other fluids; it is composed of muscle, fat, bone, etc., which may be normal or affected by various degrees of nutrition, trauma, disease, or hydration. He must determine the image details that are to be accentuated and, if necessary, make suitable adjustment in the exposure factors. No matter what departures from the normal there may be in the radiographic density of these details, they must be clearly demonstrated if a correct radiologic identification is to be made of existing disease or trauma. When an abnormal *increase* in tissue absorption takes place, the radiographic density *decreases* from the normal value. When a *decrease* in tissue absorption occurs, a corresponding *increase* over the normal in radiographic density takes place.

Evaluation should be based upon the patient's physique and upon the clinical situation. In general, it is the objective in examining new patients to make, initially, *survey* radiographs that will record all details of the anatomical area in question. The technician should be able after some clinical experience to recognize deviations from the normal, since these changes intimately affect the choice of exposure factors. The influence of disease, trauma, age, and nourishment, should be recognized early. For example, the short obese person might possess 35 per cent or more of body fat; 65 per cent of the body weight may consist of skeleton and lean body tissues containing about 73 per cent water. These tissues in a lean, well-trained athlete might contain approximately 20 per cent more water. Hence more radiation would be absorbed by the tissues and more secondary radiation produced. Obviously, the obese person would not absorb as much x-radiation as the muscular type.

INFLUENCE OF DISEASE

The total body fluid content changes with disease. In general, disease causes either demineralization (osteoporosis) of bones or an increase in mineralization (osteosclerosis). At times, both conditions may occur in the same patient. When osteosclerosis or osteoporosis exists, there may be also a loss of soft tissue substance because of dehydration, or an invasion of the soft tissues by fluids. Certain degenerative diseases frequently cause excessive fluid to accumulate in the abdomen, causing distention. This condition should not be confused with obesity, because there is usually an associated generalized *loss* of fat. Acute illness usually causes fat loss. Pathologic accumulation of fluid seems to occur more frequently than dehydration. Chronic wasting diseases diminish fat storage to a greater degree than fluid. Acute illnesses exhaust fluid. Dehydration is often seen in fever, in the mentally deranged, or in conditions associated with persistent nausea and diarrhea.

INFLUENCE OF TRAUMA

In trauma, body fluids frequently invade the injured soft tissues and create edema. With inactivity as a result of bone or joint trauma, demineralization (atrophy) of bone often takes place.

INFLUENCE OF SEX

In general, the deposition of subcutaneous fat, particularly in the pelvic, upper femoral and arm regions, is greater in the female than the male. The male musculature and bony structure is more massive than in the female. The female skull is more delicate in structure than the male.

INFLUENCE OF AGE

During the early months of a child's life, the gain in weight is rapid. Usually the child's weight doubles in the first six months and triples at the end of a year. Thence the gain in weight is slow but steady until the eighteenth year. Throughout life there is a constant flux in the mineral content of bone. During the growth period, bone formation occurs at a greater rate than bone resorption. In middle life, bone formation and resorption is in balance. The rate of bone resorption exceeds bone growth in old age. Mineralization of average living bone decreases with age. Dehydration of tissues assumes major radiographic importance in the aged since chemical as well as structural osseous changes take place. Such changes may be generally described by the term *atrophy* and are manifested by a reduction in body water and a mineral loss. The soft tissues of infants contain a greater quantity of body fluid than the adult and the aged less than the younger adult.

SOFT TISSUE-BONE RELATION

The proportion of bone to soft tissue is fairly static for a given anatomic part. If the part is naturally large, the probabilities are that the bone is large and has a proportionate amount of soft tissue covering it. The technician must judge whether the part is *naturally* small, average, or large. The aggregate of the tissues possesses a certain thickness-density ratio that influences the degree of x-ray absorption that will take place. This fact must be considered when determining the amount of penetration that is necessary to overcome, within a reasonably short exposure time, the absorbing power of the part.

BODY THICKNESS

Human beings are dissimilar in their thickness characteristics. These tend to change in varying degrees during life and in health and disease. Despite these human differences, it is possible to establish certain pattern measurements for radiographic purposes that conform to what may be termed *average*-thickness ranges. Such measurements can be standardized just as anthropologists have standardized indices of human measurement. They are an important means toward standardization of exposure factors.

METHOD FOR MEASURING THICKNESS OF PART

The type of calipers to be used for mensuration is illustrated in Figure 29. Be sure the calipers are always in good repair. All measurements should be made along the course of the projected central ray. In general the nonmovable leg of the calipers (A) is placed opposite the body entrance or exit of the central ray and the movable leg (B) closed so that it just makes contact with the skin. The calipers should not be squeezed for tissue will be displaced and a true dimension will not be obtained. This method should be employed in measuring the head and the upper and lower extremities.

Chest measurements should normally be made with the patient standing or sitting erect in a neutral or resting state. Respiration should be normal. When the central ray enters or leaves the body in the median plane, it is most important that the thickness of the tissue in the pectoral area be included. Therefore, the measurements should be made with the calipers horizontal and at the level of the sixth thoracic vertebra.

For anteroposterior projections of the abdominal structures, measurements are normally made with the patient supine and at rest. The nonmovable leg of the calipers is placed in a horizontal plane next to the skin posteriorly; the movable arm is then closed so that it just touches the anterior wall of the abdomen. With this measurement gentle palpation of the abdomen should be made to determine the presence of an unusual amount of gas or fluid. When present the technician should make allowances in the use of the MaS factor.

When making abdominal measurements with the patient erect or semierect, it should be recognized that the abdominal viscera gravitate to the pelvis thereby increasing the density of the tissues accumulated in the pelvic region.

THICKNESS RANGES

The young adult conforms to a definite physical standard and may be considered as basic for establishing average thickness ranges. For that reason, a series of average-thickness ranges has been established. Since the thickness of any body part is not necessarily an index of its physiology or its x-ray absorption qualities, it cannot be employed *per se* as an authoritative index of the radiographic density desired to be produced. Every body part consists of a proportionate amount of bone and flesh with a normal fluid content, irrespective of thickness.

Determination of Average-Thickness Ranges

Statistically, the frequency with which adult patients conform to a fairly average-thickness range for a given projection is relatively high. Since the x-ray absorption properties of human tissues are *unpredictable,* some latitude in compensating for this fact can be made. Thousands of ac-

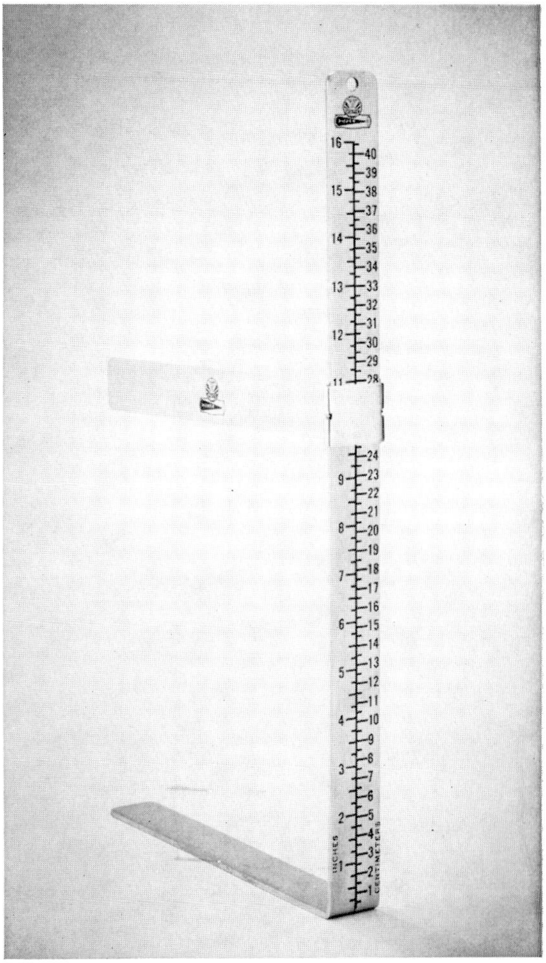

Figure 29. Photograph of type of calipers to be employed for measurement of a body part.

curate measurements of tissue thicknesses were made for various projections.* The thickness of the tissue to be traversed by the x-ray beam was always determined in the same manner and it was measured along the course of the central ray. The tissues were never compressed by the measuring calipers. In each case, the thickness of tissue was tabulated. The frequency with which various thicknesses appeared for a given projection was then statistically determined. The higher thickness frequencies for a given projection were then grouped into an *average-thickness range,* to which could be applied a common group of exposure factors with the assurance that satisfactory radiographic quality would be rendered in a high percentage of cases. It should be stated at this point that patient weight and patient height are not reliable indices of x-ray absorption and cannot be used as guides in formulating or standardizing an exposure for a given projection. A list of average-thickness ranges for various projections is shown in Table IX.

* Fuchs, A. W.: The Optimum Kilovoltage Technique in Military Roentgenography. *Am. J. Roentgenol., 50:*358-365, 1943.

Chapter 8

Function of Focus-Film Distance

A STUDY OF the influence of the focus-film distance on the radiographic image reveals three important properties: (1) its influence on radiographic density; (2) its geometric influence on the size and shape of the image of the part being examined; (3) the sharpness with which image details are rendered. The last two properties are discussed in Chapter 13. Since intensity directly influences radiographic density, any change in distance will cause a change in density when other factors are constant.

THE INVERSE SQUARE LAW

Since x-rays conform to the laws of light, they diverge as they are emitted from the focal spot, and, proceeding in straight paths, cover an increasingly larger area with *lessened* intensity as they travel from their source. This principle is illustrated in the diagram (Figure 30). It is assumed that the intensity of the x-rays emitted at the focal spot (FS) remains the same, and that the x-rays cover an area of 4 square inches on reaching the horizontal plane (C) which is 12 inches from FS.

TABLE I

MaS MULTIPLYING FACTORS FOR USE WHEN FFD IS CHANGED

Original Focus-Film Distance	*New Focus-film Distance* 20″	25″	30″	36″	40″	48″	60″	72″	
20″	1.00	1.56	2.25	3.22	4.00	5.76	9.00	12.96	*MaS Multiplying Factors*
25″	.64	1.00	1.44	2.07	2.56	3.68	5.76	8.29	
30″	.44	.69	1.00	1.44	1.77	2.56	4.00	5.76	
36″	.31	.48	.69	1.00	1.23	1.77	2.77	4.00	
40″	.25	.39	.56	.81	1.00	1.44	2.25	3.24	
48″	.17	.27	.39	.59	.69	1.00	1.56	2.25	
60″	.11	.17	.25	.36	.44	.64	1.00	1.44	
72″	.08	.12	.17	.25	.31	.44	.69	1.00	
	MaS Multiplying Factors								

When the focus-film distance (FFD) is increased to 24 inches to plane D or twice the distance between FS and C, the x-rays will cover 16 square inches—an area 4 times as great as that at C. It follows, therefore, that the intensity of the radiation per square inch on the plane at D is only one quarter that at the level C. Thus, the exposure that would be adequate at C must be increased 4 times in order to produce at D an equal radiographic density. The above computation is based on the following equation:

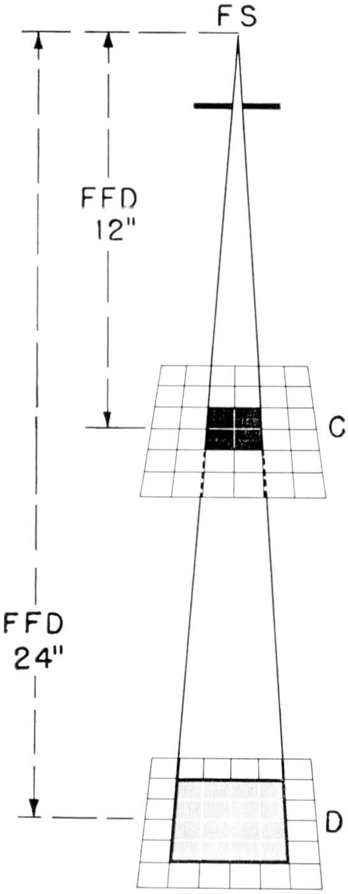

Figure 30. Diagram illustrating the inverse square law.

$$\frac{\text{Original MaS}}{\text{New MaS}} = \frac{\text{Original FFD}^2}{\text{New FFD}^2}$$

DENSITY CHANGES VERSUS FFD

Table I may be employed for determining the correct MaS multiplying factor to employ when the FFD is changed.

When radiographic density requires changing by specific amounts, there may be occasions when it is inconvenient to change the Ma or Time because of apparatus limitations. However, the FFD may be changed to secure densities of the order of ¼, ½, ¾, 1, 1½, 2, 4, 8 of the original density value. The equation for determining the new FFD is as follows:

$$\text{NEW FFD}^2 = \frac{\text{New MaS x Original FFD}^2}{\text{Original MaS}}$$

TABLE II

TABLE OF FFD VALUES TO BE USED WHEN RADIOGRAPHIC INTENSITY IS TO BE CHANGED BY SPECIFIC AMOUNTS

Original Focus-film Distance	***When Radiographic Intensity is to be Changed by***								
	¼	½	¾	1	1½	2	4	8	
25″	50″	35″	29″	25″	20″	18″	12″	9″	*New Focus-film Distance*
30″	60″	42″	35″	30″	24″	21″	15″	11″	
36″	72″	51″	42″	36″	29″	25″	18″	13″	
40″	80″	56″	46″	40″	33″	28″	20″	14″	
48″	96″	68″	56″	48″	39″	34″	24″	17″	
60″	120″	85″	70″	60″	49″	42″	30″	21″	
72″	144″	102″	83″	72″	59″	51″	36″	25″	

Table II will assist in determining directly the FFD when specific density changes are desired.

Example. If the original FFD is 36 inches and the radiographic density is to be increased by 2 without changing the MaS or KvP, what new FFD must be used:

Solution. Consulting Table II, the original FFD of 36 inches may be found under the column headed "Original Focus-Film Distance." Locate the vertical column headed by the numeral 2. The value found at the intersection of these two columns is 25 inches, which represents the new FFD.

The diminution of intensity of the x-ray beam as it travels further and further away from the focal spot in accordance with the inverse square law may be observed in the radiograph (Figure 31). This image was produced by placing one edge of a 14 x 17-inch film contained in an exposure holder at the portal of the x-ray tube. An exposure was made and the film processed. The top of the image was at the tube portal. Note the high density in this area. As the radiation coursed downward along the film, the x-ray intensity gradually diminished, hence the loss in radiographic density as the FFD increased. The difference in density along a horizontal plane through the beam from the anode to the cathode side is due to the "heel effect" (see Chapter 12).

ARITHMETICAL RELATIONS

RELATION NO. 1—TIME AND FFD

Rule. The exposure time required for a given radiographic density is directly proportional to the *square* of the focus-film distance when the remaining factors are constant. This rule may be expressed by the following formula for the purpose of solving the exposure problems:

$$\frac{\text{(E) Original Time}}{\text{(F) New Time}} = \frac{(C^2)\text{ Original FFD}^2}{(D^2)\text{ New FFD}^2}$$

Example No. 1. Assume that an exposure time of 10 seconds (E) and an FFD of 30 inches (C) have been used, and it is desired to decrease the FFD to 24 inches (D). What exposure time (F) would be required?

Solution. E, D, and C are known; F is unknown. The following working equation adapted from the above basic formula should be employed to solve the problem:

$$F = \frac{ED^2}{C^2}$$

$$F = \frac{10 \times 24^2}{30^2} = \frac{10 \times 4^2}{5^2} = 6.4 \text{ sec. Answer.}$$

Example No. 2. Assume that an exposure time of 2 seconds (E) and an FFD of 60 inches (C) have been employed in a given projection. It is desired to decrease

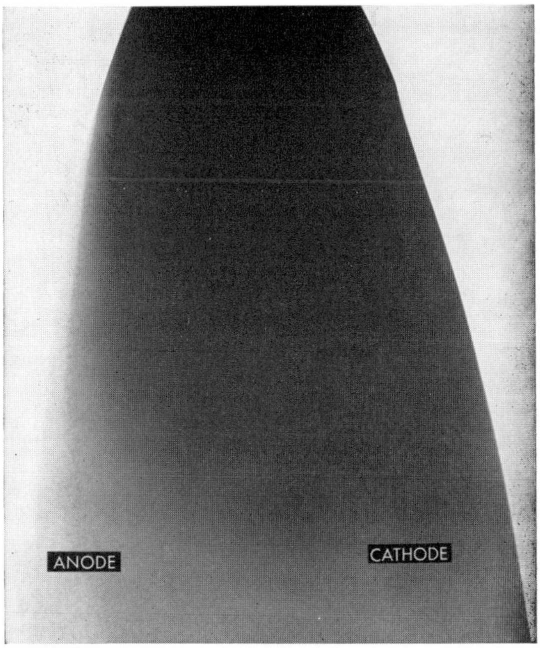

Figure 31. Flash x-ray exposure to demonstrate decrease in intensity of radiation as x-ray beam becomes remote to its source.

the time to ½ second. What FFD (D) would be required?

Solution. E, F, and C are known; D is unknown. The following working equation derived from the above basic formula may be employed for solving the problem:

$$D^2 = \frac{FC^2}{E}$$

$$D^2 = \frac{\frac{1}{2} \times 60^2}{2} = 900$$

$$D = 30 \text{ inches. Answer.}$$

RELATION NO. 2—Ma AND FFD

Rule. The Ma required for a given radiographic density is directly proportional to the *square* of the FFD when the remaining factors are constant. This rule may be expressed by the following formula for the purpose of solving exposure problems.

$$\frac{\text{(A) Original Ma}}{\text{(B) New Ma}} = \frac{(C^2)\text{ Original FFD}^2}{(D^2)\text{ New FFD}^2}$$

Example No. 1. Assume that 50 Ma (A) and an FFD of 36 inches (C) have been employed, and it is desired to increase the FFD to 72 inches (D). What milliamperage (B) would be required?

Solution. A, C, and D are known; B is unknown. The following working equation adapted from the above basic formula should be employed to solve the problem:

$$B = \frac{AD^2}{C^2}$$

$$B = \frac{50 \times 72^2}{36^2} = 50 \times 4 = 200 \text{ Ma. Answer.}$$

Example No. 2. Assume that 100 Ma (A) and an FFD of 72 inches (C) have been employed with a large focal spot x-ray tube and it is desired to change to a small focal spot using 20 Ma (B). What FFD (D) would be required?

Solution. A, B, and C are known; D is unknown. By transposition of the above basic formula, the following working equation is obtained to solve the problem:

$$D^2 = \frac{BC^2}{A}$$

$$D^2 = \frac{20 \times 72^2}{100} = \frac{103680}{100} = 1036.8$$

$$D = 32 \text{ inches (approximate). Answer.}$$

RELATION NO. 3—MaS AND FFD

Rule. The MaS required to produce a given radiographic density is proportional to the *square* of the FFD when the remaining factors are constant. This rule may be expressed by the following formula for the purpose of solving exposure problems:

$$\frac{\text{(X) Original MaS}}{\text{(Y) New MaS}} = \frac{(C^2)\text{ Original FFD}^2}{(D^2)\text{ New FFD}^2}$$

Example. Assume that an exposure of 10 MaS (X) at an FFD of 25 inches (C) is employed. The FFD is increased to 60 inches (D). What MaS (Y) must be employed to maintain the same radiographic density?

Solution. X, C, and D are known; Y is unknown. The following working equation adapted from the above formula should be used to solve the problem:

$$Y = \frac{XD^2}{C^2}$$

$$Y = \frac{10 \times 60^2}{25^2} = \frac{36000}{625} = 57.6 \text{ MaS. Answer.}$$

To facilitate the mathematics involved, Table I may be employed to determine MaS values when common FFD values are changed. For example, under the column headed "Original Focus-Film Distance" find 25 inches. Find the vertical column headed by the new FFD of 60 inches. Where these two columns intersect will be found the MaS multiplying factor 5.76. Multiply the original MaS of 10 by 5.76. The answer is 57.6 MaS.

EXPOSURE EXPERIMENTS

EXPERIMENT NO. 1—FFD-DENSITY RELATION

Purpose. To demonstrate the relation between focus-film distance and radiographic density.

Theory. Any change in FFD influences the intensity of radiation. The intensity varies inversely as the square of the FFD. Since changes in FFD produce changes in intensity, radiographic density, therefore, changes.

Procedure No. 1

1. A series of three exposures is to be made *without* an absorber on the exposure holder using the following materials and exposure factors.

Materials	Film:	Screen-type, 8 x 10-inch
	Exposure holder:	8 x 10-inch
	Cone:	To cover exposure area
Constant	Development:	5 min. 68° F.
Factors	KvP:	50
	Ma:	10
	Time:	1 sec.
	MaS:	10
	Filter:	1 mm. aluminum

Variable Factors	Exposure No.	FFD
	1	25 inches
	2	40 inches
	3	60 inches

2. Place mask on 8 x 10-inch exposure holder containing film. Directly expose each circle in sequence. Place small lead sheet over the No. 2 and No. 3 exposure holes and expose No. 1. Then cover Nos. 1 and 3 and expose No. 2, etc., until all exposures are completed. Process film.

Comment. With all other factors constant, the loss in radiographic density with increasing FFD (Figure 32 *Top*) occurs because as the FFD increases, the *intensity* of radiation reaching the film diminishes. The radiograph made at 60 inches received less intensity of radiation than the radiograph made at 25 inches and consequently shows less density.

Procedure No. 2

1. The FFD-density relation can be readily demonstrated by making a series of three pos-

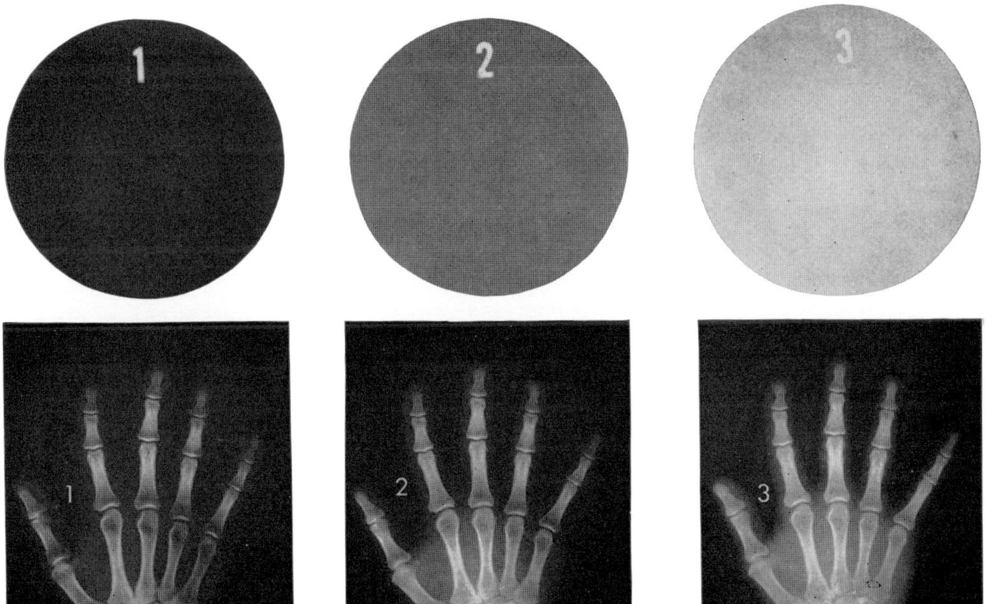

Figure 32. Demonstration of effect of FFD on radiographic density. Top, without absorber; bottom, with absorber (hand). The exposure sequence is numerically inscribed on each image.

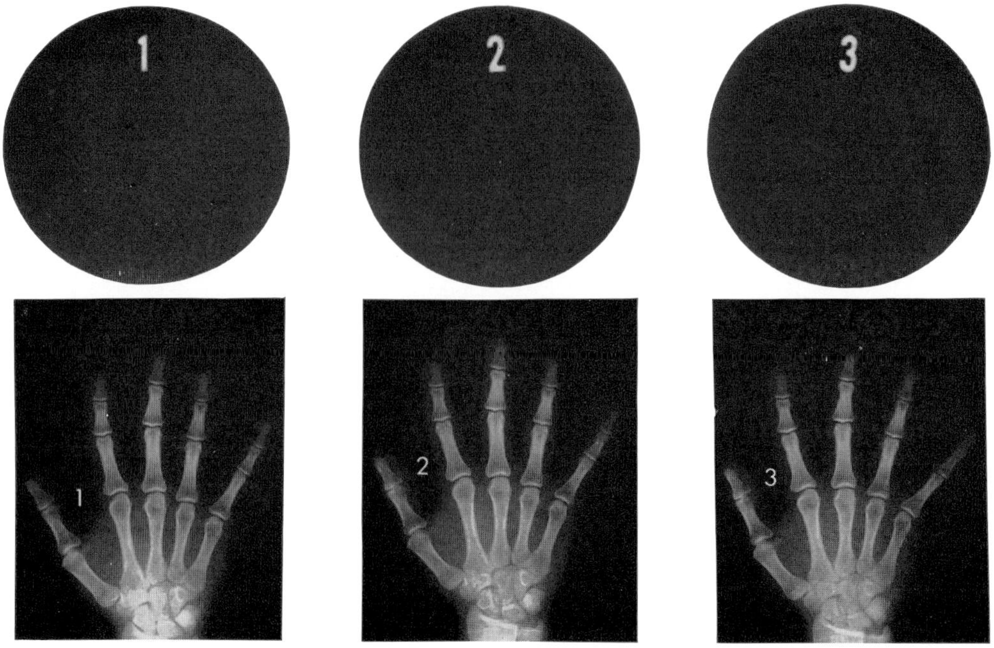

Figure 33. Demonstration of effect of the time-FFD density relation. (*Top*) without absorber; (*Bottom*) with absorber (hand). The exposure sequence is numerically indicated on each image.

teroanterior radiographs of the hand using the following materials and exposure factors:

Materials	Film:	Screen-type, 8 x 10-inch
	Exposure holder:	8 x 10-inch
	Cone:	To cover exposure area
Constant	Development:	5 min. 68° F.
Factors	KvP:	50
	Ma:	50
	Time:	1 sec.
	MaS:	50
	Filter:	1 mm. aluminum
Variable	Exposure No.	FFD
Factors	1	25 inches
	2	36 inches
	3	48 inches

Comment. As in Procedure No. 1, it may be observed that as the FFD increased, the radiographic density diminished because the intensity of the x-radiation reaching the film diminished (Figure 32, *Bottom*).

EXPERIMENT NO. 2—TIME-FFD DENSITY RELATION

Purpose. To demonstrate the interrelation of time of exposure and focus-film distance to radiographic density when all other factors are constant.

Theory. The time required for a given radiographic density is directly proportional to the *square* of the FFD when all other factors are constant.

Procedure No. 1

1. A series of three exposures is to be made *without* an object on the exposure holder, using the following materials and exposure factors:

Materials	Film:	Screen-type, 8 x 10-inch	
	Exposure holder:	8 x 10-inch	
	Cone:	To cover exposure area	
Constant	Development:	5 min. 68° F.	
Factors	KvP:	50	
	Ma:	10	
	Filter:	1 mm. aluminum	
Variable	Exposure No.	Time	FFD
Factors	1	½ sec.	25 inches
	2	1³⁄₁₀ sec.*	40 inches
	3	2⁹⁄₁₀ sec.*	60 inches

2. Place mask on 8 x 10-inch exposure holder containing film. Directly expose each circle in sequence. Place small lead sheet

* These values are approximate and serve experimental purposes within the capabilities of modern timers; very small time differences have little radiographic density effect.

over the No. 2 and No. 3 exposure holes and expose No. 1. Then, cover Nos. 1 and 3 and expose No. 2, etc., until all exposures are completed. Process film.

Comment. The experiment demonstrates that as FFD changes, the time of exposure can be used to equalize densities by applying the above theory (Figure 33, *Top*).

Procedure No. 2

1. The time-FFD relation may also be demonstrated by making a series of three posteroanterior radiographs of the hand employing the following materials and exposure factors:

Materials	Film:	Screen-type, 8 x 10-inch		
	Exposure holder:	8 x 10-inch		
	Cone:	To cover exposure area		
Constant Factors	Development:	5 min. 68° F.		
	KvP:	50		
	Ma:	50		
	Filter:	1 mm. aluminum		
Variable Factors	Exposure No.	FFD	Time	MaS
	1	25 inches	½ sec.	25
	2	36 inches	1 sec.	50
	3	48 inches	1⁸⁄₁₀ sec.	90

Comment. In comparing these radiographs, (Figure 33, *Bottom*) it may be seen that the densities are approximately the same because suitable exposure time compensation has been made for each FFD change in accordance with the inverse square law. Since the FFD has a material effect on radiographic density, it is recommended that once an FFD is established for a given projection that it should be considered a constant. When some unusual need arises for varying the FFD, the above inverse square formula should be used to equalize density.

EXPERIMENT NO. 3—Ma-FFD DENSITY RELATION

Purpose. To demonstrate the interrelation of milliamperage and focus-film distance to radiographic density.

Theory. When all other factors are constant, the milliamperage required for a given exposure is directly proportional to the square of the FFD.

Procedure No. 1

1. A series of three exposures is to be made *without* an object on the film using the following materials and exposure factors:

Materials	Film:	Screen-type, 8 x 10-inch		
	Exposure holder:	8 x 10-inch		
	Cone:	To cover exposure area		
Constant Factors	Development:	5 min. 68° F.		
	KvP:	50		
	Time:	1 sec.		
	Filter:	1 mm. aluminum		
Variable Factors	Exposure No.	Ma	FFD	MaS
	1	10	27 inches	10
	2	10	60 inches	10
	3	50	60 inches	50

2. Place mask on 8 x 10-inch exposure holder containing film. Directly expose each circle in sequence. Place small lead sheet over the No. 2 and No. 3 exposure holes while exposing No. 1, and over Nos. 1 and 3 when exposing No. 2, etc., until all exposures are completed. Process film.

Comment. These radiographs (Figure 34, *Top*) demonstrate that when No. 2 exposure is made with the same factors employed for No. 1 but the FFD increased to 60 inches, the loss in intensity at this FFD results in a marked reduction in radiographic density. Applying the above theory, the new milliamperage was found to be 50 and equalization of the density is obtained as shown in Exposure No. 3.

Procedure No. 2

1. The Ma-FFD relation can be demonstrated by making a series of three posteroanterior exposures of the hand, employing the following materials and factors:

Materials	Film:	Screen-type, 8 x 10-inch			
	Exposure holder:	8 x 10-inch			
	Cone:	To cover exposure area			
Constant Factors	Development:	5 min. 68° F.			
	KvP:	50			
	Filter:	1 mm. aluminum			
Variable Factors	Exposure No.	Ma	FFD	Time	MaS
	1	10	25 in.	2 sec.	20
	2	30	40 in.	1⁷⁄₁₀ sec.	51
	3	100	60 in.	1³⁄₂₀ sec.	115

Comment. The radiographs shown (Figure 34, *Bottom*) demonstrate that as the FFD

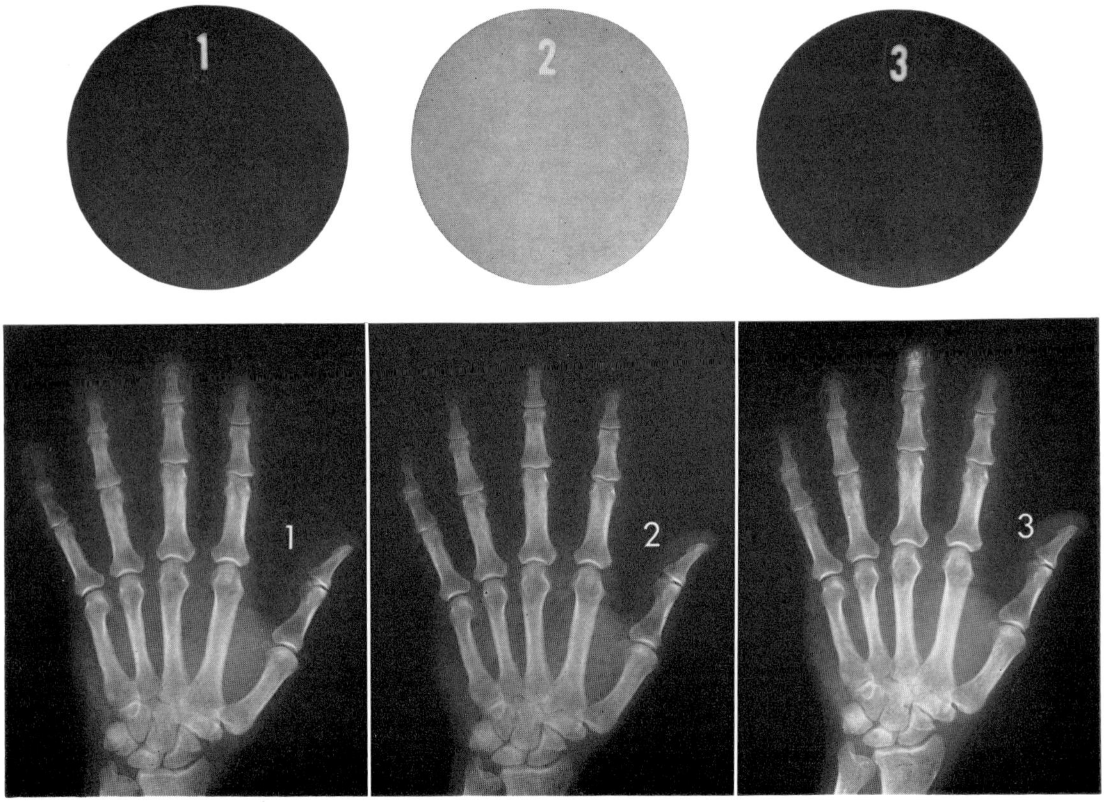

Figure 34. Demonstration of Ma-FFD relation. (*Top*) without absorber; (*Bottom*) with absorber (hand).

changes, the Ma may be used to help compensate for the normal loss in density. In standard practice, however, Ma should be established as a constant for a given projection whenever possible and its use as a variable should be limited.

SUMMARY

The influence of focus film distance and its relation to other exposure factors in altering radiographic density is summarized as follows:

FFD-DENSITY RELATION

When all factors but focus-film distance are constant, the radiographic density decreases as the FFD increases.

TIME-FFD DENSITY RELATION

The time of exposure required to produce a given radiographic density is directly proportional to the square of the FFD when all other factors are constant.

Ma-FFD DENSITY RELATION

The milliamperage required to produce a given radiographic density is directly proportional to the square of the FFD when all other factors are constant.

MaS-FFD DENSITY RELATION

The MaS required to produce a given radiographic density is directly proportional to the square of the FFD when all other factors are constant.

Chapter 9

Function of Kilovoltage

Part One

Of all the exposure factors, kilovoltage has the greatest effect on the radiographic image when all other factors remain constant. It has direct influence on the *quality* of the radiation reaching the film, i.e., by virtue of radiation wavelength. This in turn determines the radiographic contrast exhibited by the image. Kilovoltage also influences exposure latitude and radiographic density. It is a factor in the production of secondary radiation which must be suitably controlled in order to prevent

TABLE III

MaS Multiplying Factors for Use When Kilovoltage Is Changed

(*SCREEN Exposures Only*)

Old KvP	***MaS Multiplying Factor***													***Old KvP***
40	1.	.4	.23	.15	.11	.08	.064	.05	.04	.032	.025	.02	.017	**40**
45	2.5	1.	.52	.3	.22	.16	.12	.1	076	.06	.05	.04	.032	**45**
50	4.	1.7	1.	.68	.5	.35	.27	.21	.16	.13	.1	.08	.066	**50**
55	8.	2.5	1.5	1.	.74	.56	.43	.35	.28	.22	.18	.15	.12	**55**
60	10.	4.	2.3	1.5	1.	.78	.6	.46	.37	.3	.25	.2	.17	**60**
65	12.	5.	3.	2.	1.4	1.	.8	.62	.5	.4	.32	.26	.21	**65**
70	16.	7.	4.2	2.6	2.	1.4	1.	.8	.6	.5	.39	.31	.25	**70**
75	20.	9.	5.4	3.5	2.5	1.8	1.3	1.	.76	.6	.47	.38	.3	**75**
80	24.	11.	6.6	4.5	3.2	2.3	1.7	1.3	1.	.8	.6	.47	.37	**80**
85	28.	13.	8.	5.4	4.	2.9	2.2	1.7	1.3	1.	.8	.64	.5	**85**
90	34.	15.	9.	6.2	4.5	3.4	2.6	2.	1.6	1.25	1.	.8	.64	**90**
95	48.	18.	11.	7.8	5.6	4.2	3.2	2.5	2.	1.6	1.3	1.	.8	**95**
100	60.	22.	13.	9.	6.8	5.	3.8	3.	2.4	1.9	1.5	1.2	1.	**100**
	40	**45**	**50**	**55**	**60**	**65**	**70**	**75**	**80**	**85**	**90**	**95**	**100**	
	New Kilovoltage													

in some measure its fogging action on the film.

Progress in radiography has been occasioned by the pioneer use of the higher kilovoltages because with low current apparatus, penetrating radiation was a paramount necessity. With the development of higher powered equipment and faster photographic plate and film emulsions, the trend swung to the use of lower kilovoltages, high Ma values and high emulsion contrast. Diagnostically, this technic had many disadvantages for an insufficient number of image details were visible in the radiograph. Now the trend fortunately is back to the use of higher kilovoltages, small MaS values and lower patient dosages with the production of better diagnostic images. However, the use of higher kilovoltages in radiography caused the factor of secondary radiation to assume great importance. Greater efficiency in the use of cones and grids then becomes quite necessary. A complete understanding of the effects of kilovoltage and companion factors on the quality of the radiograph must play an important part in the training of those who make radiographs.

ARITHMETICAL RELATION

RELATION NO. 4—KvP-MaS AND DENSITY

Theory. Radiographic density varies greatly with the KvP. In medical radiography, there is no precise mathematical method for determining KvP-MaS density ratios. Such factors as the thickness and density of the body tissues to be examined,

TABLE IV

MaS MULTIPLYING FACTORS FOR USE WHEN KILOVOLTAGE IS CHANGED

(*DIRECT Exposures Only*)

Old KvP	*MaS Multiplying Factor*													*Old KvP*
40	1.	.42	.26	.18	.13	.1	.08	.06	.05	.04	.032	.026	.021	**40**
45	2.3	1.	.62	.45	.32	.24	.19	.15	.12	.1	.08	.064	.051	**45**
50	3.7	1.6	1.	.7	.5	.4	.3	.24	.19	.15	.12	.1	.082	**50**
55	5.4	2.3	1.5	1.	.74	.56	.43	.35	.27	.22	.18	.14	.12	**55**
60	7.5	3.2	2.	1.4	1.	.78	.6	.48	.37	.3	.24	.2	.16	**60**
65	9.8	4.1	2.6	1.8	1.3	1.	.8	.62	.48	.4	.32	.26	.22	**65**
70	12.5	5.3	3.3	2.3	1.7	1.3	1.	.8	.62	.52	.42	.35	.28	**70**
75	16.	6.6	4.2	2.9	2.1	1.6	1.3	1.	.8	.6	.54	.44	.35	**75**
80	20.	8.5	5.4	3.7	2.7	2.1	1.6	1.3	1.	.81	.66	.54	.45	**80**
85	26.	11.	7.	4.8	3.5	2.7	2.	1.6	1.3	1.	.82	.68	.54	**85**
90	30.	13.	8.	5.6	4.2	3.2	2.5	1.9	1.6	1.25	1.	.84	.7	**90**
95	35.	14.	9.	6.2	4.6	3.5	2.8	2.2	1.8	1.5	1.2	1.	.84	**95**
100	40.	16.	10.	7.	5.2	4.	3.2	2.6	2.1	1.7	1.4	1.2	1.	**100**
	40	**45**	**50**	**55**	**60**	**65**	**70**	**75**	**80**	**85**	**90**	**95**	**100**	
	New Kilovoltage													

the characteristics of the x-ray apparatus, and whether the film is used with or without intensifying screens exert pertinent influences. Fairly close approximations between KvP and other exposure factors have been of necessity established by empirical means—by trial and error. There are two procedures that may be followed in estimating the KvP required for a given density change or for determining the approximate change in MaS required to compensate a density change in KvP. One is for screen exposures and the other for direct exposures.

Tables III and IV were developed empirically from radiographs of living subjects on screen-type film. By the use of MaS multiplying factors, approximate MaS values may be obtained for changes in the KvP range of 50 to 100 in increments of five. Since the film response to x-ray exposure differs when screens are used and when direct exposure is employed, two tables of values are required. Table III is for screen exposures and Table IV for direct x-ray exposures. Some MaS values derived from these tables may require the use of a time value that is not within the practical scope of the timer. It is then necessary to employ the *nearest* practical value. The resulting density difference is usually so small that it often is not recognizable. In most instances the derived MaS values are approximations and, if necessary, only slight alterations need be made for a given projection and body tissue. X-ray generators may differ in the manner in which their x-ray outputs vary with KvP and due to calibration differences. Tables cannot, therefore, be expected to apply accurately to *all* generators but they can provide a close guide to an anticipated value.

TABLE V

MaS MULTIPLYING FACTORS FOR USE WHEN KvP IS CHANGED UPON DIRECT EXPOSURE WITH SCREEN-TYPE FILM. THIS TABLE APPLIES WHEN *No Absorber* IS EMPLOYED

Old KvP	***MaS Multiplying Factor***													***Old KvP***
40	1.	0.68	0.5	0.42	0.35	0.29	0.235	0.2	0.175	0.155	0.14	0.13	0.125	**40**
45	1.47	1.	.73	.62	.51	.42	.34	.29	.26	.23	.2	.19	.18	**45**
50	2.	1.36	1.	.84	.7	.58	.47	.4	.35	.31	.28	.26	.25	**50**
55	2.4	1.6	1.2	1.	.83	.69	.56	.48	.41	.37	.33	.31	.3	**55**
60	2.8	1.9	1.4	1.2	1.	.83	.67	.57	.5	.44	.4	.37	.36	**60**
65	3.4	2.3	1.7	1.4	1.2	1.	.81	.68	.6	.53	.48	.44	.43	**65**
70	4.2	2.8	2.1	1.8	1.5	1.2	1.	.85	.74	.65	.61	.55	.53	**70**
75	5.	3.4	2.5	2.1	1.75	1.45	1.17	1.	.87	.77	.7	.65	.62	**75**
80	5.7	3.88	2.85	2.4	2.	1.65	1.34	1.14	1.	.88	.8	.74	.71	**80**
85	6.4	4.38	3.16	2.8	2.26	1.87	1.51	1.29	1.12	1.	.9	.84	.8	**85**
90	7.1	4.85	3.57	3.	2.5	2.07	1.68	1.43	1.25	1.1	1.	.93	.89	**80**
95	7.6	5.23	3.84	3.23	2.69	2.23	1.8	1.54	1.34	1.19	1.08	1.	.96	**95**
100	.8	5.32	4.	3.36	2.8	2.32	1.88	1.6	1.4	1.24	1.14	1.04	1.	**100**
	40	**45**	**50**	**55**	**60**	**65**	**70**	**75**	**80**	**85**	**90**	**95**	**100**	
	New Kilovoltage													

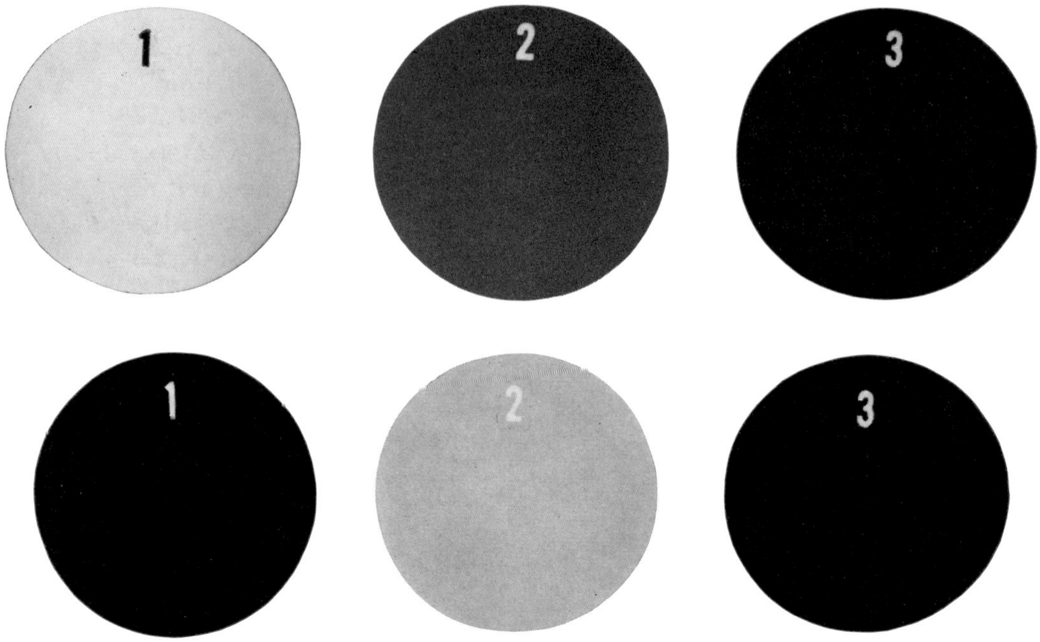

Figure 35. Demonstrates the KvP-density relation when no absorber is used.

It is quite important to remember that when kilovoltage is employed to change radiographic density, radiographic contrast and the quantity of secondary radiation generated also change.

Example 1. Assume that 70 KvP was used in making a posteroanterior view of the hand employing screen-type film in an exposure holder (direct exposure radiography). The MaS was 15 and the FFD, 36 inches. Because of an excessively long scale of contrast present, it was desired to reduce the KvP to 50. What would be the new MaS value when this radiograph was remade?

Solution. Consult Table IV. In the left- or right-hand vertical column, locate the original KvP value of 70. Locate the new KvP of 50 in the horizontal row at the bottom of the Table. Follow the column upward in which the numeral 50 appears. Where it coincides with the 70-KvP horizontal row will be found the multiplying factor 3.33. This value should be multiplied by the original MaS to provide an answer of 49.5 MaS. Practically, this value cannot ordinarily be secured on modern x-ray control panels and the nearest practical value should, therefore, be used, i.e., 50 MaS.

Example 2. Assume that 55 KvP was used in making a posteroanterior view of the chest employing 10 MaS at a 72-inch FFD. Average speed intensifying screens were used. It is desired to penetrate the chest more thoroughly and to lengthen the scale of contrast so that more structural details will be clearly shown in the image. A KvP of 80 was selected to accomplish the desired result. What MaS value should be employed at the new KvP?

Solution. Consult Table III. In the left-hand column, locate the original KvP value of 55. Pass the finger horizontally across the chart until it reaches the column of multiplying factors indicated by the new KvP of 80 at the bottom of Table III. Multiply this factor of 0.33 by the original MaS of 10. The answer is 3.33 MaS.

EXPOSURE EXPERIMENTS

EXPERIMENT NO. 4—KvP-DENSITY RELATION

Purpose. To demonstrate the relation between kilovoltage and radiographic density when no absorber (object) is placed on the film.

Theory. Radiographic density increases as the kilovoltage increases and vice versa, when other factors are constant.

Procedure

1. A series of three exposures should be made *without an object* on the exposure holder using the following materials and exposure factors.

Materials	Film:	Screen-type, 8 x 10-inch
	Exposure holder:	8 x 10-inch
	Cone:	To cover exposure area
Constant	Development:	5 min. 68° F.
Factors	FFD:	36 inches
	Ma:	10
	Time:	2 sec.
	MaS:	20
	Filter:	1 mm. aluminum
Variable	Exposure No.	KvP
Factors	1	40
	2	60
	3	80

2. Place mask on 8 x 10-inch exposure holder containing screen-type film. Directly expose each circle in sequence. Place small lead sheet over the No. 2 and No. 3 exposure holes and expose No. 1. Then, cover No. 1 and No. 3 and expose No. 2, etc., until all exposures are completed. Process film.

Comment. It may be noted (Figure 35) that as the kilovoltage increases, the radiographic density increases when the remaining factors are constant and no absorber is on the film.

EXPERIMENT NO. 5—KvP-DENSITY RELATION

Purpose. To demonstrate the relation between kilovoltage and radiographic density when a homogeneous absorber of varying thickness is used.

Theory. When an absorber is placed on the film, the x-ray *absorption properties* of the material composing the absorber as well as its thickness are factors that cause variation in the radiographic densities.

Procedure

1. A series of six radiographs of a long step-wedge containing a number of aluminum steps, 1 millimeter in thickness, should be made using the following materials and exposure factors. The exposure of the first step is adjusted to obtain a light gray tone—a translucent density.

Materials	Film:	Screen-type, 10 x 12-inch
	Exposure holder:	10 x 12-inch
	Cone:	To cover exposure area
Constant	Development:	5 min. 68° F.
Factors	FFD:	36 inches
	Ma:	10
	Time:	2 sec.
	MaS:	20
	Filter:	1 mm. aluminum
Variable	Exposure No.	KvP
Factors	1	40
	2	50
	3	60
	4	70
	5	80
	6	90

2. Place step-wedge on 10 x 12-inch exposure holder containing screen-type film. Directly expose each film in sequence until all exposures are completed. Process films.

Comment. The quantity of silver deposit in each image that represents the first step of the wedge is dependent in degree upon the quantity of remnant radiation emerging from the wedge to expose the film, and its wave length (Figure 36). The density of the first step in each radiograph increases with each advance in kilovoltage indicating that greater image densities are obtained because of the greater penetrating quality of the radiation. Note that the density of the sixth step in each radiograph differs widely as the kilovoltage is advanced; at the lower kilovoltages very little silver is deposited to represent the various steps because most of the radiation is absorbed, whereas at the higher values, a larger

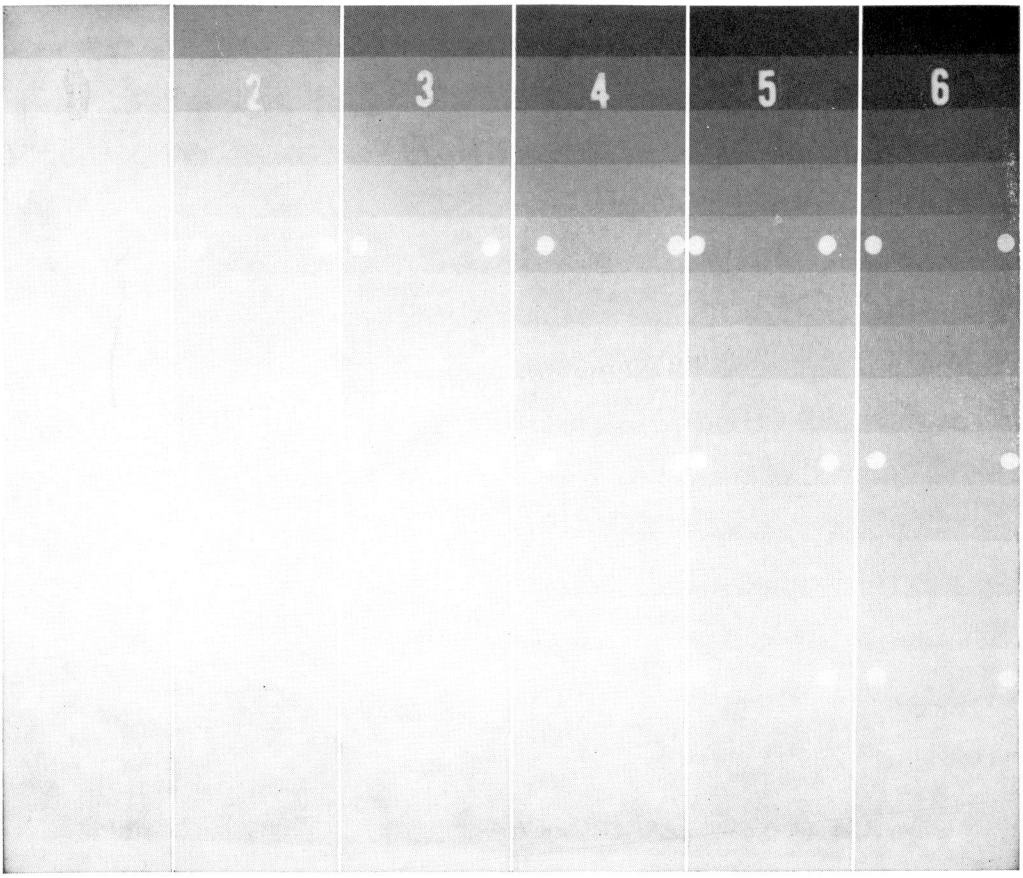

Figure 36. Demonstrates the KvP-density relation when an absorber of varying thickness is used. Numerals indicate exposure sequence.

amount of silver causes all steps to become visible since *less* radiation is absorbed. As compared to the situation in Experiment No. 4, it is here demonstrated that the *thickness* of any homogeneous object placed on the film has direct influence in *decreasing* the intensity of the radiation reaching the film. The variation in the intensities of the remnant beam reaching the film results in a series of radiographic densities of varying tone value that constitute a radiographic image of the *entire* wedge only at the higher kilovoltages. At the lower kilovoltages, an entire image of the wedge was not secured because the long wave length radiation was absorbed by the thicker sections of the step-wedge and little remnant radiation reached the film to produce a satisfactory image. Note that all steps of the wedge are not shown in the 40-KvP image, nor do they all show in the 60-KvP image; but all steps show when 90 KvP is used because of the increase in x-ray output and diminished absorption of x-rays by the step-wedge (penetration).

EXPERIMENT NO. 6—KvP-DENSITY RELATION

Purpose. To demonstrate that radiographic densities increase as the kilovoltage increases when an absorber (hand) containing structures of varying absorption properties is employed.

Procedure

1. A series of four posteroanterior radiographs of the hand should be made employing the following materials and factors:

Materials	Film:	Screen-type, 8 x 10-inch
	Exposure holder:	8 x 10-inch
	Cone:	To cover exposure area
Constant	Development:	5 min. 68° F.
Factors	FFD:	36 inches
	Ma:	100
	Time:	0.2 sec.
	MaS:	20
	Filter:	1 mm. aluminum
Variable	Exposure No.	KvP
Factors	1	40
	2	50
	3	60
	4	70

2. Expose all films in 8 x 10-inch exposure holder and in sequence. Process films.

Comment. In this series of radiographs (Figure 37) the over-all density of the radiographs increases with the KvP. The over-all density of the No. 3 radiograph made with 60 KvP is greater than that of No. 1 made with 40 KvP. Successive increases in kilovoltage cause corresponding increases in density due to greater tissue penetration, since less radiation is absorbed by the tissues and more reaches the film because of the shorter wave lengths. However, it should be noted that in each radiograph less radiation emerged from those portions of the hand representing the bones than from those representing the flesh —less silver deposit is rendered in the bone images than that representing the adjacent soft tissues because bone absorbs a greater amount of radiation than does soft tissue.

EXPERIMENT NO. 7—KvP-MaS DENSITY RELATION

Purpose. To demonstrate that radiographic densities can be equalized when MaS is used as a compensator for changes in kilovoltage where an absorber (object) is *not* used.

Theory. The rate of increase in radiographic density, as the kilovoltage increases, is not proportional but advances in a rather complex manner. *Note.* MaS multiplying factors that may be employed (when *no* absorber is used) for various changes in kilovoltage are contained in Table V. They are to be used for determining approximately correct MaS values.

Procedure

1. A series of three exposures should be made *without* an object on the exposure holder using the following materials and exposure factors:

Materials	Film:	Screen-type, 8 x 10-inch	
	Exposure holder:	8 x 10-inch	
	Cone:	To cover exposure area	
Constant	Development:	5 min. 68° F.	
Factors	FFD:	36 inches	
	Filter	1 mm. aluminum	
Variable	Exposure No.	KvP	MaS
Factors	1	40	10
	2	60	3.5
	3	80	1.75

2. Place mask on 8 x 10-inch exposure holder containing film. Directly expose each circle in sequence. Place small lead sheet over the No. 2 and No. 3 exposure holes and expose No. 1. Then, cover No. 1 and No. 3 and expose No. 2, etc., until all exposures are completed. Process film.

Comment. These radiographs (Figure 38) demonstrate that as the kilovoltage was increased comparable densities were secured when the MaS values were adjusted in accordance with Table V and no absorber was employed.

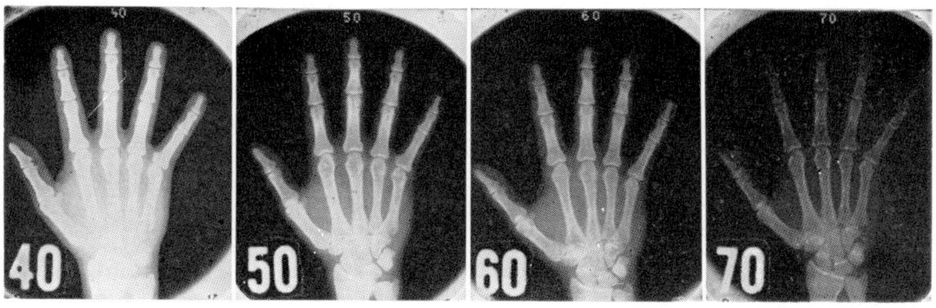

Figure 37. Demonstrates KvP-density relation. Kilovoltages employed for each exposure are inscribed on the various images.

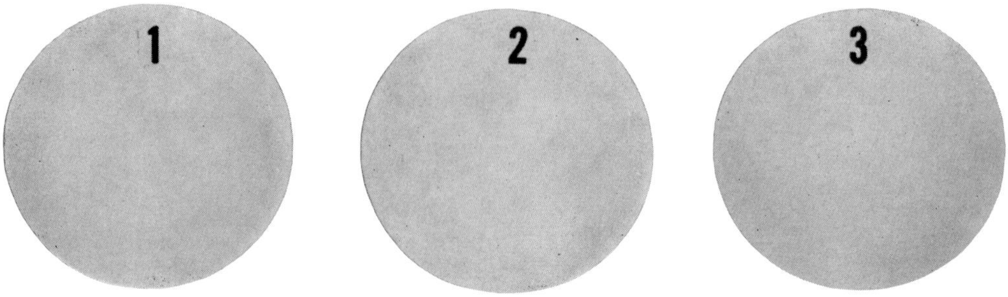

Figure 38. Demonstration of KvP-MaS relation. Exposure sequence is numerically shown on each image.

EXPERIMENT NO. 8—KvP-MaS DENSITY RELATION

Purpose. To demonstrate that equalization of image densities with all kilovoltages cannot be attained in an absorber (step-wedge) because of varying absorption by different thicknesses.

Procedure

1. A series of six radiographs of a long step-wedge should be made employing the following materials and exposure factors:

Materials	Film:	Screen-type, 10 x 12-inch	
	Exposure holder:	10 x 12-inch	
	Cone:	To cover exposure area	
Constant	Development:	5 min. 68° F.	
Factors	FFD:	36 inches	
	Filter:	1 mm. aluminum	
Variable	Exposure No.	KvP	MaS
Factors	1	40	120
	2	50	50
	3	60	30
	4	70	20
	5	80	15
	6	90	12.5

2. Place wedge on 10 x 12-inch exposure holder filled with screen-type film and expose in sequence until all exposures have been completed. Process films.

Comment. In this series of radiographs (Figure 39 *Top*) the densities representing the first step of the wedge are approximately equalized at all kilovoltages in accordance with use of above MaS values, largely derived from Table IV. In comparing the density of step No. 6 at various kilovoltages, it may be noted that the density obtained with 40 KvP is considerably less than that attained with 90 KvP. The differences in density are attributable to the differences in thickness and the increasing intensity and penetrating power of the x-radiation as the kilovoltage is increased. Since the absorption properties of the step-wedge exert a definite influence on radiographic density, the MaS must be adjusted to suit the over-all density and thickness as the kilovoltage changes. The loss in density at the lower kilovoltages is due to lack of intensity and, penetration of the step-wedge. As soon as *adequate* penetration and intensity is secured with the higher kilovoltages, densities representing all portions of the step-wedge can be seen. To secure all image details of an absorber, it is necessary that the

→

Figure 39. Step-wedge radiographs illustrating the KvP-MaS density relation. (*Top*) Normal exposure. (*Bottom*) overexposure. The exposure sequence is numerically indicated on each image. *Note:* Normal exposure shows that many details are absent when using the lower kilovoltages. When the over-all density is increased by over-exposure, details in the thinner portions of the wedge are obscured by excessive densities and little gain is achieved in showing details of the heavier portions when the lower kilovoltages are employed.

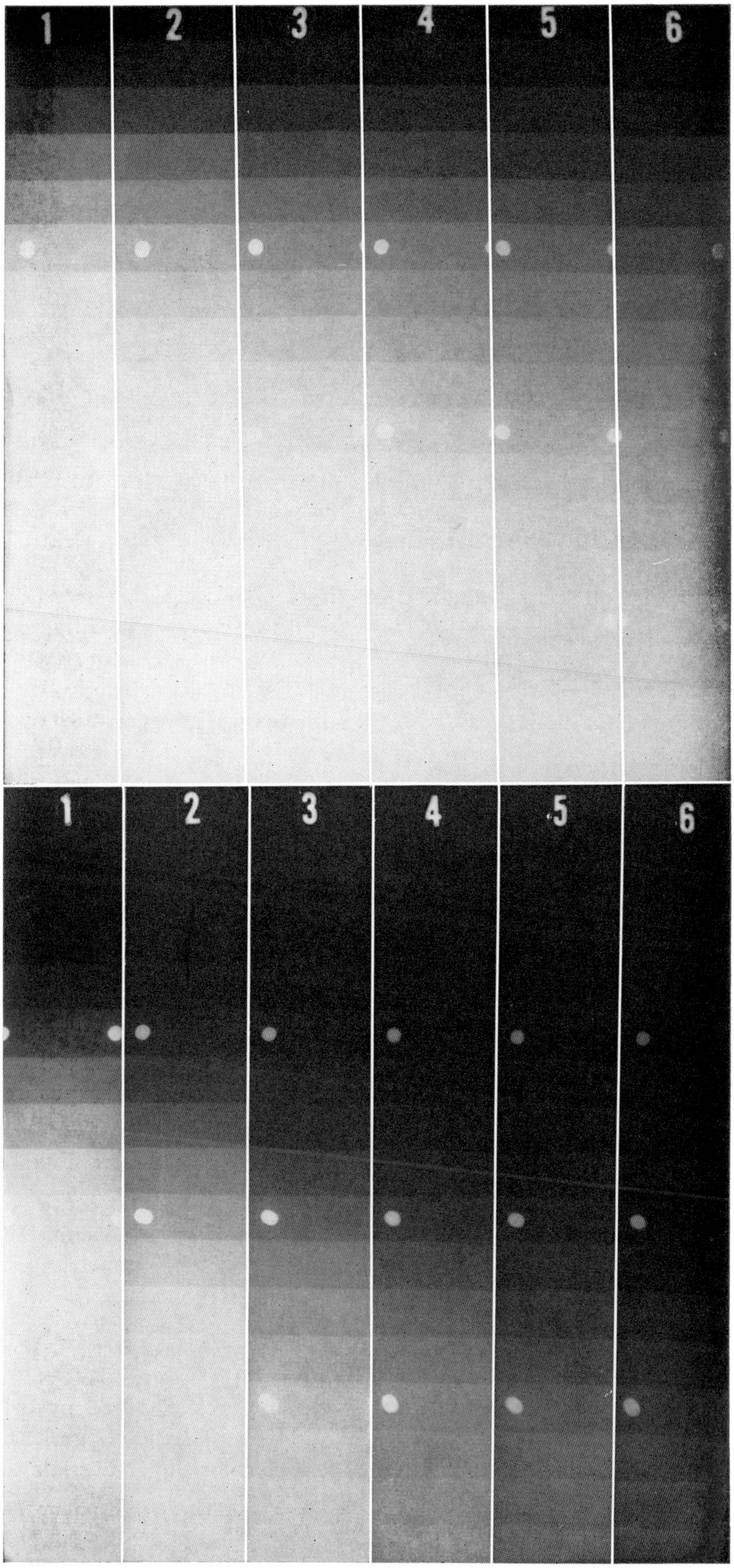
1
2
3
4
5
6
1
2
3
4
5
6

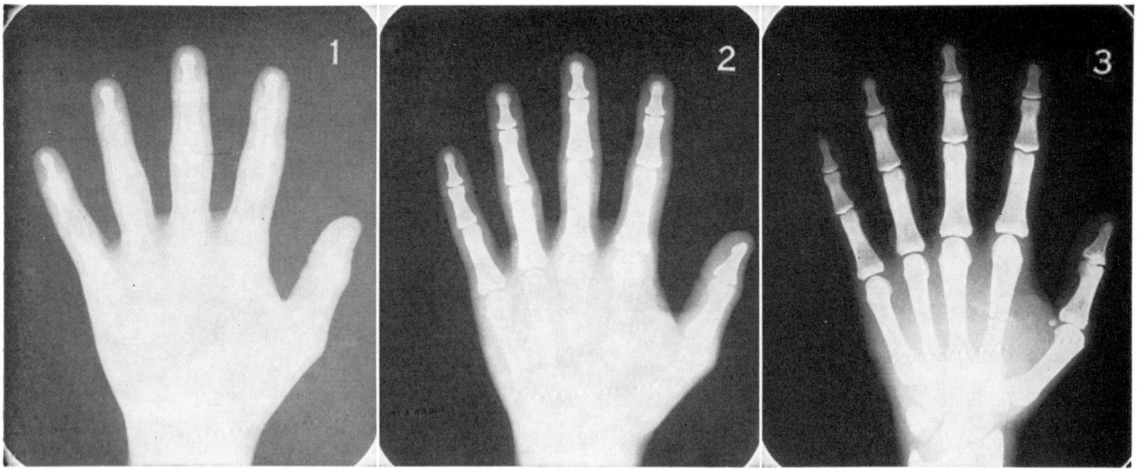

Figure 40. Direct-exposure radiographs of the hand made with insufficient KvP. Numerals indicate exposure sequence.

wave length of the radiation assures adequate penetration.

EXPERIMENT NO. 9—KvP-MaS DENSITY RELATION

PART ONE

Purpose to demonstrate (1) that overexposure does not compensate for insufficient kilovoltage at the lower KvP values and (2) that at the higher kilovoltages overexposure obliterates details, when an absorber such as a step-wedge is exposed.

Procedure

1. Duplicate exposures employed in making radiographs for Experiment No. 8, except that all MaS values should be multipled by 5.

Variable Factors	Exposure No.	KvP	MaS
	1	40	600
	2	50	250
	3	60	150
	4	70	100
	5	80	75
	6	90	62.5

Comment. In this series of radiographs (Figure 39 *Bottom*) it may be noted that the excess in MaS has caused overexposure (opaque silver deposits) in all images of the thinner portions of the step-wedge although more satisfactory densities are shown in the images of the thicker steps of the step-wedge when the higher kilovoltages are used. However, the image of the *entire* step-wedge is not shown in a single radiograph at any kilovoltage because of overexposure. The 40-KvP radiograph shows about two-thirds of the steps because of insufficient penetrating power, even though the MaS value is impractical. At the higher kilovoltages (60-100), the images of the steps of the thin portion of the step-wedge are lost due to high silver deposits. It may be seen, therefore, that any *blanket* increase in the quantity of radiation cannot compensate for insufficient kilovoltage at the lower values; whereas at the higher values opaque silver deposits tend to obliterate details when overexposures are present.

PART TWO

Purpose. To demonstrate that no practical amount of MaS will compensate for insufficient kilovoltage (penetration) when a human hand is employed as the absorber.

Procedure

1. A series of three posteroanterior radiographs of the hand * should be made employing the following materials and factors:

* Use left hand for exposure Nos. 1 and 2; right hand for exposure No. 3.

Materials	Film:	Screen-type, 8 x 10-inch
	Exposure holder:	8 x 10-inch
	Cone:	To cover exposure area
Constant	Development:	5 min. 68° F.
Factors	FFD:	36 inches
	KvP:	30
	Filter:	1 mm. aluminum
Variable	Exposure No.	MaS
Factors	1	120
	2	240
	3	480

Comment. In this series of radiographs (Figure 40) the kilovoltage provided little penetrating radiation. With increasing MaS values, proper density values that would demonstrate details in the entire image were not obtained. As the MaS increased, opaque silver deposits obscured details in the phalanges and insufficient silver in the carpal region did not provide satisfactory image detail. This experiment demonstrates that *impractical* MaS values should never be used in an effort to compensate for insufficient kilovoltage.

EXPERIMENT No. 10—KvP-MaS DENSITY RELATION

Purpose. To demonstrate (1) that radiographic densities vary in silver deposit when an absorber (body part) containing various structures is exposed with changing kilovoltages; and (2) that satisfactory *over-all* densities can be made comparable by using MaS to compensate for the density effect of changing kilovoltage, provided the radiation penetrates the structures.

Procedure

1. A series of four posteroanterior radiographs of the hand should be made employing the following materials and factors:

Materials	Film:	Screen-type, 8 x 10-inch	
	Exposure holder:	8 x 10-inch	
	Cone:	To cover exposure area	
Constant	Development:	5 min. 68° F.	
Factors	FFD:	36 inches	
	Filter:	1 mm. aluminum	
Variable	Exposure No.	KvP	MaS
Factors	1	50	50
	2	60	32
	3	70	18
	4	80	14

Comment. In this series of radiographs (Figure 41) the *over-all* densities of the radiographs are approximately equal. Because of varying absorption factors of the structures within the hand, different densities in each image comprise the requisite details for radiologic purposes. The MaS values for changes in kilovoltage were derived from Table 4.

EXPERIMENT NO. 11—KvP-CONSTRAST RELATION

Purpose. To demonstrate the influence of kilovoltage on radiographic contrast.

Theory. As kilovoltage increases and the MaS is adjusted to secure approximate equalization of translucent densities of a given body part, radiographic contrast decreases.

Procedure

1. A series of four posteroanterior chest radiographs of average thickness (22-23 cm.) should be made employing the following materials and exposure factors:

Materials	Film:	Screen-type, 14 x 17-inch	
	Screen:	Average speed	
	Cone:	To cover exposure area	
Constant	Development:	5 min. 68° F.	
Factors	FFD:	72 inches	
	Filter:	1 mm. aluminum	
Variable	Exposure No.	KvP	MaS*
Factors	1	50	20
	2	60	8.33
	3	80	3.33
	4	100	1.66

Comment. In this experiment (Figure 42) a circular area about 2 inches in diameter over the inferior portion of the right upper lobe of the lung was selected as a density guide since it possesses average pulmonary tissue density. As the kilovoltage was increased, the MaS was adjusted so that translucent densities in this area of each radiograph showed essentially the same details. With each successive rise in kilovoltage, details of heavier and more dense tissue structures gradually made their appearance in the entire images, indicating gradual penetration by the more abundant shorter wave length x-rays.

* To offset the influence of increasing kilovoltages on density, the MaS values were selected to produce translucent densities as computed from Table III.

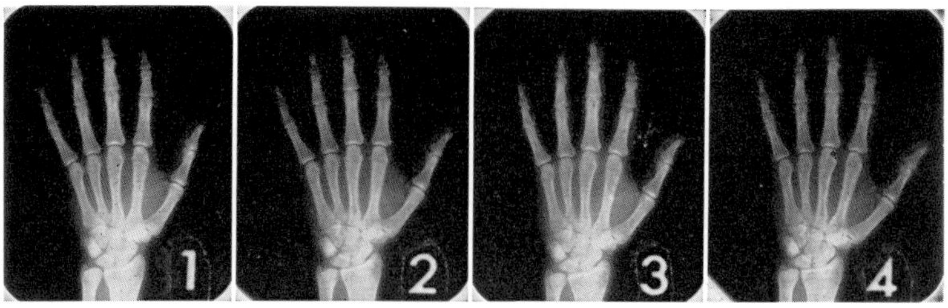

Figure 41. Direct-exposure radiographs of the hand to demonstrate the KvP-MaS Relation. Exposure sequence is numerically indicated on each image. Note contrast change with increase in KvP.

The 80-KvP radiograph demonstrates all essential thoracic detail. No added diagnostic features become visible when 100 KvP is employed. However, unmistakable evidence of an unduly long scale of contrast is shown in this radiograph. Note that many details are absent in the 50-KvP radiograph that are visible in the 80-KvP radiograph particularly those portions of the image that represent thick structures. In other words, as the kilovoltage increases, more densities become visible—the contrast scale becomes longer—up to a certain point (80 KvP). Above this level, the scale of contrast is much too long. The experiment demonstrates that kilovoltage is the factor of radiographic contrast, i.e., kilovoltage controls the scale of radiographic densities by means of which image details become visible. This fact is further substantiated in Chapter 10.

PART TWO

It was demonstrated in Part One that kilovoltage exercises considerable influence on the radiographic image. A more detailed study of its various effects in medical radiography will help the technician to appreciate its value in achieving good radiographic quality. Commonly, low kilovoltages have been employed, resulting in images deficient in details; also injudicious use of the higher kilovoltages has resulted in fogged or high-density images in which details have been obscured by excessive silver deposits or by a degradation of contrast.

It has been shown that the x-radiation must be of the correct wave length if a satisfactory image is to be produced. Since the kilovoltage regulates the wave length—hence the penetrating power of the radiation—the higher the KvP within the medical range, the less radiation is absorbed by tissues and the more radiographically effective it becomes. The *range* of these densities is regulated by the kilovoltage. Representative examples in medical radiography will better serve to illustrate the several effects that kilovoltage exercises on the radiographic image.

KILOVOLTAGE AND DENSITY

It was shown in Part One that, as kilovoltage increases and all other factors remain constant, radiographic density increases.

Small KvP Changes

Small changes in kilovoltage have little radiographic effect since the wave length is not appreciably changed.

Example 1. The above facts may be illustrated by a series of posteroanterior views of the hand (Figure 43) made on direct exposure in 1-KvP steps from 45 to 54 KvP; all other factors were constant: 40 MaS; 36-inch FFD. Radiographs were developed for 5 minutes at 68° F. in rapid

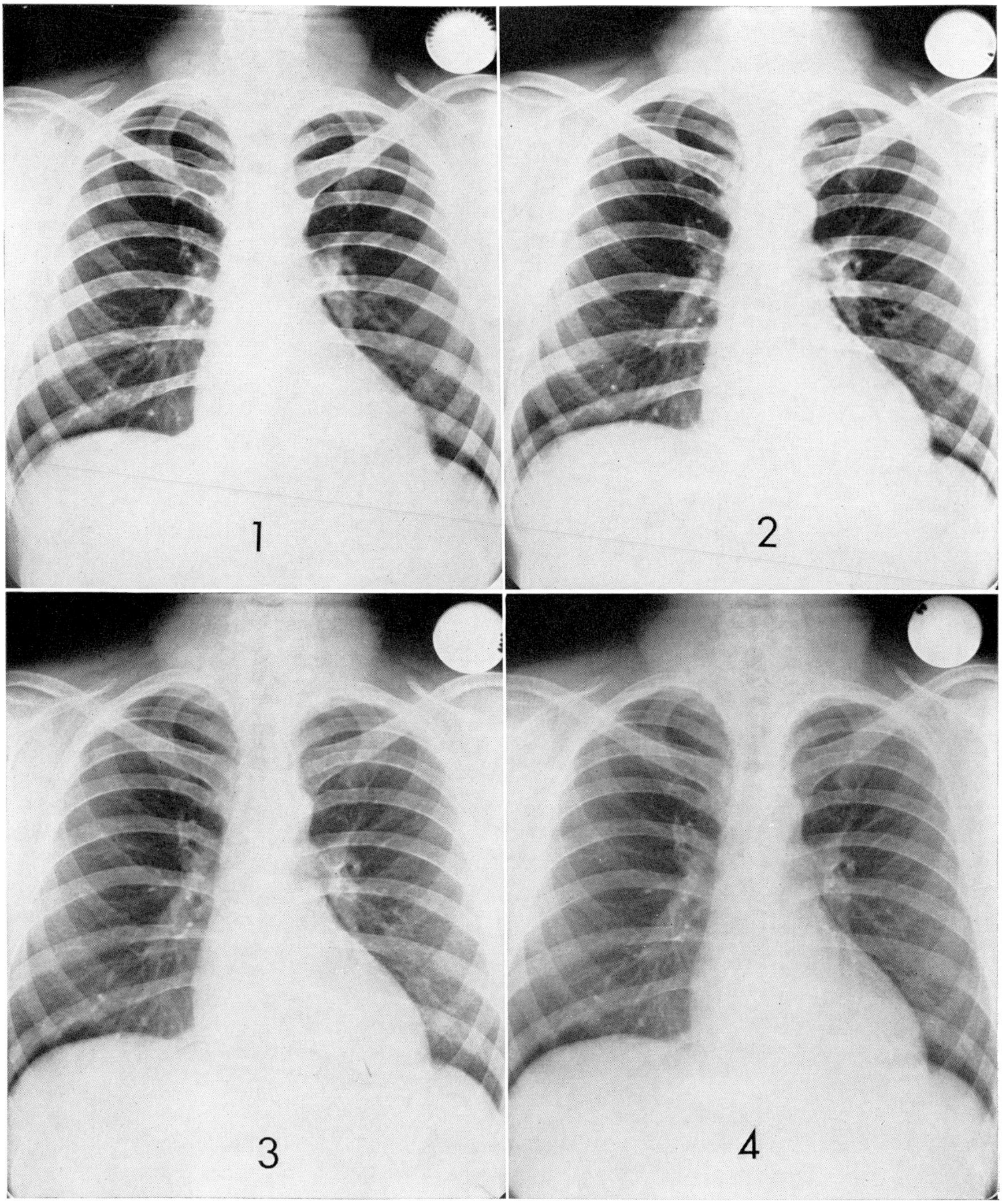

Figure 42. Posteroanterior screen radiographs of the chest that demonstrate the KvP-contrast relation. Exposure sequence is indicated numerically on each radiograph.

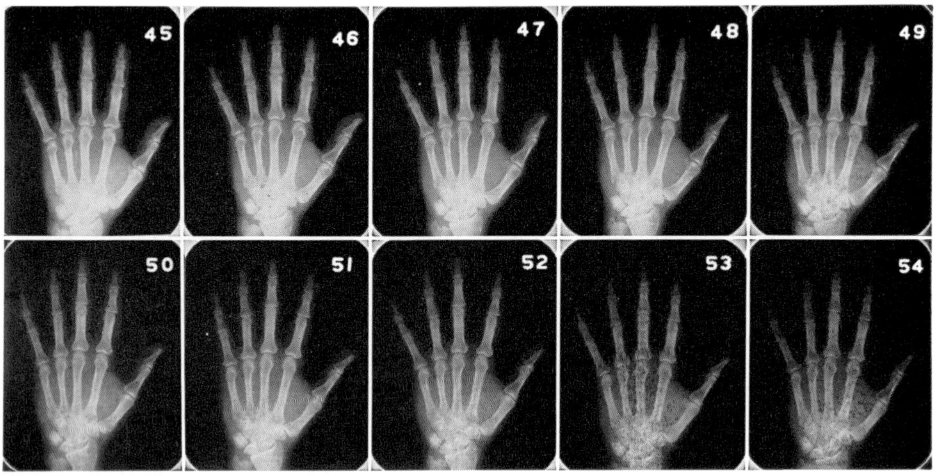

Figure 43. Direct exposure radiographs of the hand that demonstrate the effect on radiographic density with small changes in KvP. Kilovoltage values are indicated on each image.

x-ray developer. Comparison between the densities produced at 45 and 46 KvP shows no discernible difference; the densities produced at 45 and 50 KvP demonstrate visual differences, as do those between 49 and 54 KvP. Changes in kilovoltage of 1 or 2, or even 3, do not demonstrate definite visual density differences. It requires approximately a 5 KvP change to obtain any appreciable change in density.

Example 2. A series of posteroanterior screen exposures of the chest, Figure 44, illustrates further the influence of small kilovoltage changes. Exposures were made employing a range of 75 to 84 KvP in 1-KvP steps; all other factors were con-

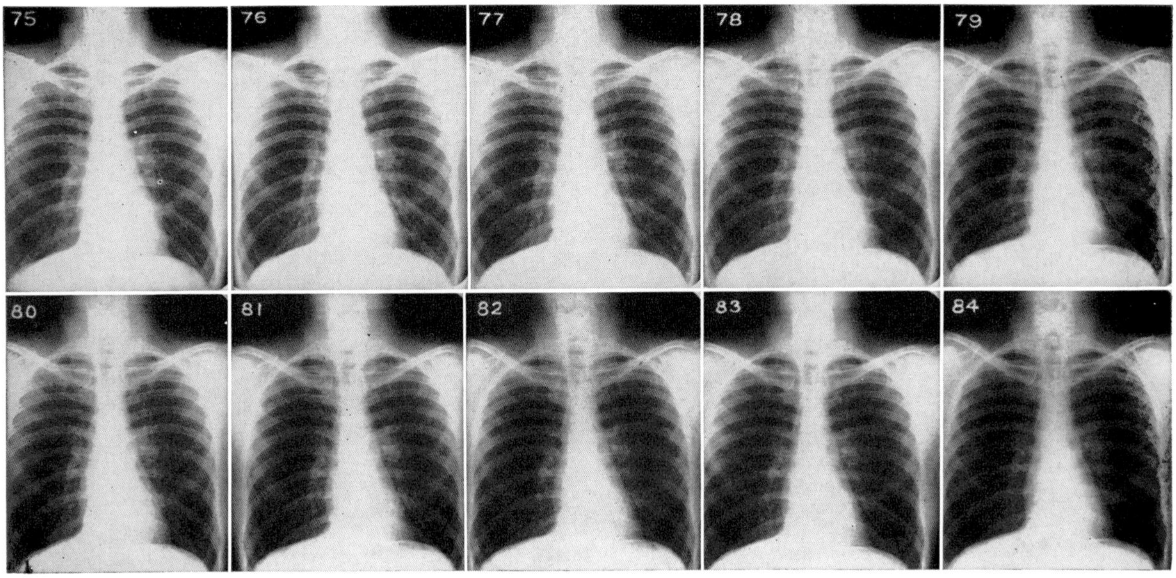

Figure 44. Screen exposures of the chest to demonstrate the density effect with small changes in kilovoltage. The respective KvP value used for each radiograph is shown on the image.

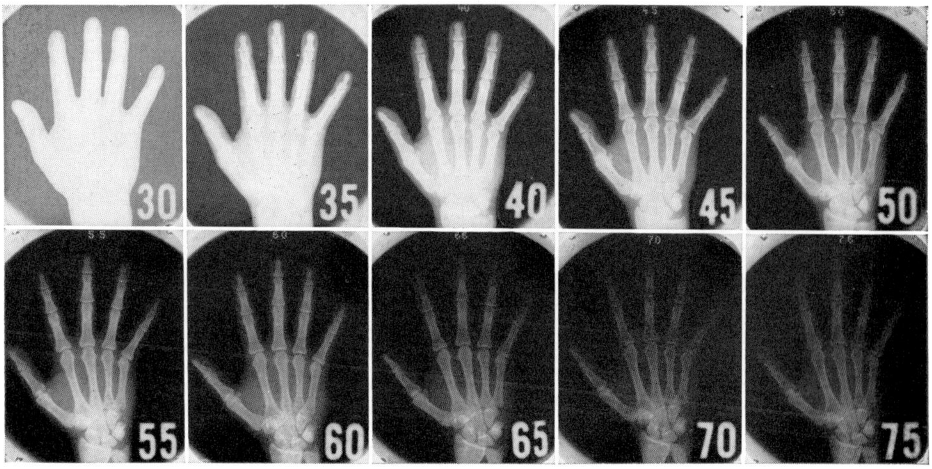

Figure 45. Demonstrates KvP-Density changes. Kilovoltages employed in making the radiographs are inscribed on the respective images.

stant: 2.5 MaS; 72-inch FFD. Comparison of the densities in the 75- and 76-KvP images shows little difference. The same holds true in the 83- and 84-KvP radiographs. A definite difference exists, however, between the 75- and 80-KvP and the 79- and 84-KvP images. A positive difference exists between the densities seen in the 75- and 84-KvP radiographs. Hence, there is no advantage to be derived by changing KvP in increments less than 5.

Large KvP Changes

It was demonstrated above that small changes in kilovoltage have negligible effect on density. The following examples exhibit the effect of larger changes when (1) direct exposure, (2) screen exposure, and (3) grid exposures are made.

Example 1. The series of direct exposure posteroanterior radiographs of the hand (Figure 45) were made in 5 KvP increments from 30 to 75 KvP. All other factors were constant for each radiograph; 45 MaS; 36-inch FFD. Note that the increase in density between each increment of 5 KvP is appreciable between 30 and 55 KvP. The density change between increments above 55 KvP is small. Note that, as overexposure occurs by reason of the accelerated density effect at the higher kilo-

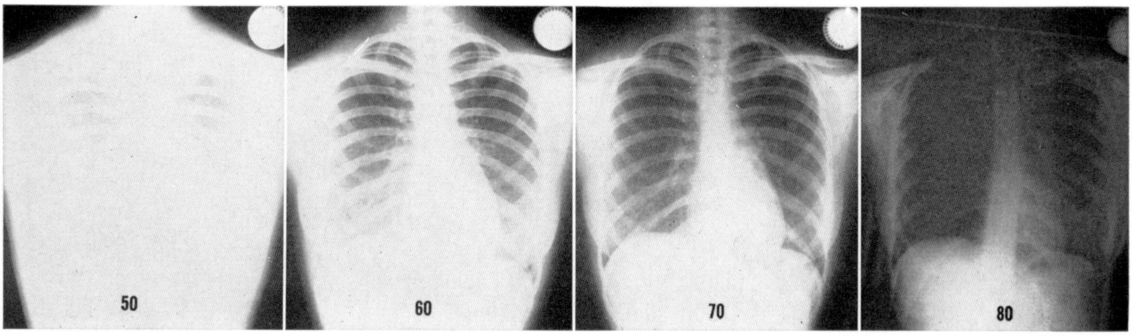

Figure 46. Screen radiographs of the chest to show influence of larger KvP increments on over-all density. Respective kilovoltages employed are shown on the radiographs.

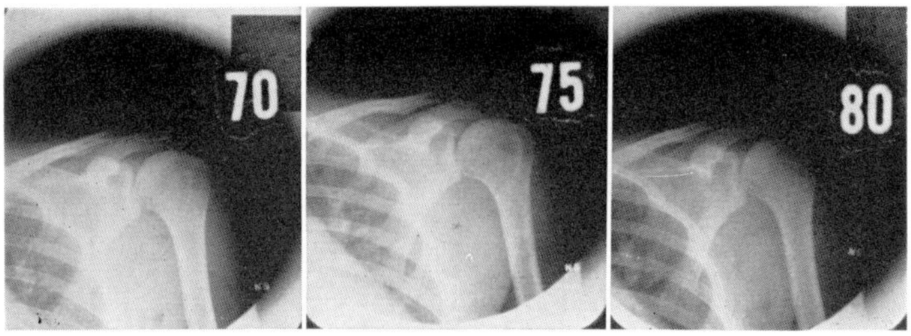

Figure 47. Direct exposure radiographs of the shoulder made with a grid to show influence of larger KvP increments on density. Kilovoltages employed are shown on the radiographs.

voltages, the scale of image contrast also lengthens unduly.

Example 2. This series of screen posteroanterior chest radiographs (Figure 46) was made in increments of 10 from 50 to 80 KvP. All other factors were constant for each radiograph: 10 MaS; 72-inch FFD; average-speed screens. The increase in kilovoltage produces an increase in density. The transition in densities, however, is more exaggerated than in Example 1 because screen contrast was introduced. At the higher KvP values fog begins to appear because of overexposure.

Example 3. A series of three grid radiographs of the shoulder (Figure 47) was made with direct-exposure film employing 70 to 80 kilovolts in increments of five. All other factors were constant: 200 MaS; 36-inch FFD; P-B (Potter-Bucky) grid (8-1). The increase in density between the 70- and 80-KvP films is not as great as that exhibited between the KvP increments in Example 2, for the density changes are due to the influence of kilovoltage. Because a Potter-Bucky grid was employed, the low level of secondary radiation reaching the film contributed only a negligible amount of fog density.

Comment. The appearances of all the above images are characteristic of the manner in which they were produced. In Examples 1 and 2, some fog veils the images when kilovoltages above 60 are employed. In Example 3, fog density is very low because the grid was able to cope with existing secondary radiation.

KvP and Secondary Radiation Fog

The relation of KvP to secondary radiation fog is discussed in Chapter 10.

Compensation for KvP-Density Effect

In the preceding text it was shown that density increases with the kilovoltage. Accurate adjustment of the MaS cannot be established mathematically because the thickness and tissue density of the human body exercises an unpredictable absorption influence. However, the MaS multiplying factors listed in Tables III and IV when correctly applied for various changes in KvP, yield usable MaS values. The following examples illustrate how MaS may compensate for KvP-density changes in medical radiography (see Experiment 10, also).

Example 1. A series of posteroanterior screen radiographs of the chest (Figure 48) was made with a range of 45 to 100 KvP. The MaS was adjusted to compensate for the increasing KvP-density effect with the assistance of Table III; the translucent over-all density of the upper right pulmonary area was used as a guide in adjusting MaS values. The over-all density values in all radiographs of this area are relatively equal.

Example 2. A series of three radiographs of the pelvis (Figure 49) was made with 60 KvP and 150 MaS; 65 KvP and 125

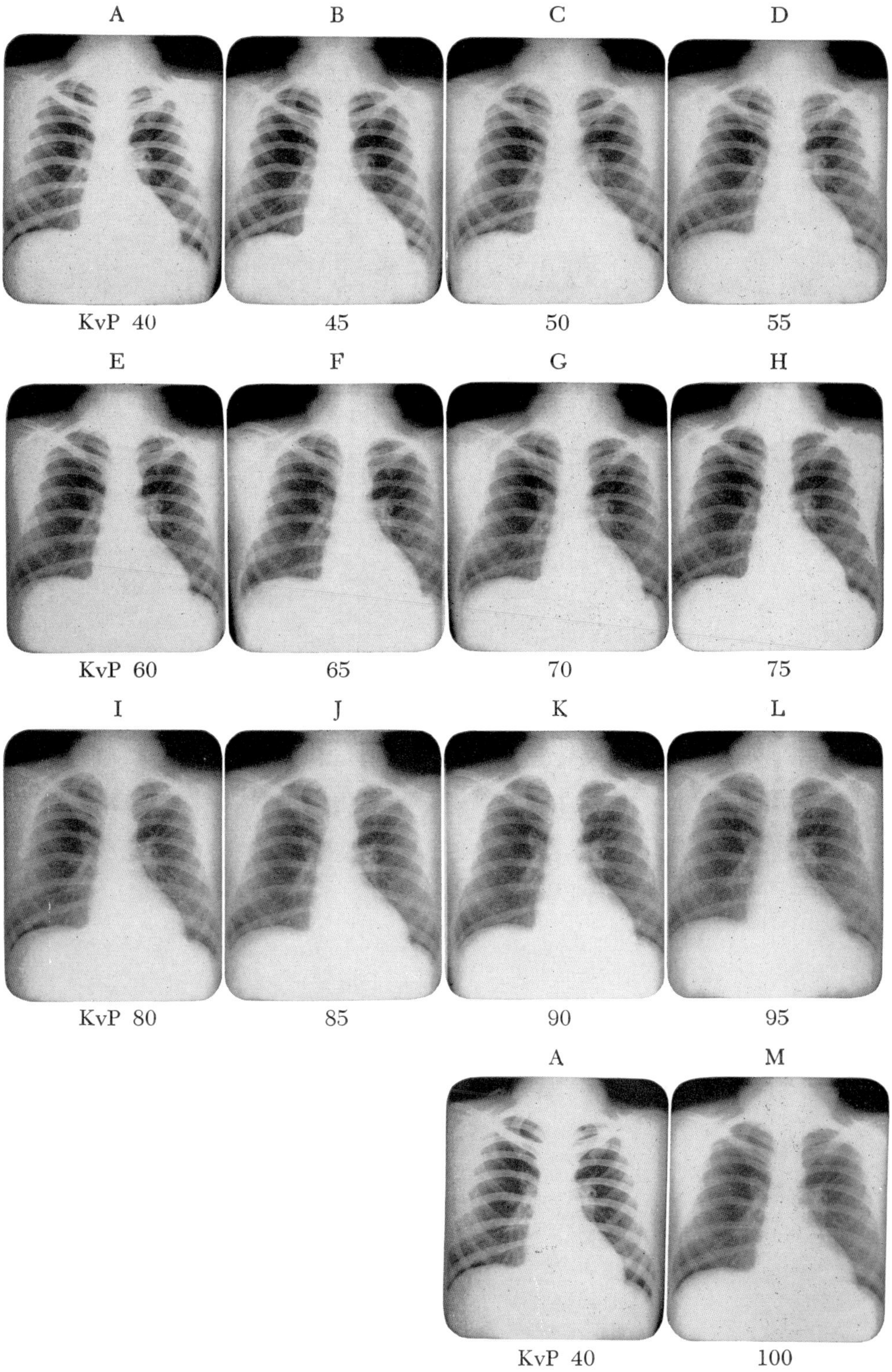

Figure 48. Series of screen radiographs of the chest in which the MaS was decreased in compensation for increasing KvP-density effect. The kilovoltages employed are shown under radiographs. Note that the contrast scale becomes longer with the advance in kilovoltage. Compare the short-scale contrast of the 40-KvP radiograph with the long-scale contrast of the 100-KvP radiograph. MaS Factors: Radiograph A, 70; B, 40; C, 20; D, 10; E, 8.3; F, 6.3; G, 5; H, 4.12; I, 3.3; J, 2.5; K, 2; L, 1.6; M, 1.6.

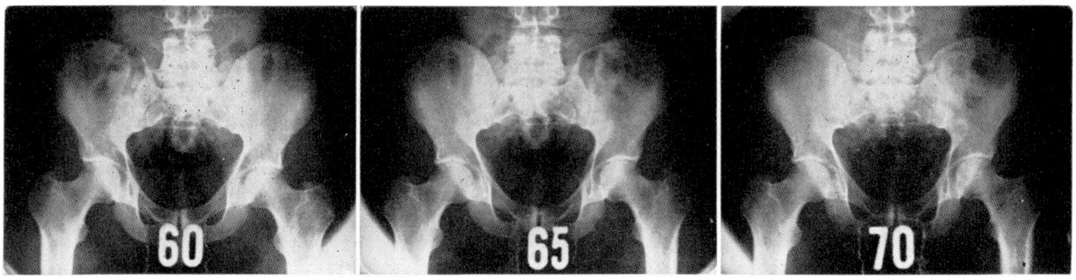

Figure 49. Radiographs of the pelvis made at various kilovoltages with corresponding changes in MaS to equalize densities. Kilovoltages employed are numerically shown on the respective images.

MaS; 70 KvP and 90 MaS; a Potter-Bucky grid; and screens. The MaS values were adjusted so that the over-all densities in all three radiographs were approximately equal.

Example 3. This example demonstrates quite well that when secondary radiation is efficiently controlled, MaS can easily compensate for the density effect of kilovoltage. Two posteroanterior screen radiographs of the skull (Figure 50) were made with 80 KvP (*Left*) and 100 KvP (*Right*); grid (8-1); and 36-inch FFD. Equalization of densities was secured by adjusting the MaS. The longer scale contrast of the 100 KvP radiograph makes it more informative than the 80 KvP film.

Comment. Note that as the kilovoltage increased, the MaS values became greatly reduced, thereby diminishing the radiation dose to the patient. The lower MaS values also contribute increased image sharpness since patient movement is virtually eliminated.

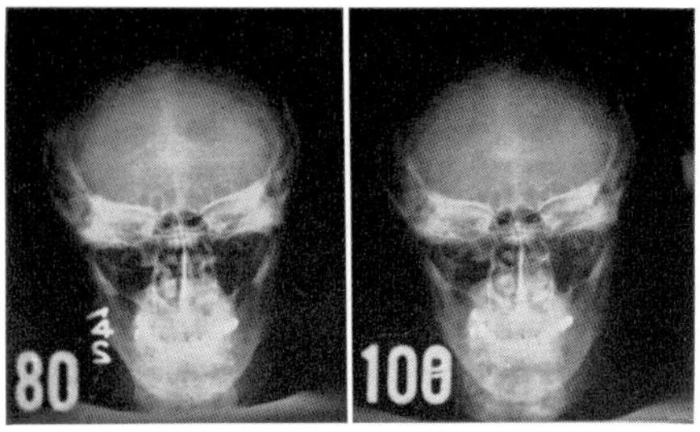

Figure 50. Two posteroanterior screen-grid radiographs of the skull demonstrating that when secondary radiation is controlled, the MaS can compensate for the density effect of kilovoltage and kilovoltage changes can influence the scale of contrast.

Overexposure with Kilovoltage

Overexposure with KvP frequently occurs when greater than necessary kilovoltages are employed. The over-all density present has a characteristic appearance of a high, translucent over-all density, (Figure 51 *Left*). The contrast scale is degraded and detail is partially or totally obscured. Usually, a simple reduction of 10 to 20 kilovolts will correct the appearance appreciably (Figure 51 *Right*). On occasion, it may be necessary to adjust the MaS factor slightly to obtain an over-all density more in keeping with the preferred radiographic quality. In order to avoid overexposure due to KvP, it would be well to adhere closely to the optimum kilovoltages listed for various routine projections (Tables XI-XV).

Underexposure with Kilovoltage

Underexposure due to inadequate KvP is the result of lack of penetration and is characterized by blank transparent areas without silver deposit and other areas possessing very high densities. Very few intermediate tones of density are present. An increase of 15 to 20 kilovolts will usually produce sufficient penetrating radiation to enable the technician to obtain the necessary detail, provided some slight adjustment of the MaS is also made. Again, the use of optimum kilovoltages will assist in avoiding gross errors as can be seen in radiograph 2 or 3 (Figure 40).

MaS Cannot Compensate for Insufficient KvP

No practical amount of MaS can ever compensate for the loss in penetrating power of radiation because of inadequate kilovoltage. Excessive MaS values are dangerous to the patient and are not justified in medical radiography. All medical radiography can be adequately performed within a range of 50 to 100 KvP. It is well to remember that when a kilovoltage is to be assigned to a given projection, one must think of it in relation to *tissue penetration*, and whether the radiation will penetrate the part and provide remnant radiation of a quality and quantity that will produce a satisfactory image. The following example will illustrate the futility of employing an inadequate kilovoltage.

Example. A series of direct-exposure posteroanterior radiographs of the hand on screen-type film (Figure 52), was made to determine an MaS value that would produce a translucent image of all structures in the hand. For the initial radiograph 45 MaS was used at an FFD of 36 inches. The kilovoltage applied was 30. For each succeeding exposure, the MaS was doubled in an attempt to produce an image with the required concentration and distribution of silver deposit. A final MaS value of 1440 was employed, but the image was still unsatisfactory. The lack of penetrating radiation in sufficient quantity made the objective entirely hopeless. By exposing the hand with 50 KvP, 50 MaS, and an FFD of 36 inches, a diagnostic image (G) was obtained. Obviously an MaS of 1440 at 30 KvP was a most impractical exposure since the diagnostic objective was not attained. Opaque densities obscured detail in the phalanges and insufficient silver in the carpal area prevented details being seen in that region. However, the 50-KvP radiograph provided an image in which *all* densities were translucent and details in the entire image were

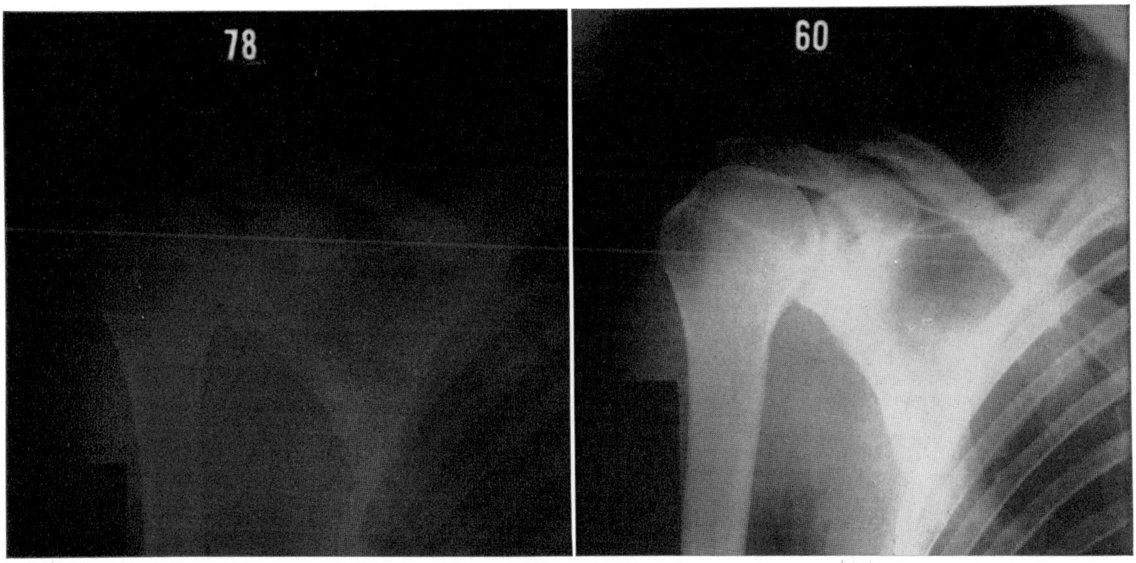

Figure 51. Radiographs of the shoulder showing effect of KvP overexposure. Kilovoltages are numerically indicated on each image. Note fog on radiograph made with 78 KvP.

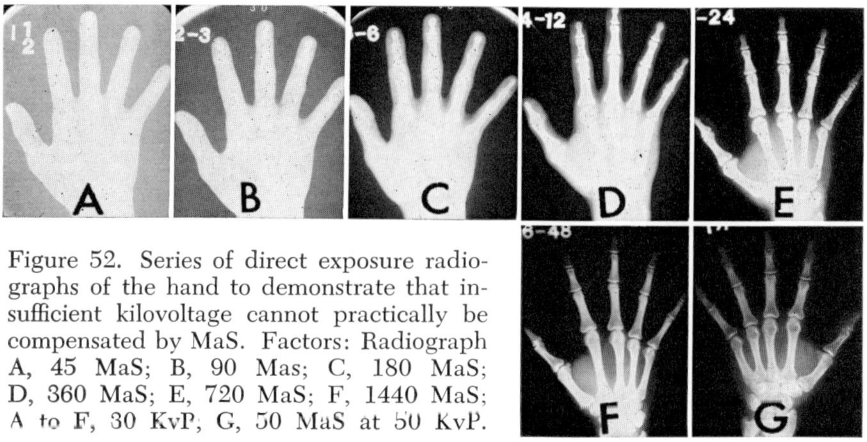

Figure 52. Series of direct exposure radiographs of the hand to demonstrate that insufficient kilovoltage cannot practically be compensated by MaS. Factors: Radiograph A, 45 MaS; B, 90 Mas; C, 180 MaS; D, 360 MaS; E, 720 MaS; F, 1440 MaS; A to F, 30 KvP; G, 50 MaS at 50 KvP.

clearly recorded when a comparatively short exposure was employed.

KILOVOLTAGE AND CONTRAST

It was demonstrated in Part One that, when control of exposure time and secondary radiation was exercised, kilovoltage became the factor of radiographic contrast. Since the visualization of detail is dependent upon radiographic contrast, it is obvious that kilovoltage becomes an important factor in detail delineation. Radiographic details cannot become visible unless the radiation is able to penetrate the part being examined. As previously demonstrated, if remnant radiation is absent, so are details. When the radiation is optimum for a given part, numerous details become visible because of the large number of small density differences (Figure 53). The following exposition will demonstrate the multi-effects of kilovoltage on contrast in the projection of various body parts.

Contrast Without Fog

The influence of kilovoltage on contrast can be demonstrated by a series of radiographs of a dry skull (Figure 54). The absence of soft tissues in the specimen eliminates in large measure the influence of secondary radiation on the image. The images, therefore, may be considered substantially free of secondary radiation fog. The radiographs were exposed in 5 KvP increments from 45 to 100 KvP. The density effect of each kilovoltage was offset by compensating MaS. As a guide in MaS compensation, a step-wedge was recorded in each radiograph—the density of its third step being used as a "control." This density was maintained constant for all kilovoltages. The procedure made it possible to demonstrate the contrast characteristics of each skull image produced by each advance in kilovoltage.

In the 45-KvP film, very high image densities are exhibited and there are also areas in which no details appear because of a lack of sufficient silver deposit. Penetrating radiation was needed to traverse the thicker and denser structures, such as the jaws, pars petrosae, and superior portions of the vault. As the kilovoltage was advanced, some details in these latter structures begin to appear. At 90 and 100 KvP, all structures are thoroughly penetrated and all radiographic details are visible. In comparing the 45-KvP and 100-KvP radiographs, a difference in "brightness" of the images is manifest. The lower kilovoltage film attracts the eye at once because of its brilliance. The eye ignores the fact that a large number of details representative of the anatomy are absent. The few details that are adequately recorded are composed of rather heavy silver deposits and a *rapid* fall-off in image density occurs in areas representing the thicker or denser anatomical structures. Also, the distribution is unequal. At 100 KvP, there is a uniform distribution of translucent densities over the entire image. This radio-

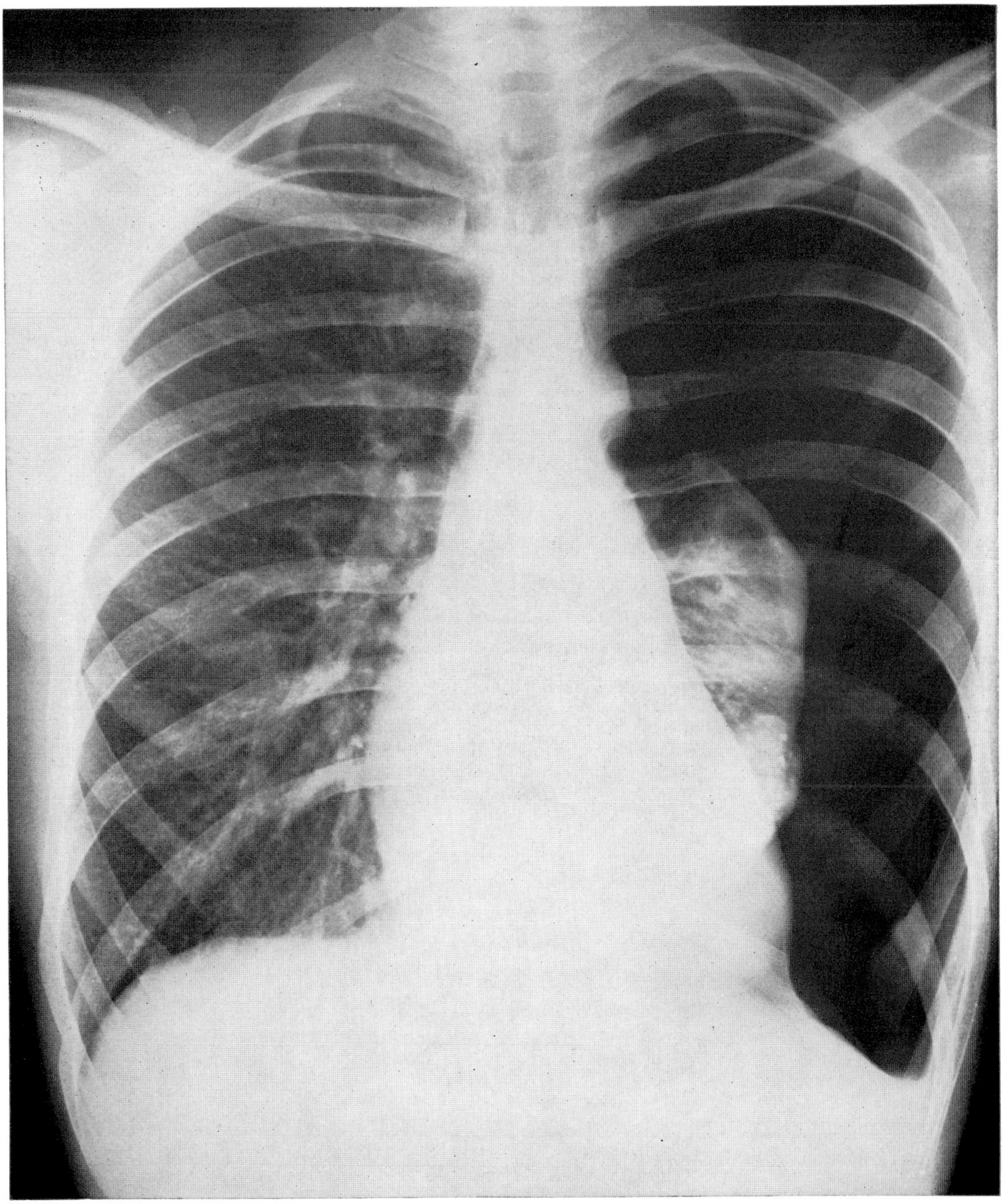

Figure 53. Radiograph of the chest that demonstrates the wide range of radiographic densities that are required for diagnostic purposes. This radiograph exhibits long-scale contrast.

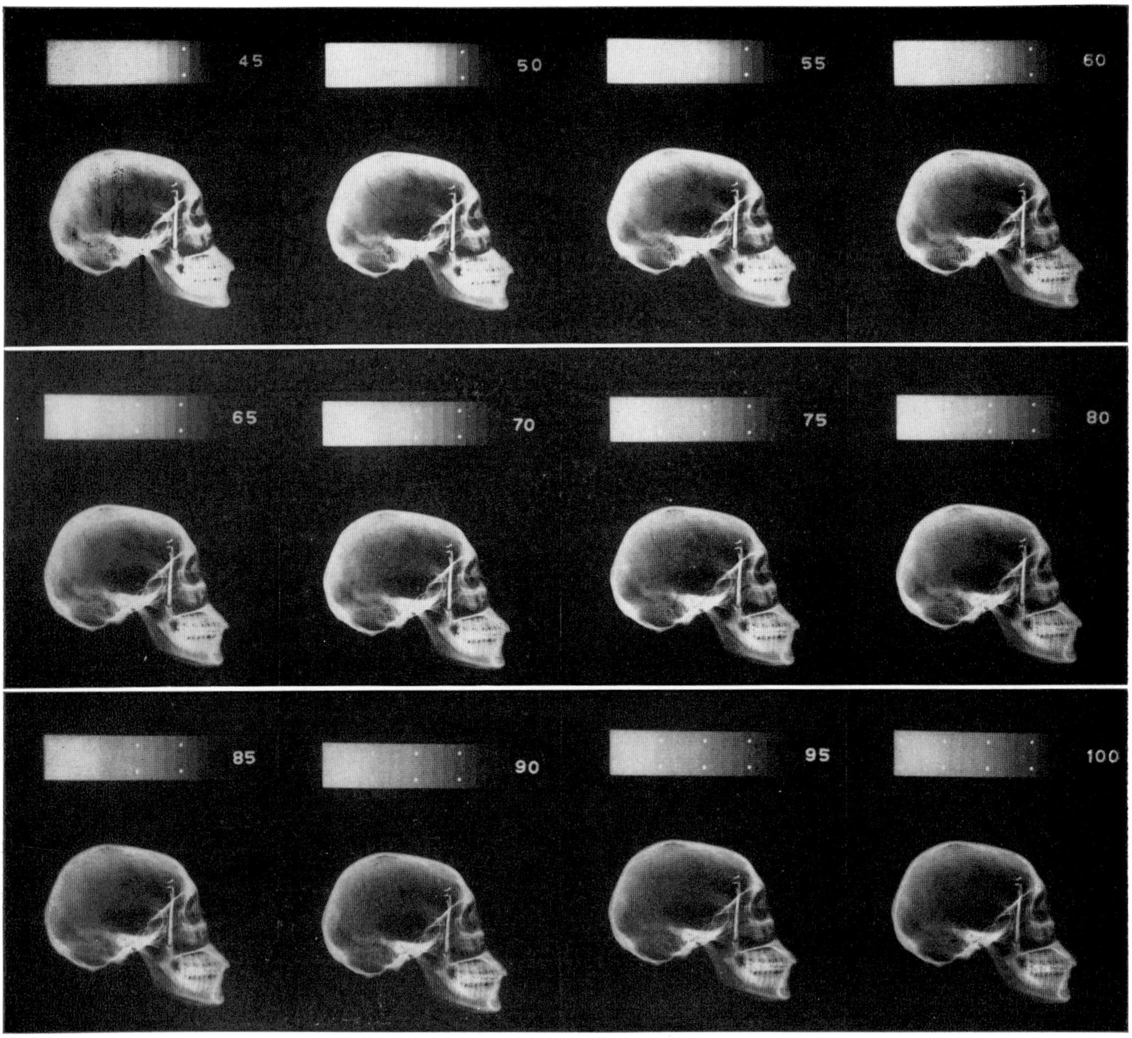

Figure 54. Direct exposure radiographs of a dried skull demonstrate the influence of kilovoltage on contrast and its relation to the visualization of detail. Kilovoltages are shown on each image.

graph has a lower level of "brightness," but the image contains an abundance of details which are so necessary for diagnostic purposes. Whenever great "brightness" or brilliance of an image immediately attracts the eye, short-scale contrast exists as shown in the 45-KvP film. Whenever a lower level of brightness exists and the image contains an abundance of details, long-scale contrast exists as shown in the 100-KvP film. The former is to be avoided and the latter to be attained.

Comment. From this demonstration it may be seen that, when secondary radiation is efficiently controlled, kilovoltage becomes the factor of radiographic contrast. The same conditions may be exhibited by the series of posteroanterior screen chest radiographs shown in Figure 48. A low level of secondary radiation fog is present, however, due to the fluid content of the living tissues of the thorax. Note that in both examples, the contrast scale lengthens as the KvP rises. Also, the radiographs exhibiting the greatest number of details are made with low MaS and higher

KvP values. Examples of long contrast scale radiographs are shown in Figure 16.

KILOVOLTAGE AND EXPOSURE LATITUDE

When a body part is radiographed, the absorption properties of the tissues are largely unpredictable. Naturally, the question arises as to how great an error can be made in the exposure factors without degrading radiographic quality. The term "correct exposure" does not necessarily mean that there is only one exposure factor that will produce the best diagnostic image. Depending upon the kilovoltage used, it may actually mean that many different exposures can be employed to yield radiographs that are diagnostically acceptable to the radiologist. This phenomenon is linked to what is known as *exposure latitude*—an important element in any standardized exposure system.

Exposure Latitude

Exposure latitude may be defined as the range between the minimum and maximum exposure that will produce a scale of translucent densities acceptable for diagnostic purposes. As previously demonstrated, the scale of image densities is determined by the kilovoltage employed. Hence, exposure latitude varies with the kilovoltage applied.

Wide Exposure Latitude

When optimum kilovoltage values are used, the exposure latitude is wide because long-scale contrast is produced in the image which can compensate at times for wide errors in MaS. The large number of densities of small tonal differences produced by the more penetrating radiation serves to retain image details even to the extremes of tissue thickness; that is, details in the *thin and thick* portions of the part may be shown.

Example 1. In a series of anteroposterior direct-exposure radiographs of the elbow (Figure 55) 60 was considered to be the optimum kilovoltage; the FFD was 30

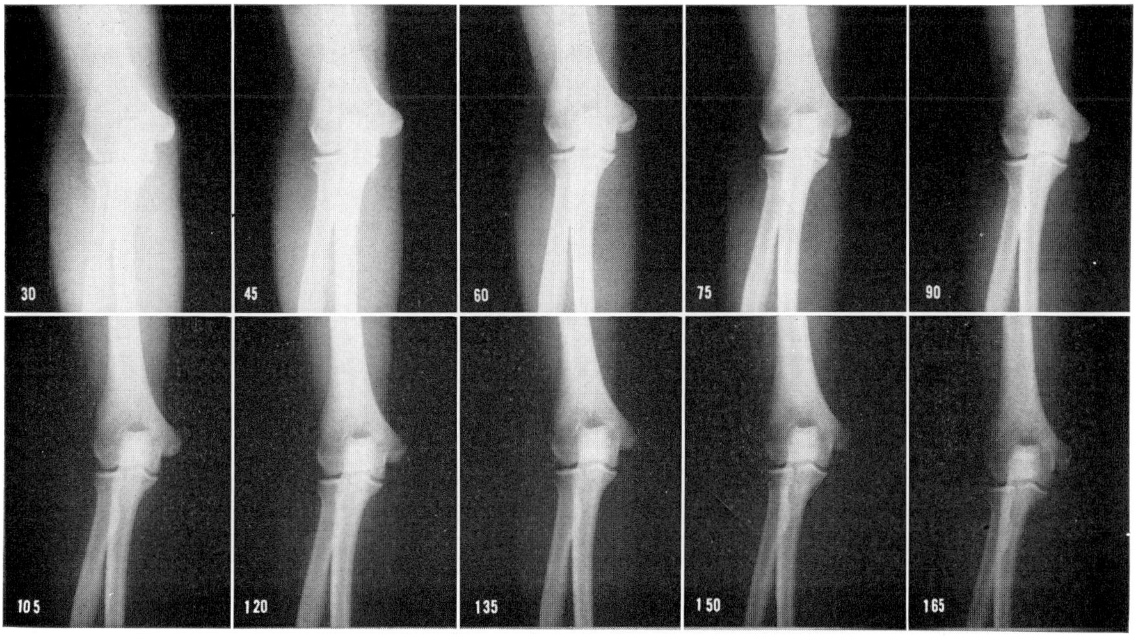

Figure 55. Direct exposure radiographs of the elbow demonstrating exposure latitude. Respective MaS values are inscribed on each image.

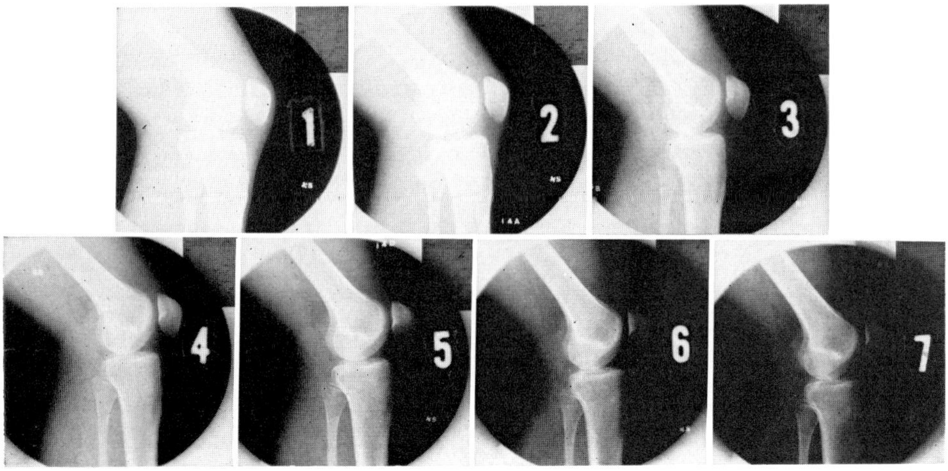

Figure 56. Series of lateral views of the knee to demonstrate latitude. The range between 37.5 and 100 MaS (Nos. 3-6) may be considered the exposure latitude in this case.

inches; the MaS was varied in steps of 15 MaS from 30 to 165 MaS. The exposure latitude in this series may be considered to be between 60 and 150 MaS. The selection of this range was based upon the fact that visualization of all required details was attained in the images although they possessed varying degrees of density. The extremes in density shown in this range, however, are not to be recommended for routine radiography. Selection of the optimum density may easily be made by choosing three adjacent radiographs in the series that approach nearest to the required density–75, 90, and 105 MaS. A desirable density may be considered as produced by about 90 MaS.

Example 2. A demonstration of wide exposure latitude using 80 KvP, direct exposure film and a Potter-Bucky diaphragm (8-1) is shown in Figure 56. A series of lateral exposures of a 10 centimeter knee were made employing MaS values of: (1) 12.5; (2) 25; (3) 37.5; (4) 50; (5) 75; (6) 100; and, (7) 125. FFD: 36 inches. Radiographs Nos. 1 and 2 may be considered as underexposed; No. 7 as overexposed. Radiographs Nos. 3 to 6 may be considered to possess diagnostic densities and the latitude is 37.5 to 100 MaS. Between these values lies the correct exposure; that is, approximately 75 MaS as represented by radiograph No. 5.

Example 3. A series of screen-grid anteroposterior radiographs of the lumbar vertebrae (Figure 57) was made using 70 KvP; 36-inch FFD; and 20 to 70 MaS in increments of 10 MaS. The latitude may be considered to be in the 20 to 60 MaS range. The optimum density was produced with 40 MaS.

Comment. Examples 2, 3, and 4 demonstrate the influence of MaS on density in three exposure categories when the x-rays penetrated the part. Since the kilovoltage was optimum for the projections illustrated, any degree of density could be obtained over a wide range simply by varying the MaS without disturbing the kilovoltage. All optimal densities were produced with low exposure values which were practical in their application. Since long-scale contrast is present in the image, wide exposure latitude exists.

Narrow Exposure Latitude

Exposure latitude is usually narrow when short-scale contrast prevails, as produced by the lower kilovoltages. The small number of usable densities present requires that the exposure be more nearly correct to obtain densities that are representative of the thinnest or the thickest portions of the part. The scale of contrast, however, is seldom such that all desired tissues are shown in the same image, particularly of a subject that contains a number of structural details of widely different tissue densities or thicknesses. Also, the MaS values required are usually so great as to be impractical in application.

Example 1. A series of direct-exposure posteroanterior radiographs of the hand (Figure 52) was made with 30 KvP; 36-inch FFD; and 45 to 1440 MaS—the MaS values were doubled in each case. Note that the high contrast prevents equal rendition of all densities—some are excessive, others weak, despite the impractical exposure values.

Example 2. A series of screen postero-anterior radiographs of the chest (Figure 58) made with 50 KvP; 72-inch FFD; and 5, 10, and 20 MaS in increments obtained by doubling the MaS, demonstrates the wide differences in densities secured because the kilovoltage was too low for this body part and, consequently, short-scale contrast prevailed. The nearest approach to a desirable image was obtained with 20 MaS—another impractical exposure.

Example 3. A series of three screen-grid lateral radiographs (Figure 59) of the skull was made with 55 KvP; 36-inch FFD; and 50, 100, and 150 MaS. Note that the 50-MaS image is underexposed (the image of the vault contains little silver); the 100-MaS radiograph shows the facial bones with excessive silver deposits although the pars petrosae are not penetrated; and the 150-MaS image shows opaque silver deposits in the facial area, the vault is well shown but the pars petrosal area was not recorded. The extremes of short-scale contrast are exhibited in this image—opacities and transparencies that make only a small portion of the image fully informative.

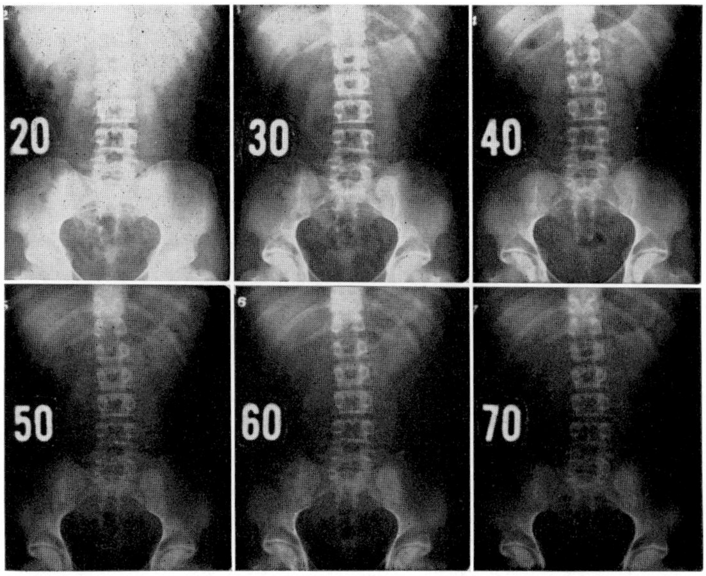

Figure 57. Anteroposterior screen-grid radiographs of the lumbar vertebrae to demonstrate exposure latitude at 70 KvP and 36″ FFD. Respective MaS values are shown on the radiographs. The exposure latitude lies in the range of 20-60 MaS.

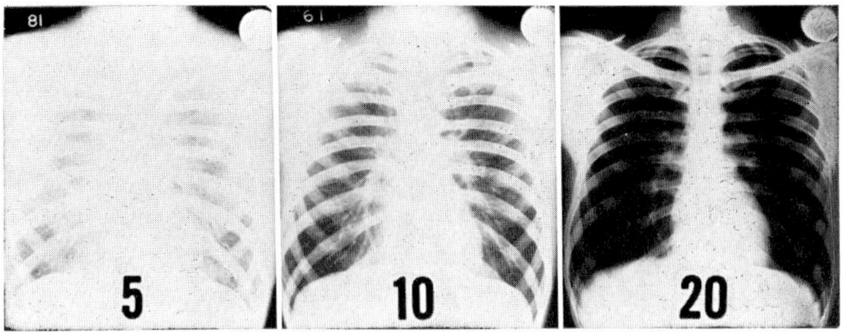

Figure 58. Posteroanterior screen exposures of the chest at 50 KvP. Respective MaS values are shown on each image. Note large differences in over-all density that occurs when MaS is changed—a characteristic of short-scale contrast.

CONTRAST VERSUS EXPOSURE LATITUDE

The close relationship between contrast and exposure latitude may be observed by a study of Figure 60. This relationship obviously is dependent upon the factor of kilovoltage.

Example. In Figure 60, radiographs (A-E) were made with 50 KvP at 72″ FFD and a cone. MaS: (A) 7.5; (B) 10; (C) 13.3; (D) 20; (E) 30. Radiographs (F-J) were made with 80 KvP at 72″ FFD and a cone; MaS: (F) 2.5; (G) 3.3; (H) 4.16; (I) 5; (J) 6.6.

Radiographs A-E

Note that, as the MaS increased, the over-all density of the image increased; (D) and (E) contain opaque silver deposits and details are obscured. When the density level became satisfactory and the silver deposits were translucent as shown in (B) or (C), there was an absence of silver to depict details in the denser tissue areas despite the fact that MaS values of 10 or 13.3 were employed. The dosage values were too high. The contrast differences were so great that one could safely assume that many of the finer details were being lost due to lack of tissue penetration in (A) and to silver opacities in (D) and (E). This is a condition typical of short-scale contrast. The exposure latitude was constricted between (B) and (C) which is too narrow a range for good chest radiography. Secondary radiation fog was no problem at this KvP.

Radiographs F-J

As the MaS increased, the over-all density increased; all silver deposits were

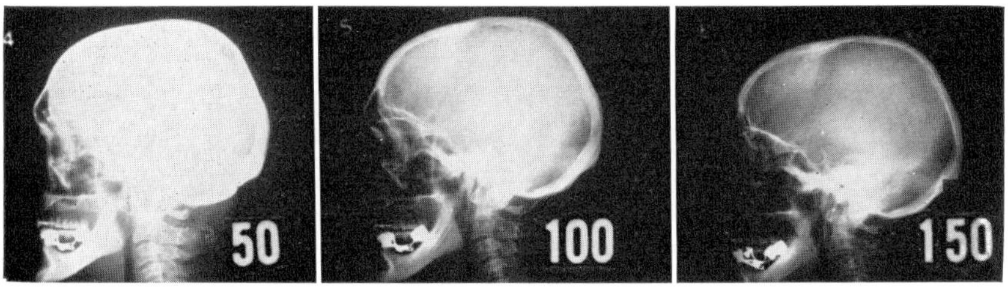

Figure 59. Lateral screen-grid radiographs of the skull at 55 KvP. MaS values are indicated on each image. Note highlights that are devoid of details and opacities that obscure details—characteristics of short-scale **contrast.**

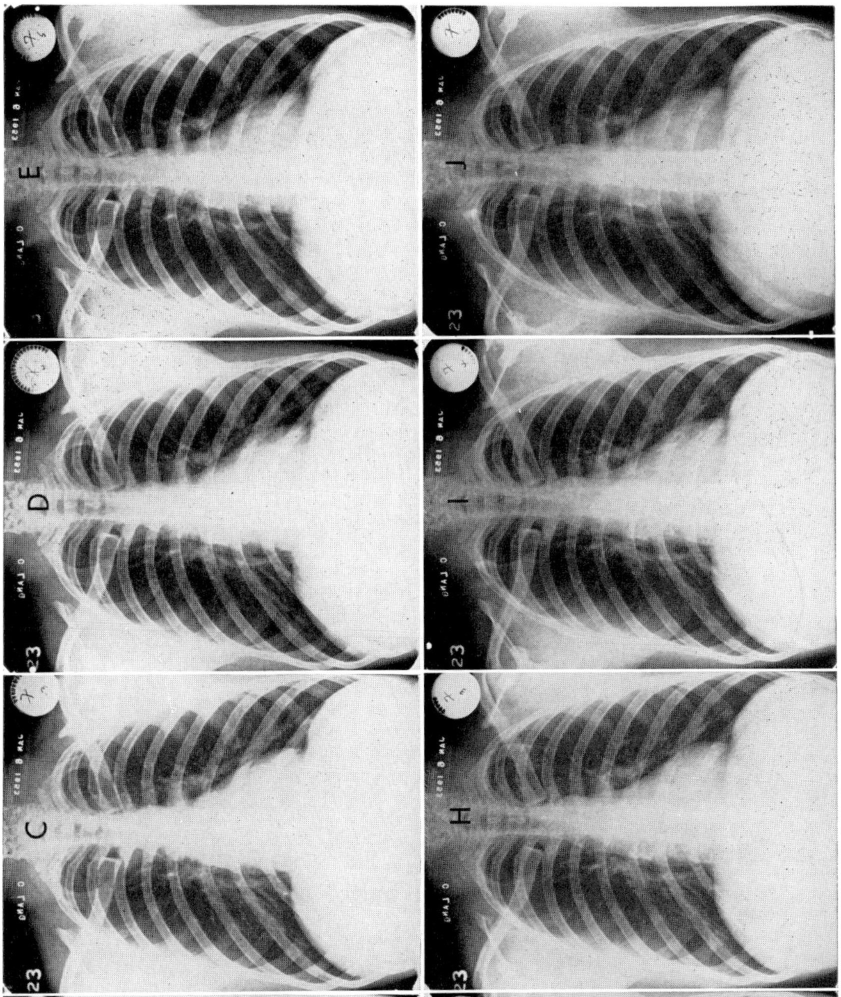

Figure 60. Two series of posteroanterior screen-radiographs of a 23 cm. chest (unretouched) that serve as a study in radiographic density, contrast, and exposure latitude. Note shorter scale of contrast in A to E as compared to the longer contrast scale in F to J.

translucent even in (J), which exhibits some secondary radiation fog due to overexposure. In (F), minimal silver deposits demonstrate details that are absent in (A). All essential details are recorded with varying levels of over-all density in (F) to (I), which is typical of long-scale contrast images. The density of (J) is a bit excessive and some details are obscured because of overexposure. The exposure latitude is wide, as represented by radiographs (F) to (I). All MaS values are small and the dosage minimal. Radiograph (G) may be considered as having received the correct exposure. Some secondary radiation fog is present but its level is within diagnostic acceptability. All exposure times were such as to reduce the effect of respiratory or cardiac motility to a minmum—hence greater sharpness of detail was obtained than in (A-E).

Comment. The examples cited above demonstrate that when the kilovoltage is not adequate to provide radiation that penetrates all portions of the part being examined, no practical amount of MaS can compensate for the lack of image density representing the thicker structures. When short-scale contrast prevails, the resulting narrow exposure latitude prevents the rendition of a large number of densities for diagnostic use. The lower kilovoltages overemphasize the less dense tissue areas with high densities, while the heavier tissue areas are weakly recorded with thin densities or transparencies.

Recommendation. A technician operating with an optimum kilovoltage technic is more likely to produce greater uniformity of radiographic results than one who uses a relatively low, variable kilovoltage technic. In fact, the latitude available at the higher kilovoltages is the very factor that permits consistency in radiographic results obtained with a fixed kilovoltage technic.

Rule

The following general rule may be considered basic: *The longer the scale of radiographic contrast, the greater is the exposure latitude.*

USE OF HIGHER KILOVOLTAGES

The use of the higher kilovoltages provides greater exposure efficiency in radiography for the following reasons:

1. Anatomical details in all tissue thicknesses are rendered as translucent densities. The relative absorption properties between bone and flesh are reduced making possible visualization of more structural details. Soft tissue detail is as good, if not better, than that produced by the lower kilovoltages because shorter exposures tend to reduce motion unsharpness. At lower kilovoltages, bone detail often tends to obscure details of soft tissues that lie behind the bone. Complete penetration of bone by higher kilovoltages reveals soft tissue details that are often not visible at lower kilovoltages. The greater penetration effected by higher kilovoltage radiation makes possible the rendition of a greater number of anatomical details than when lower kilovoltages are employed.
2. Greater image sharpness is obtained because shorter exposures may be employed with smaller focal spots.
3. The radiation dose to patients is reduced as the kilovoltage level increases because the body absorbs less radiation than at the lower kilovoltages. More radiation can, therefore, reach the film to expose it, and exposures can be reduced.
4. Heat production in the x-ray tube is reduced because smaller energy loads (MaS) can be employed, thereby increasing x-ray tube life. As the kilovoltage increases, tube efficiency increases. There is more x-radiation per watt of electric power consumed when using the higher kilovolt-

ages than there is when using the lower kilovoltages. A correct exposure may therefore be produced with less heat generated in the tube.

5. Greater exposure latitude may be secured. As the kilovoltage increases, exposure latitude increases because of the narrowed absorption range of body tissues created by virtue of complete penetration. Details become visible in tissues of wide density and thickness. The absorption range is greater when the lower kilovoltages are employed. Consequently, exposure latitude is decreased and longer exposures are required.

6. The higher kilovoltages make possible the use of many radiographic technics that, heretofore, have been deemed too difficult to perform.

7. When the source of electric power is variable or is in a state of constant flux, the higher kilovoltages make possible more satisfactory bed-side radiography.

8. As a matter of economics, the use of higher kilovoltages causes x-ray tubes to last longer.

SUMMARY

The influence of kilovoltage and its relation to other exposure factors in altering radiographic density and contrast is summarized as follows:

KvP-DENSITY RELATION

When all other factors are constant, density changes with the KvP.

KvP-TIME RELATION

With changes in KvP, the time of exposure must be adjusted to compensate for the density influence of KvP; Tables III and IV assist in this operation.

KvP-Ma RELATION

It is impractical in routine radiography to employ this relation. The effects are the same, however, as the KvP-Time Relation.

KvP-FFD RELATION

In practical radiography, the need for using this relation is extremely rare.

KvP-PENETRATION RELATION

By virtue of its control of x-ray wave length (quality of radiation), KvP governs the degree of x-ray penetration of body tissues.

KvP-FOG RELATION

KvP has direct influence on the production of secondary radiation generated in the tissues; hence, KvP influences the amount of secondary radiation fog produced on the radiographic image. The greater the kilovoltage, the greater the amount of secondary radiation generated in the tissues.

KvP-CONTRAST RELATION

KvP has a direct bearing upon the contrast scale; as KvP changes, contrast changes. The lower the kilovoltage employed, the shorter the scale of contrast; the higher the kilovoltage, the longer the scale of contrast.

KvP-LATITUDE RELATION

Because of its control over radiographic contrast, KvP regulates exposure latitude.

Chapter 10

Secondary Radiation Fog

Part One

On foggy days, details of the out-of-doors are obscured. The mist in the air scatters the light more or less evenly over a landscape so that it may be difficult to differentiate one object from another. However, on a clear day the same landscape can be seen distinctly. When a primary beam of x-rays traverses an object, some of the x-rays are absorbed while others pass directly through it; a considerable percentage, however, is scattered in all directions by the atoms of the material struck—very much as light is dispersed by a mist. These scattered rays comprise what is known as *secondary radiation* and are radiographically effective. Secondary radiation strikes the film from all directions and produces a fairly uniform deposit of silver over an *entire* image. This veil of silver overlays the image density produced by the remnant radiation and is, in reality, a *supplemental* density known as secondary radiation *fog*. When fog is present, the effect is as if image details were being viewed through a mist. In other words, the quality of the image is degraded. Radiographic examples of secondary radiation fog are shown in Figure 61. Observe (1) the characteristic dull gray appearance of the images and (2) the absence of important details.

The role of secondary radiation in producing an image may be easily demonstrated (Figure 62). When a block of wood is placed on the x-ray table at a 45° angle it can be irradiated by a vertical x-ray beam. At right angles to the beam a lead tunnel is aligned with one end opposite the wooden block. At the other end of the tunnel a cassette is placed with an object in front of it. The piece of wood is then exposed. The secondary radiation produced in the wood emanates in all directions and some of it travels down the tunnel to expose the film. The tunnel protects the cassette from primary radiation. Therefore, the image is produced solely by secondary radiation. A diagram of the arrangement and a radiograph made of a metal grill exposed by the secondary radiation is shown as Figure 62.

Virtually the whole question of radiographic quality is related to the effect of secondary radiation fog on the visualization of detail. Its effect is greatest on those elements of an object that are farthest from the film. Visibility of these details may be greatly lessened and on occasion they may not even appear in the image. By controlling the amount of secondary radiation reaching the film during an exposure, details become more pronounced with resultant improvement in image quality. Rendition of all anatomic details, then, becomes more in accord with the actual absorption properties of the tissues irradiated. Also, reduction in fog makes possible easier visualization of details representing small differences on tissue absorption.

The secondary radiation reaching the film has more of the quality of the longer wave lengths (lesser penetration) than the remnant radiation. Its intensity is modified either (1) by the *absorbing action* of the tissues through which it must pass, or (2) by the *distance* from the film to its origin

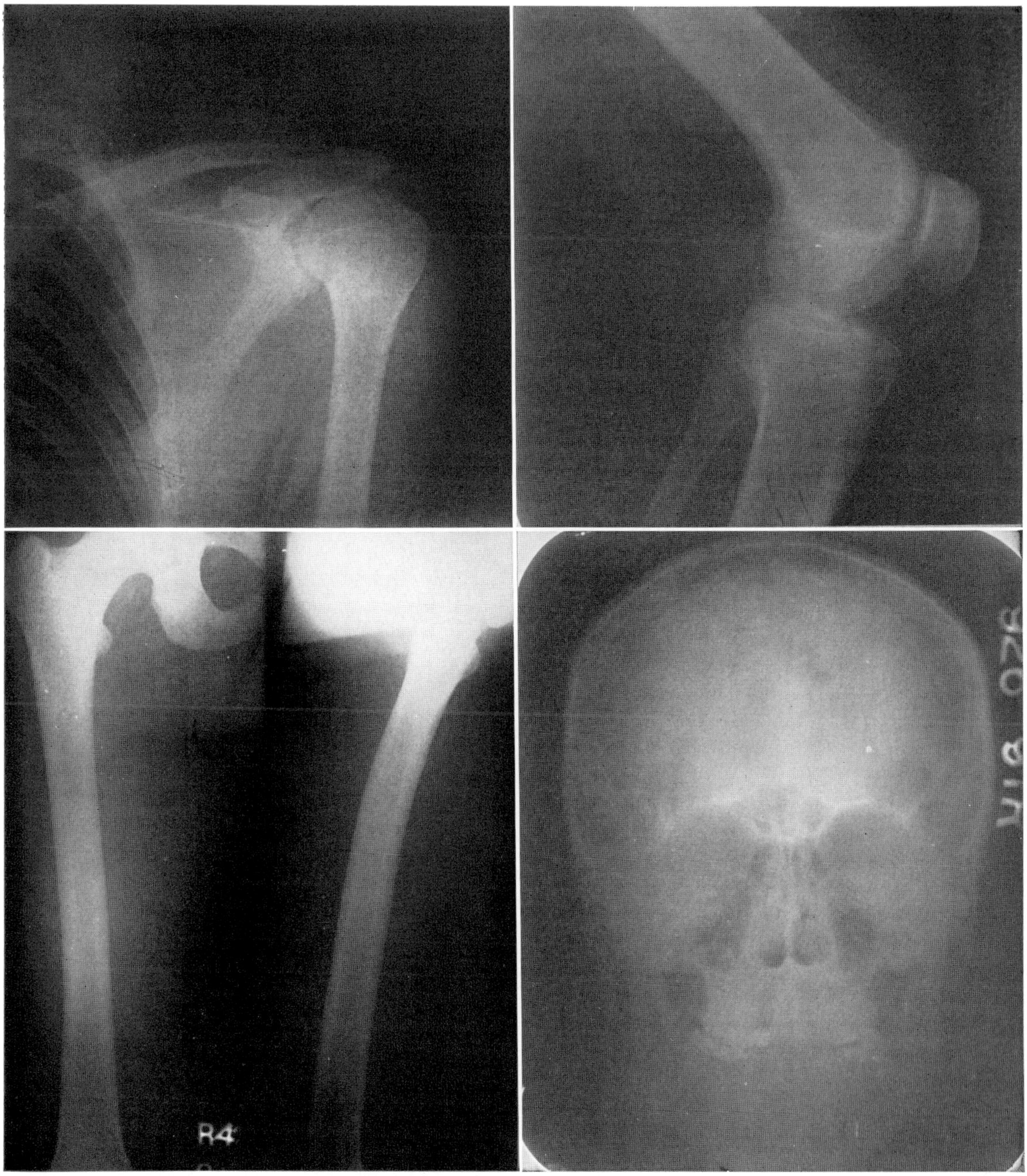

Figure 61. Radiographs that exhibit evidence of secondary radiation fog. Note similarity of image appearance and general loss in detail visualization because of degradation of contrast.

in the tissues. Secondary radiation originates from a multiplicity of sources and is, therefore, unfocused and aberrant. Even with present-day accessories, it is not always possible to control it completely. The supplemental density superimposed by this radiation on the image is like a veil; it actually increases the over-all density of the image and limits the ability to see radiographic details clearly. In fact a desirable range of densities (contrast) is usually destroyed and important detail is obscured.

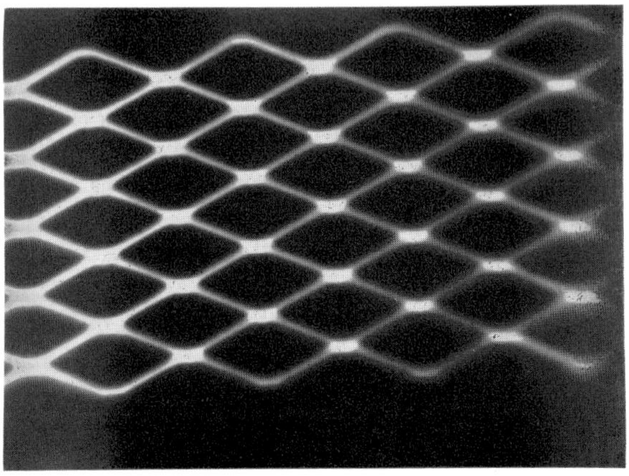

Figure 62. Diagram of arrangement for exposing an x-ray film only with secondary radiation generated by a block of wood. (*Top*, page 101) A radiograph of the metal grill is shown above.

EMISSION OF SECONDARY RADIATION

The emission of secondary radiation and its influence on the image may be simulated radiographically by the use of paraffin—a material that generates large quantities of secondary radiation. A block of paraffin 2½ x 6 x 10-inches may be used for this purpose.

Three principal conditions under which secondary radiation fog may be produced on film are illustrated by the series of diagrams and radiographs shown in Figures 63 and 64.

WHEN OBJECT IS NEAR FILM

When a metal disc or coin is placed on a film and the paraffin block is placed *over* it (Figure 63A), an x-ray exposure will produce a radiograph in which the image of the disc is relatively free of fog. The secondary radiation generated by the emitter could not sufficiently undercut the coin to fog its image. However, the film areas outside the coin image are fogged. This example demonstrates that the image of elements in an emitter that are *close* to the film is less affected by secondary radiation fog. A radiograph illustrating this fact is shown as (Figure 64A).

WHEN OBJECT IS DISTANT

When the emitter is placed on the film and the disc is mounted on its top (Figure 63B), the radiograph will show the image of the disc to be fogged by the secondary radiation that undercuts the object. This diagram and radiographic example (Figure 64B) demonstrate that images of objects, in or on an emitter, located at a distance from the film will be fogged when the emitter is adjacent to the film.

WHEN OBJECT AND EMITTER ARE DISTANT

When the emitter together with the disc on its top is moved away from the film (Figure 63C), the degree of fog in the image will be *less* than that shown in Radiograph (B) (Figure 64), since the secondary radiation reaching the film has been diminished by reason of its greater distance from its source. Therefore, by in-

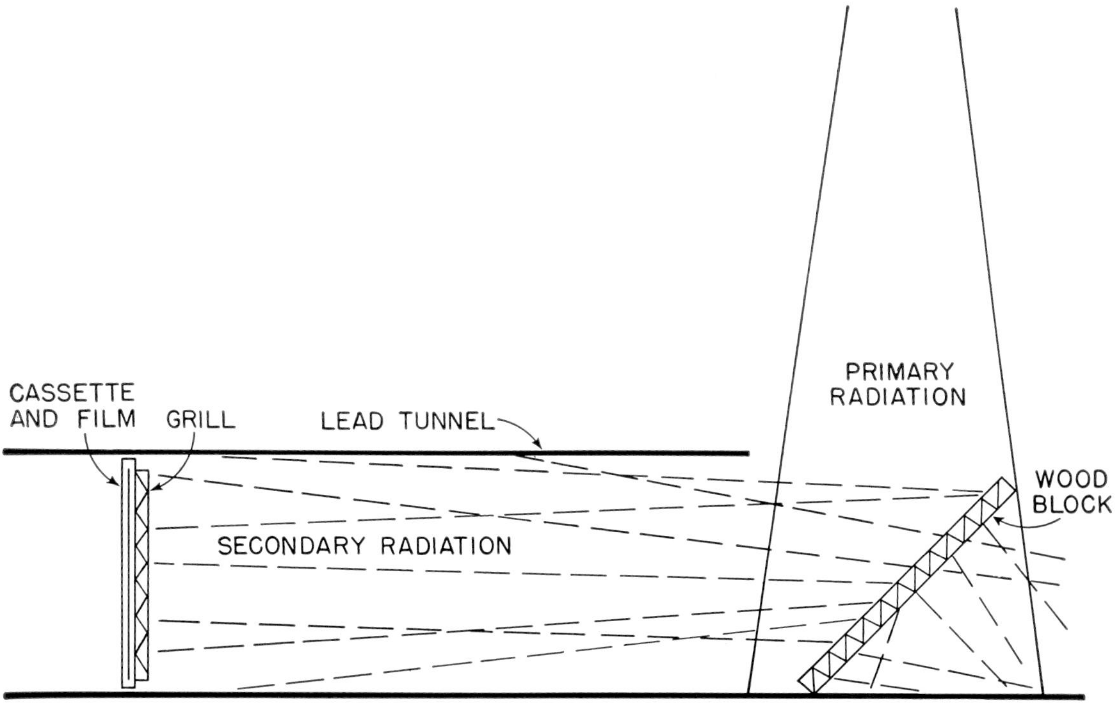

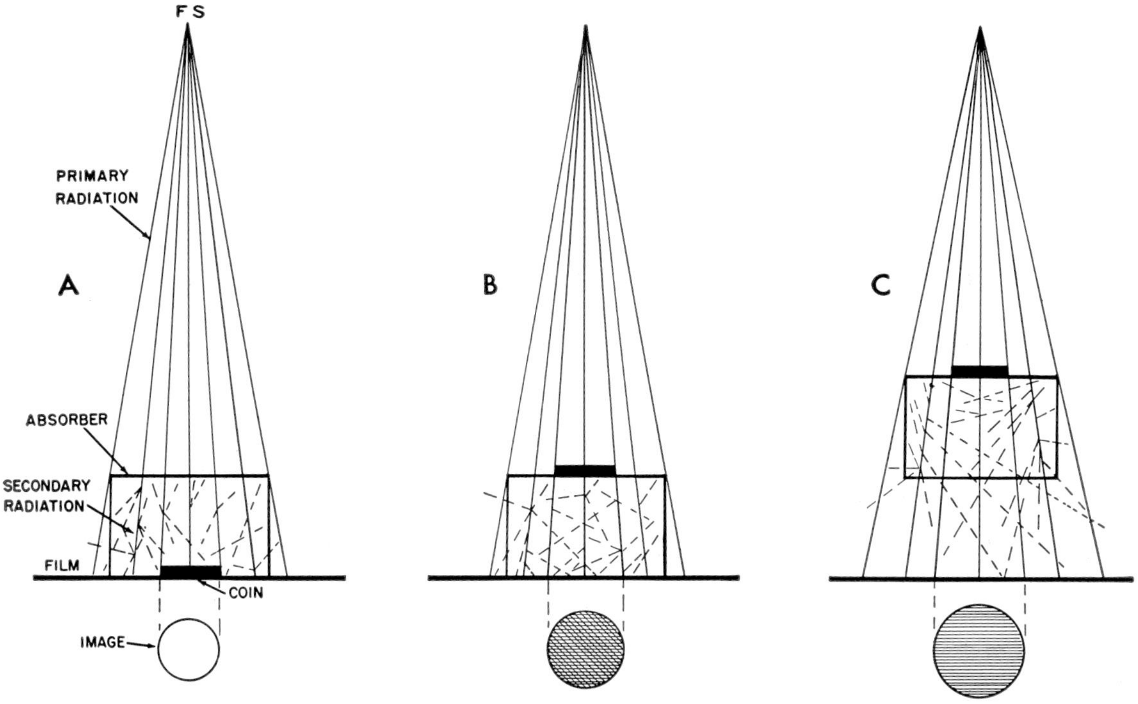

Figure 63. Diagrams that demonstrate the effect of secondary radiation from an emitter (paraffin block) on the radiographic image of a coin or metal disc. (A) When the disc is placed on the film and under the emitter, the image is not fogged. (B) When the disc is on top of the emitter, the image becomes fogged. (C) When the disc and emitter are moved away from the film, the fog density is reduced (see Figure 64).

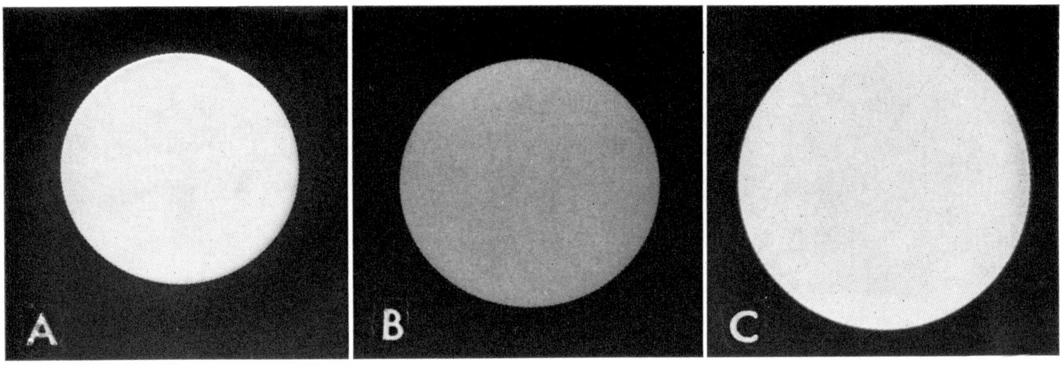

Figure 64. Radiographs of discs demonstrating effects diagrammatically shown in Figure 63. (A) disc on film; (B) disc on emitter (OFD 2.5 inches); (C) disc and emitter 5 inches above film.

creasing the distance between the emitter-disc combination and the film, the *intensity* of the secondary radiation reaching the film diminishes.

INFLUENCE OF TISSUES

The quantity of secondary radiation emitted by the human body depends upon the tissue thickness and its density as well as the kilovoltage employed. The larger and/or denser the part, the greater is the secondary radiation and vice versa. Matter of high atomic weight (bone) emits a relatively small amount of secondary radiation, whereas matter of low atomic weight (muscle) emits large quantities. The human body is composed largely of matter of low atomic weight containing fluids of various kinds. Each individual tissue is an emitter of secondary radiation. The amount emitted, however, is dependent upon its fluid content (hydration).

TYPES OF TISSUE

Since the structural composition and thickness of a normal body part are relatively constant, the amount of secondary radiation emitted by that part may be considered as a constant for a given kilovoltage. For example, the leg is composed of bone, muscle, fat, skin, circulatory vessels, etc., and the amount of secondary radiation that can be emitted by these, or any other tissues, is virtually unpredictable when variable kilovoltages are employed in exposure. Only a gross estimation can be made, but sufficient experience sometimes enables a technician to approximate the choice of correct exposure factors with the use of various fog-controlling accessories. Wherever there is a physiologic departure from the normal, the possible adverse effects of increased secondary radiation must be considered. For example, as a result of injury or disease, an invasion of fluid into a knee joint increases the amount of scattering material than in a normal knee; consequently, it is logical to use a grid as well as a cone in radiography of the part.

TISSUE THICKNESS

The problem of secondary radiation fog increases in proportion to the thickness of the part. It has been found that the radiation emerging from a tissue thickness of 6 inches may assume a ratio of secondary radiation to remnant radiation of 5 to 1, and with greater thicknesses it may rise to 10 to 1.

Thin Body Parts

In posteroanterior radiographs of the hand, the emission of secondary radiation is negligible compared to the intensity of the remnant radiation. This may be demonstrated by a series of four radiographs of the hand, Figure 65, wherein the exposure factors were constant, the only variant being the diameters of the cones. When the image contrast of the details surrounding the distal end of the third metacarpal in each radiograph is compared, no visible change in density or contrast is discernible. Since the amount of secondary radiation generated is small, the tissues absorbed most of it and little emerged to produce noticeable fog in the image. If the quantity of secondary radiation had been greater, each change in the cone diameter would have shown a reduction in image density. The fact that only a negligible amount of secondary radiation is emitted may be further illustrated by a series of posteroanterior radiographs of the hand, Figure 66, made at different object-film distances but with constant exposure factors. A cone was not employed. Note that the over-all densities of these radiographs are similar. If fog had been present, the densities would have diminished as the OFD (object-film distance) increased in accordance with the inverse square law. Note that images became magnified as the OFD was increased. Secondary radiation in varying degree is always present when any exposure is made and *cones should always be used to keep the fog level to a minimum, irrespective of the projection employed.*

Thick Body Parts

Secondary radiation emitted by the tissues in radiography of a heavy body part may be considerably greater than the remnant radiation reaching the film. For example, a radiograph of the pelvis made with an unrestricted x-ray beam and without screens, cone or grid, Figure 67, A, shows an image in which almost total obliteration of detail occurred due to the presence of a heavy veil of fog. For a second radiograph, Figure 67, B, intensifying screens were employed. The shorter exposure permitted by the screens reduced the amount of remnant and secondary radiation reaching the film but the residual fog density still degrades the scale of contrast. A cone, screens, and a Potter-Bucky diaphragm were then employed to further reduce the amount of secondary radiation and make possible better visualization of details, Figure 67, C, with adequate contrast.

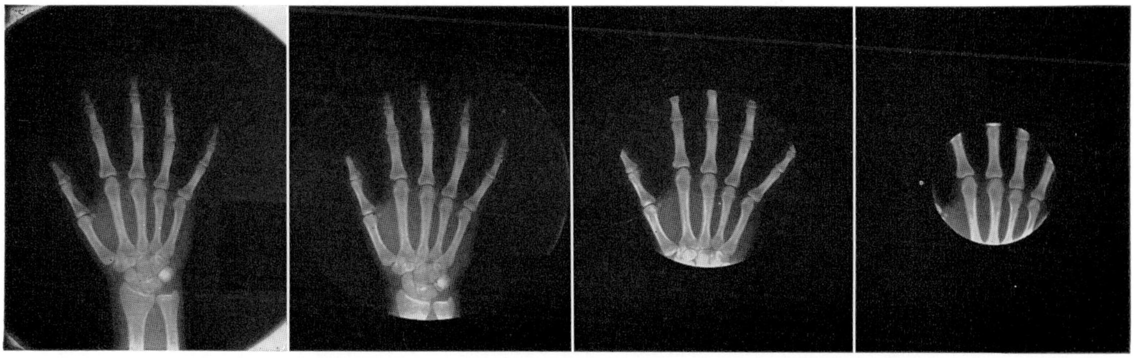

Figure 65. Series of radiographs of the hand to demonstrate the influence of the size of cones on these images. The three images to the right are masked to facilitate image comparison.

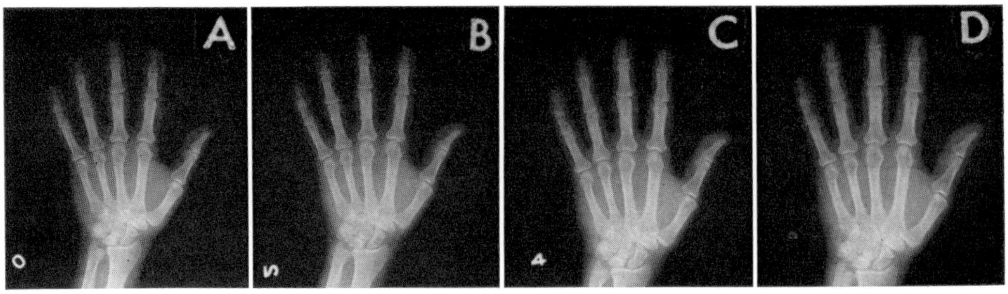

Figure 66. Series of radiographs of the hand made without cones wherein the OFD has been varied. Note comparable densities in all images. Radiograph (A) no OFD; (B) 2 inches; (C) 6 inches; (D) 8 inches.

INFLUENCE OF KILOVOLTAGE ON FOG

The characteristics of the primary radiation can be changed by kilovoltage with the result that control over secondary radiation fog becomes effective and image quality is favorably influenced. Secondary radiation as an image-forming entity is quite important as the kilovoltage is increased, for the quantity of fog produced may reach a point where it exceeds many times the density produced by the remnant radiation. Under these circumstances, the density produced by the remnant radiation is almost completely submerged in the radiograph because of the predominance of fog. In fact, it becomes virtually impossible on occasion to determine the quantity of silver deposited by the action of the remnant radiation when the radiograph is overexposed. The more that detail is veiled by fog, the less it is affected by any change in kilovoltage, focal spot, or exposure time. Kilovoltage, of course, is not entirely responsible for the production of secondary radiation because the thickness and hydration of the irradiated tissues also have a direct influence—the thicker the tissues, the greater the amount of secondary radiation produced.

Demonstration No. 1. The influence of kilovoltage on the emission of secondary radiation and its fogging effect on the image is illustrated by a series of radiographs shown in Figure 69. The arrangement of a paraffin block to be used as the emitter of secondary radiation, a dried femur, and a slab of ⅛-inch lead and a lead sheet barrier in relation to an x-ray film is shown in Figure 68. The dried femur and lead produce such small quantities of secondary radiation within the 40 to 100 KvP range that neither can be considered an effective emitter. A sheet of ⅛-inch lead when wrapped around the emitter on three sides served as a barrier to the sec-

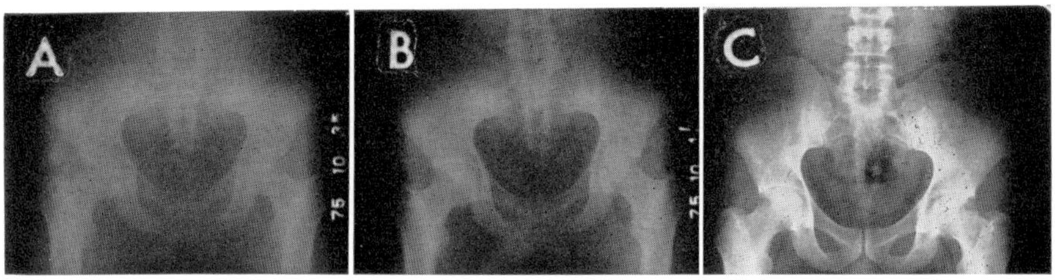

Figure 67. Radiographs of the pelvis demonstrating effect of direct exposure (A), screen exposure (B), and screen-grid exposure (C).

ondary radiation that would reach the film on one side upon exposure. Radiographs A-D, Figure 69, were made with the bone and lead sheet placed on *top* of the emitter, thereby creating a 2.5-inch OFD for these objects. The lead strip and the femur were permitted to project over the lead barrier on both sides of the paraffin block as shown in Figure 68. The radiographs were made with a constant MaS factor of 40. The KvP employed for radiograph A was 40; B, 60; C, 80; and D, 100.

Comment. The radiographs A-D demonstrate that as kilovoltage increases and all other factors are constant: (1) radiographic density and fog increase in the presence of an emitter of secondary radiation and (2) full penetration is effected at 60 KvP. In each radiograph, there are six image areas (1, 2, 3, 4, 5, 6) that should be observed as the kilovoltage is increased and all other factors remain constant.

1. Area 1 is that portion of the image of the femur that is covered by the image of the paraffin emitter. It is affected by the increasing density effect of the kilovoltage and the secondary radiation emitted by the paraffin block. As the kilovoltage increases, the density of this area increases. The ease with which details are visualized becomes less and less until they are virtually obliterated by the excessive density in the 100-KvP film (D).
2. Area 2 is that portion of the image of the femur that projects over and *beyond* the lead barrier. Since the lead barrier prevents secondary radiation from affecting this portion of the image of the femur, the increased density is solely due to the increased kilovoltage. This area becomes overexposed in the 100-KvP radiograph (D).
3. Area 3 is that portion of the image of the lead strip covered by the image of the paraffin emitter. Because the object-film-distance of the lead strip is 2.5 inches, secondary radiation undercuts the lead and this image area becomes fogged. In the 40-KvP radiograph (A) there is only small evidence of fog in this area. As the kilovoltage increases, as shown in radiographs B, C, and D, the fog becomes greater. Because the lead strip is not penetrated by the primary radiation, the silver deposit in this image area may be entirely attributed to exposure by secondary radiation.
4. Area 4 is that portion of the image of the lead strip that extends beyond the lead barrier. No appreciable change in density of this image area occurs because no primary radiation penetrates the lead and no secondary radiation reaches this image area from the emitter.
5. Area 5 is that portion of the image of the femur projecting over the *unshielded* side of the emitter. Details in the femur image nearest the emitter are fogged, but the fogging effect diminishes as the bone becomes more remote to the emitter. Here, the inverse square law has an opportunity to become effective in reducing the fogging action of the secondary radiation.
6. Area 6 is that portion of the image representing the lead strip that projects

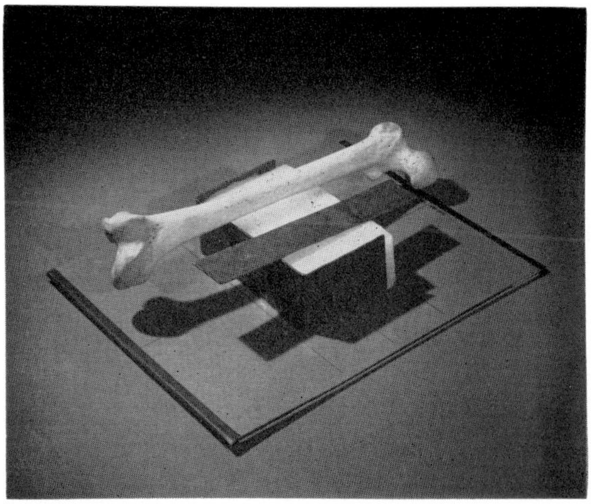

Figure 68. Photograph of a paraffin emitter and associated objects used to illustrate the influence of kilovoltage on the generation of secondary radiation.

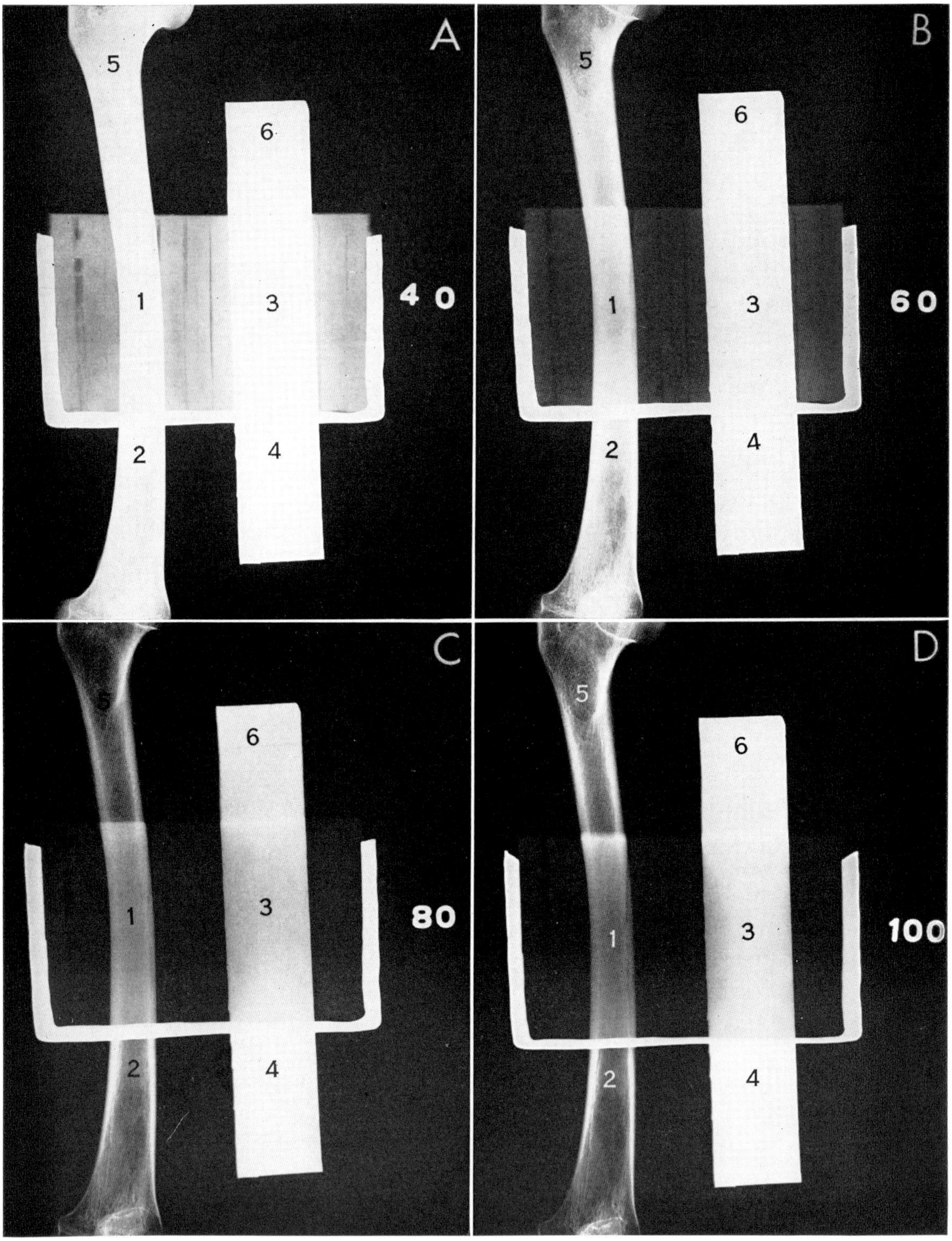

Figure 69. Radiographs of paraffin emitter and associated objects. Kilovoltages employed are inscribed on each radiograph.

over and beyond the unshielded side of the emitter. The diminution in fogging by undercutting as the strip becomes more remote is shown. The condition is similar to that shown for area 5 except for the fact that details are not present in the image area.

Demonstration No. 2. In medical radiography it can also be shown in a series of posteroanterior chest radiographs, Figure 70, that as the kilovoltage advances, radiographic density and fog increase. This series of radiographs was exposed with a range of 60 to 100 KvP in increments of 10 KvP. The MaS and all other factors were constant. The emitter of secondary radiation in this case is a human thorax.

Comment. In the radiograph made with 60 KvP, the kilovoltage is relatively low, and no perceptible fog is shown in the image. Most of the silver image was produced by remnant radiation. In the 80-KvP radiograph, the over-all density has increased and the fog-density begins to be observed. The combined densities rapidly gain in silver concentration as the kilovoltage advances further. From the appearance of the radiograph made with 90 and 100 KvP, it can readily be seen that fog-density is abundant.

Demonstration No. 3. The paraffin block, femur, and lead strip combination described in Demonstration No. 1 may again be employed, using the arrangement shown in Figure 68. The resulting radiographs A-D, Figure 71, were made within the 40-100 KvP range in increments of 20 KvP. To equalize the density effect of KvP, the MaS was reduced for each radiograph. The MaS values were estimated by employing the multiplying factors contained in Table IV.

Comment. In Areas 1 and 3 of radiographs A to D, Figure 71, the same relative degree of fogging was obtained. Area 1 is affected by the density influence of kilovoltage as well as fog. Note the relative freedom from fog in Area 2 in the radiographs made with all kilovoltages

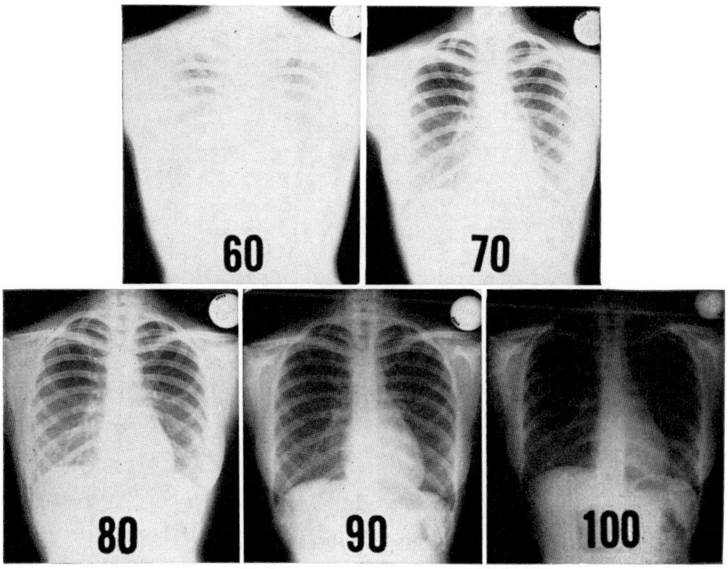

Figure 70. Series of chest radiographs demonstrating that as the kilovoltage advances and all other factors are constant, radiographic density increases. Numbers on respective images indicate the applied kilovoltages.

when compared with Area 1. Details are also more readily visible in Area 2 than in Area 1 in the radiographs made at any kilovoltage because the contrast has not been degraded by fog-densities. The images of Area 2 exhibit a longer scale of contrast as the kilovoltage is advanced. At 40 KvP the contrast is short-scale; as the kilovoltage increases, the contrast scale becomes longer, but not to a point where difficulty in discerning details occurs. This condition indicates that when secondary radiation is controlled, any desired contrast scale can be obtained with kilovoltage, provided penetration is obtained. Kilovoltage, therefore, becomes the factor of radiographic contrast. Note that the quantity of fog in Area 3 is approximately the same at all kilovoltages. Area 4 is relatively fog-free in all radiographs.

Proof that the origin of the secondary radiation in the paraffin block can be demonstrated by a radiograph, Figure 71, E, made with 100 KvP in which fog is eliminated by the use of a Potter-Bucky grid (8-1). Compare this radiograph with the fogged areas in the 100 KvP radiograph (D).

Demonstration No. 4. In medical radiography conditions comparable to those cited in Demonstration No. 3 can be illustrated by posteroanterior radiographs of the chest made with a range of 40 to 100 KvP in increments of 5, Figure 48. The over-all density effect of KvP was compensated by employing MaS values derived by the use of Table III. Note that all radiographs are relatively free from fog and the images are rendered more nearly in accordance with their true tissue-absorption patterns which makes possible the selection of any scale of contrast to suit diagnostic needs. However, the 90- and 100-KvP radiographs K and M show a small amount of fog. Therefore, radiograph (I) seems to possess the most desirable diagnostic properties. The optimum KvP value for posteroanterior chest radiography would then seem to be 80 KvP.

Summary. Demonstrations 1 through 4 illustrate that (1) as kilovoltage is increased, secondary radiation fog as well as over-all density increases; (2) when secondary radiation is controlled efficiently, kilovoltage becomes the factor of radiographic contrast; and (3) when MaS compensates for the over-all density effect of the increased kilovoltage, the low level of image fog is relatively the same, irrespective of the kilovoltage.

PART TWO

CONTROL OF FOG

There are several ways in which secondary radiation fog on the image may be controlled. Methods of control are based on the proper use of exposure factors employing grids and/or cones.

KILOVOLTAGE

The prevalent custom of reducing the kilovoltage as a means of reducing fog ignores the fact that image details distant from the film may still be fogged. Given correct exposure, structures nearer the film are usually rendered with satisfactory contrast and sharpness because only a small amount of secondary radiation can undercut them. The lower kilovoltages help to increase the contrast of the nearer structures, but may not render the more distant structures equally well. The use of low kilovoltage as a means of controlling the amount of fog often results in the use of insufficient penetrating radiation. The employment of higher kilovoltages, on the other hand, is accompanied by appre-

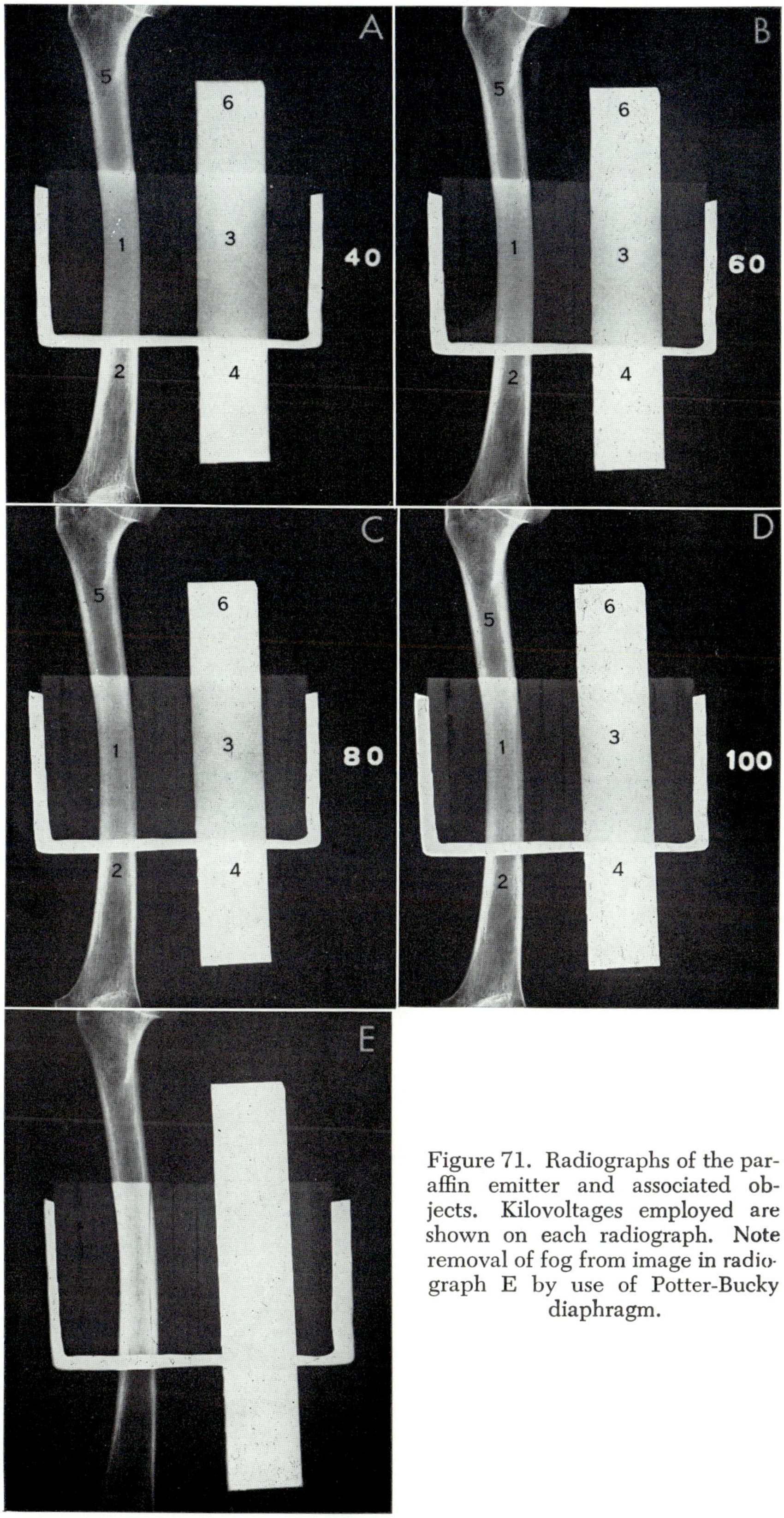

Figure 71. Radiographs of the paraffin emitter and associated objects. Kilovoltages employed are shown on each radiograph. Note removal of fog from image in radiograph E by use of Potter-Bucky diaphragm.

Clarence W. Donnelly, R.T. (ARRT)

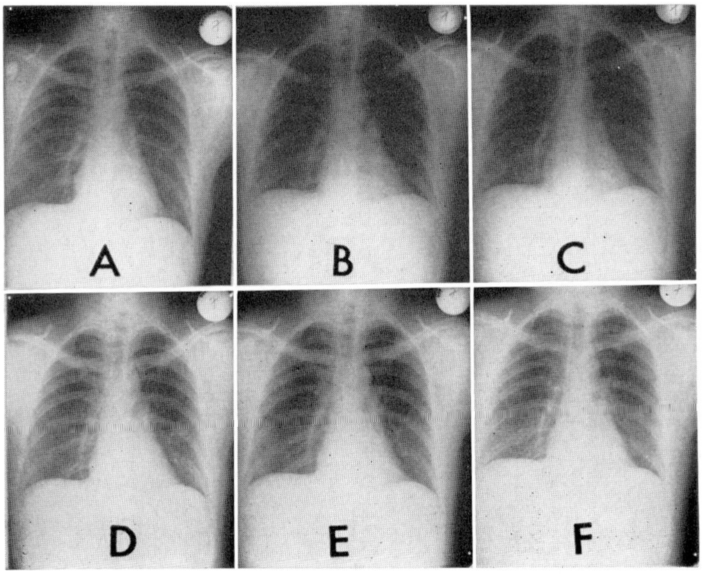

Figure 72. Series of posteroanterior screen radiographs of chest showing examples of the effects of overexposure and correct exposure when using the higher kilovoltages.

ciable amounts of secondary radiation depending upon the volume and density of the tissue irradiated but penetration of the tissue is accomplished. In practice for a given projection, therefore, there is an upper limit to the kilovoltage that can be used and still secure good quality radiographs; and, there is also a lower limit that insures penetration of the structures when a practical exposure time is employed. Between these limits is an optimum kilovoltage that assures penetration of the structures with a minimal though acceptable fog level for all thicknesses of a given part.

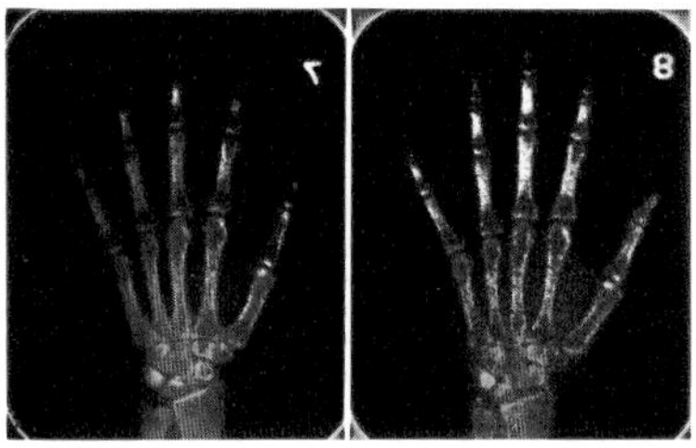

Figure 73. Two posteroanterior radiographs of the hand wherein the image on the left is overexposed and the one to the right is correctly exposed.

These image characteristics, naturally, are premised upon efficient control of secondary radiation and a standardized processing procedure.

Higher Kilovoltages

Radiographs made with the higher kilovoltages often exhibit excessive densities (overexposure). The heavy densities in the image make it difficult to determine how much is due to overexposure by remnant radiation or simply by uncontrolled secondary radiation. Rather than disturb the basic contrast provided by the kilovoltage employed, the easiest initial procedure to employ in making correction for the high density is to halve the MaS. Thus, the overall density will be reduced to a value that may be correct or enable one to judge the nature of any further adjustment.

Example. The posteroanterior screen radiographs of the chest, Figure 72, A-F, demonstrate a typical example of the condition described above. Radiograph A was made with 80 KvP and 6.66 MaS; B, with 90 KvP and 5 MaS; C, with 100 KvP and

3.33 MaS; all at a 72-inch FFD. Note the heavy densities shown in each radiograph. When all the MaS values were halved and the KvP remained constant, as shown in radiographs D to F, the overexposures were corrected and the over-all density was reduced to an acceptable level. By using this rule of thumb method of halving the MaS when overexposure occurs or of doubling the MaS when underexposure exists, an image more in keeping with the desired result can be obtained. If the quality is not exactly satisfactory, an additional small MaS adjustment should usually provide the desired result. The KvP need not necessarily be reduced.

Lower Kilovoltages

When lower kilovoltages are employed and the part is penetrated, overexposure does not become complicated by the presence of an excessive quantity of secondary radiation fog. It is therefore only necessary to halve the MaS value to obtain an approximately correct density, or to make a further small adjustment of the MaS in order to secure the best quality. The KvP should not be changed.

Example. Two posteroanterior radiographs of the hand, Figure 73, were made employing 50 KvP and 100 MaS, Left, and 50 MaS Right. The first radiograph, Left, is definitely overexposed. The appearance of the image is such that the technician can readily recognize that the fog level is so low or non-existent that the increased density must be due to an excess of MaS. By halving the MaS, a satisfactory image, Right, is obtained and exhibits satisfactory radiographic quality.

CONES

Cones or aperture diaphragms, Figure 74, are radiographic accessories *important* in the control of secondary radiation fog. By limiting the size of the x-ray beam by a cone or aperture diaphragm, less tissue is irradiated and less secondary radiation is emitted to fog the film. The closer the cone is to the part and film, the smaller the area irradiated, with resulting reduction in the quanity of secondary radiation reaching the film. Because the use of cones invariably improves radiographic contrast and detail is more easily visualized, a cone should always be used for *all* projections whether or not a grid is employed.

Ratio of Secondary to Remnant Radiation

The ratio of secondary to remnant radiation emitted by thin parts, such as the hand, is small, irrespective of the size of the field, because of the small amount of tissue irradiated. This does not hold true for the thicker and more dense structures. This fact is demonstrated in a series of diagrams and posteroanterior screen radiographs of the frontal sinuses, Figure 75, wherein radiographs A to C were exposed with the same factors.

Radiograph A was made *without* a cone; note the high image density that is largely attributable to fog generated by the neck and shoulder girdle. Radiograph B was

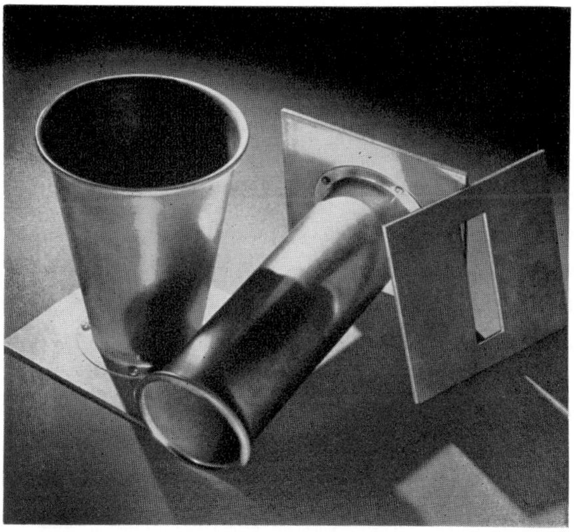

Figure 74. Cones and aperture diaphragm.

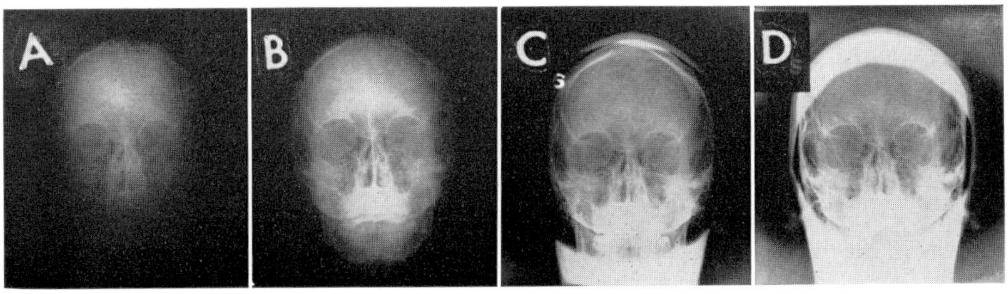

Figure 75. Series of posteroanterior screen-radiographs of the frontal sinuses which were all exposed with the same factors. Radiograph A, made without a cone; B, made with a large cone; C, made with a smaller cone; D, made with a cone of correct size. Note that, as the cone size was reduced, the quantity of secondary radiation became less, hence the fog density became virtually nil when the correct cone-grid combination was employed as shown in Figure 78.

made with a large cone and the fog is somewhat reduced because the tissue in the shoulder girdle has not been irradiated. Radiographs C and D were made with smaller cones and the fog density has been greatly reduced. The visibility of details is greatly improved because the small cone limits the *amount* of tissue irradiated; hence the quantity of secondary radiation is greatly diminished. When the entire area of any film is to be exposed, always use a cone that, at least, restricts the diameter of the beam to equal the diagonal of the film area.

Coning Small Areas

When the anatomical area is small, a cone should be used that is small enough to include just the area of interest. Coning a small area without changing the exposure factors will usually produce an image in which fog has been lessened, although the over-all density may not always be at a satisfactory level, Figure 75, D. An increase in MaS is then necessary. If a cone and grid is to be employed, the exposure time should be increased approximately 3 times to compensate the absorption factor of the grid, Figure 78D. When a small area of a given heavy part is to be more closely examined using a small cone, a reduction of kilovoltage provides shorter-scale contrast so that accentuation of the tissue components will occur. This is obviously predicated upon the use of a kilovoltage less than the initial value, yet of a wave length that will suitably *penetrate* the part. An increase in MaS must accompany the reduction in kilovoltage in order to provide adequate density. In many instances this procedure is not as successful as the use of higher kilovoltage and a grid.

Calculation of Cone Coverage

When a new or an unfamiliar cone is employed, it is advantageous to know the size of the field that it will cover at different focus-film distances as measured along the course of the central ray (CR), Figure 76. This information can be calculated from a few measurements. Measure the distance from the focal spot of the tube to the lower rim of the cone (CY). Next, measure the diameter of the *lower* opening of the cone (AB). From the following formula, the diameter of field coverage (DE) can be computed.

Formula: $$DE = \frac{CR \times AB}{CY}$$

Example. A new cone has been obtained. The diameter of the cone at its lower rim is 5 inches (AB) and the distance from the focal spot to the rim of the cone is 15 inches (CY). What is the diameter of the field coverage (DE) at an FFD of 36 inches (CR)? When the foregoing values are substituted in the formula, the answer may be derived as follows:

Solution: $DE = \frac{36 \times 5}{15}$

$DE = 12$ inches. Answer.

Aperture Diaphragm

When a suitable cone is not available for a given projection, an aperture diaphragm should be used. Such diaphragms may be cut in a piece of 1/16-inch or 1/8-inch lead sheet. Let us assume a situation in which the diameter of an aperture is to be determined that will cover a given area of film at a given distance employing the following formula:

Formula: $AB = \frac{DE \times CY}{CR}$

Example. It is desired to cut an aperture that will limit the x-ray beam to a 10-inch coverage (DE) of an 8 x 10-inch film at an FFD of 40 inches (CR). The distance from the focal spot to the lead diaphragm is 4 inches (CY). What is the diameter of the aperture (AB) to be cut in the lead diaphragm?

Solution: $AB = \frac{10 \times 4}{40}$

$AB = 1$ inch. Answer.

GRIDS

Until Gustav Bucky invented the grid diaphragm in 1913, the only control for secondary radiation was by means of various shaped single- and double-aperture diaphragms and cones inserted at the portal of the x-ray tube. Although these devices proved of value large amounts of secondary radiation could not adequately be controlled in radiography of thick body tissues.

The grid as Dr. Bucky invented it was not too practical at first because it was used in a stationary position and the grid pattern on the radiograph was quite coarse. However, it was for Dr. Hollis Potter of Chicago to solve the problem and place the Bucky grid on a practical basis. This was accomplished by *moving* the grid during the exposure and making the grid strips thinner. By moving the grid during the exposure, all grid lines were blurred out of the image. The first commercial moving grid was announced in 1920 and became known as the Potter-Bucky diaphragm. The necessity for elimination of secondary radiation fog from the radiograph with its resultant improvement in contrast and enhancement in diagnostic quality was ably presented by R. B. Wilsey

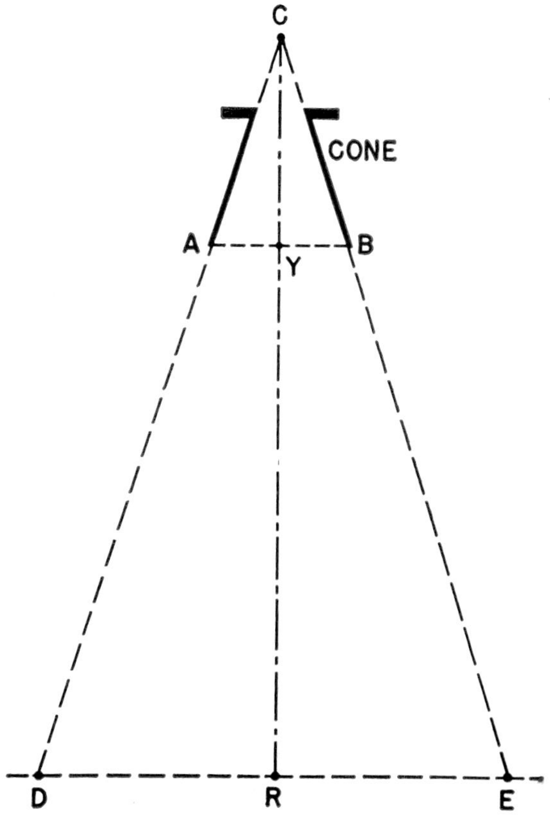

Figure 76. Diagram illustrating method for calculating cone coverage.

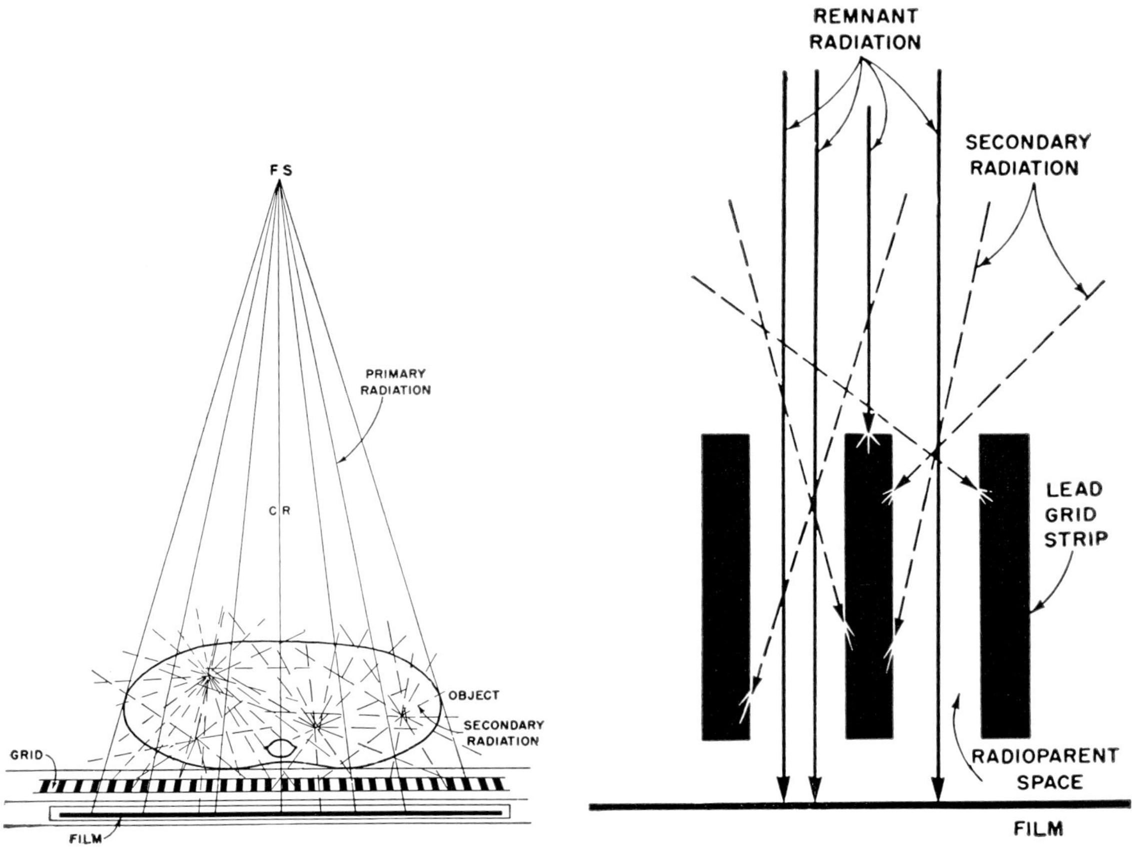

Figure 77. Diagrams illustrating: (*Left*) function of Potter-Bucky diaphragm in absorbing secondary radiation before it reaches the film; (*Right*) details of grid construction.

of the Kodak Research Laboratories. His data presented in 1920 provided the scientific basis for the application of the Potter-Bucky diaphragm to practical radiography. Wilsey's data and Potter's diaphragm marked one of the few milestones in the search for better radiographic results.

The use of the Potter-Bucky diaphragm required that the exposure be increased four times or more. However, since its first inclusion in radiographic technic, the use of faster films and screens, higher kilovoltages and improvement in grid design has reduced this requirement to about two times.

The function of the Bucky grid is to absorb secondary radiation emitted by body tissues before it reaches the film. This required that the grid be placed *between* the patient and the film. The grid composed of alternate strips of lead is separated by a radiotransparent substance; the strips are approximately .005 inch thick. In use, the focused remnant radiation passes *between* the strips to reach the film, Figure 77. Since secondary radiation is unfocused and is emitted in all directions, it is largely absorbed when it strikes the lead strips.

Types of Grids

There are two types of grids: stationary and moving. The later is known as a Potter-Bucky diaphragm. When a modern stationary grid is used, an image of the grid strips appears on the radiograph as a number of evenly spaced fine lines. In grids containing 60-80 lines to the inch, the grid lines are barely perceptible at normal viewing distances. However, recent improvements in design have made possible grids containing 110 lines to the inch which are virtually invisible at similar viewing distances. They offer little or no problem from a diagnostic standpoint. Radiographs made with a moving grid, Figure 78, do not show images of the grid strips because they are blurred into the background because of grid movement. The moving grid is used extensively for routine radiography. The stationary grid is more frequently employed in those situations where it is difficult or impossible to use the moving grid.

Grid Ratio

The efficiency of the grid in absorbing secondary radiation is determined by the *grid ratio* which is the relation of the depth of the radiotransparent space between the lead strips, to its width. For example, an 8-1 grid ratio means that the spaces are tall and narrow and that the depth is 8 times the width. The 8-1 ratio grid has great efficiency because only secondary radiation that is traveling approximately parallel to the primary radiation can reach the film; in most instances, this amount is relatively small. In general, a grid ratio of 16-1 is still more efficient, but it requires great accuracy in positioning the patient and x-ray tube to the grid and care in selecting the correct focus-film distance. With lower grid ratios, less fog is eliminated but greater latitude in positioning and focus-film distance is permissible.

The approximate percentages of secondary radiation absorbed by grids of various ratios are: 8-1, 90 percent; 6-1, 85 percent and 5-1, 75 percent.

Necessity for Increasing Exposure

When the grid is employed, it is necessary to increase the MaS over that employed when a grid is *not* used, because the density effect of the secondary radiation is lost and some absorption by the grid of the remnant radiation takes place. The amount of increase in MaS is dependent upon the grid ratio, and the approximate increase required is about 3-6 times the initial MaS value.

When secondary radiation is removed by the use of a grid, the density produced by the remnant radiation is often found to be insufficient to produce a satisfactory image. Radiography of the sinuses employing various size cones and a Potter-Bucky grid demonstrates a progressive reduction of fog as shown in Figure 78. To bring the density level of D to a satisfactory point, it would be necessary to increase the intensity of remnant radiation by additional MaS. Use of the grid to

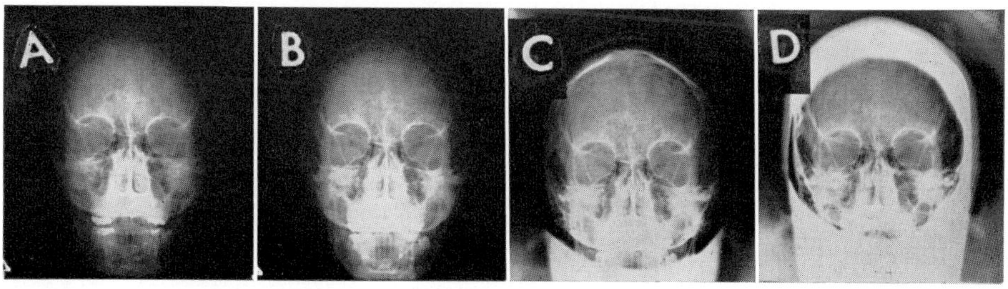

Figure 78. Screen-grid radiographs of the sinuses using an 8-1 grid ratio Potter-Bucky diaphragm and exposed with the same factors. A, employing no cone; B, large cone; C, 8-inch cone; D, 6-inch cone. Factors: 70 KvP; 60 MaS; 36-inch FFD; average speed screens. Note that, as the anatomic area is restricted by the cone, the over-all density of the image decreases.

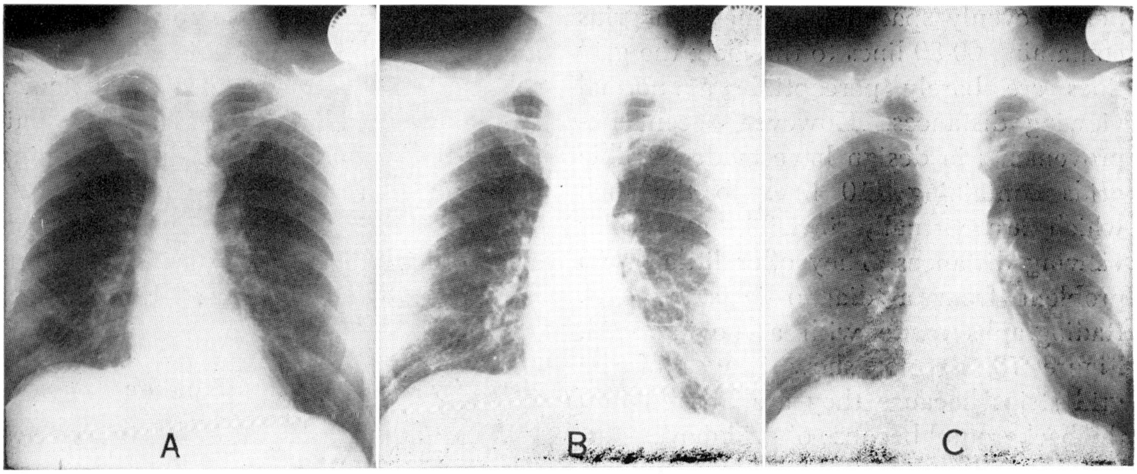

Figure 79. Three posteroanterior screen radiographs of a 28-cm. chest illustrating the manner in which contrast is affected when using a stationary grid with 80 and 100 KvP.

remove fog from images of thick dense parts is ideal as long as the radiation penetrates the part.

Grid and Contrast

Image contrast is reduced by secondary radiation fog and is increased in proportion to the amount of secondary radiation eliminated. Employment of a grid normally shortens the contrast scale so that images are produced exhibiting higher contrast; the greater the grid ratio, the higher is the contrast obtained. For example, a radiograph made with a 4-1 grid ratio has lower contrast than one made with an 8-1 ratio because of the lower efficiency of the 4-1 grid in fog cleanup. This can be offset by using higher kilovoltages with higher ratio grids to obtain images with a longer and more satisfactory contrast scale. In general, detail sharpness is lessened because of the space occupied by

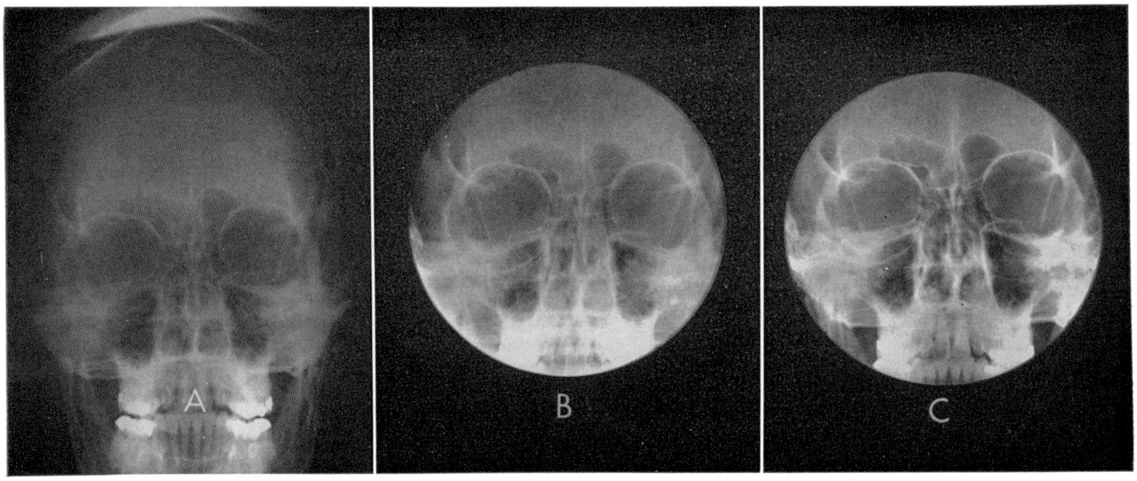

Figure 80. Posteroanterior screen radiographs of the frontal sinuses. Factors: 70 KvP, 36-inch FFD, average-speed screens. Radiographs A and B, 15 MaS; radiograph C, 62.5 MaS, stationary grid.

the grid thereby increasing the OFD but this situation is offset by the increase in contrast.

Examples of Fog Control Employing Grids

Example 1. The manner in which contrast is affected when using a stationary grid is illustrated, Figure 79, A-C. A posteroanterior radiograph (A) of a 28-cm. chest was made employing the following factors: 80 KvP; 4.125 MaS; 72-inch FFD; and average-speed screens. This radiograph exhibits definite evidence of secondary radiation fog. Another radiograph (B) was made using the same factors but with a stationary grid and an MaS of 13.3. Note that fog has disappeared and the contrast is relatively greater. Because of this greater contrast which might tend to obscure some details, it would be more practical to employ 100 KvP to lengthen the scale of contrast as is shown in radiograph (C). Here, better diagnostic quality exists because of the longer scale of image contrast obtained and also because a shorter exposure time was used (3.33 MaS).

Example 2. Posteroanterior screen radiographs of the frontal sinuses, Figure 80, A-C, were made. Radiograph A was made with a large cone—the high density is due to excessive secondary radiation fog. Radiograph B was made with a small cone of correct size—definite improvement in image quality is apparent. For radiograph C, a cone of correct size and a stationary grid was employed—the cone reduced the amount of tissue irradiated, thereby reducing the secondary radiation emitted and the grid absorbed most of the secondary radiation that might have reached the film. This teamwork resulted in good radiographic quality.

Example 3. Two posteroanterior screen radiographs of a muscular 25-cm. chest are shown in Figure 81. Radiograph A exhibits some evidence of fog even though a cone of correct size and 80 KvP were employed with 5 MaS. Effective reduction of the fog, radiograph B, was obtained by using a stationary-type grid, 100 KvP and 5 MaS for this radiograph. Similar results on a 22-cm. chest are shown in Figure 82. Radiograph A was made without a grid at 80 KvP; radiograph B, with a grid and 100 KvP.

Example 4. Two lateral screen radiographs of a 34-cm. chest are illustrated in Figure 83. Radiograph A was exposed with 90 KvP, 15 MaS, 72-inch FFD, and, as can be noted, the image is veiled with fog; radiograph B was made with a stationary grid at 100 KvP. To compensate for removal of the secondary radiation and some of the remnant radiation by the grid, it was necessary to increase the MaS to 40. This radiograph demonstrates good image quality.

OBJECT—FILM DISTANCE

The radiographic appearance of body parts is influenced with respect to secondary radiation fog by their distances from the film.

When Part is Close to Film

An area of the lung that possesses greater tissue density than that surrounding it, for example, will usually absorb the bulk of the secondary radiation emit-

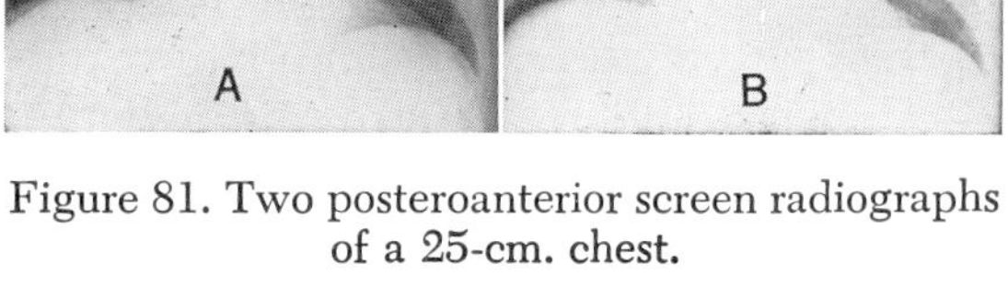

Figure 81. Two posteroanterior screen radiographs of a 25-cm. chest.

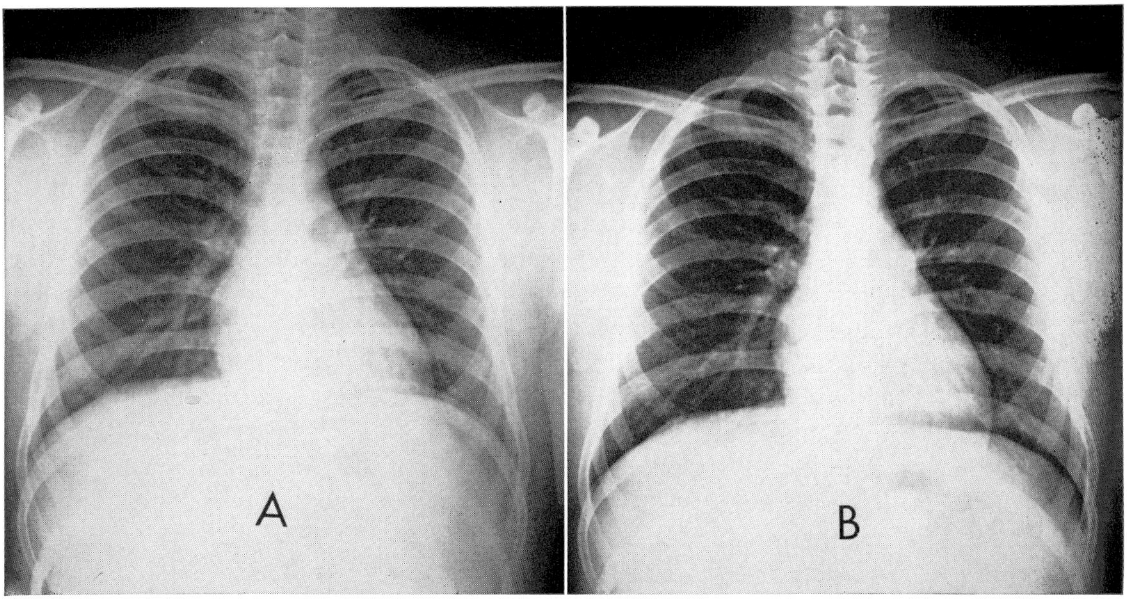

Figure 82. Two posteroanterior screen radiographs of a 22-cm. chest.

ted by surrounding tissues if it is located *near* the film; and its image will be relatively free from fog. A similar lesion farther away will be undercut by secondary radiation and will therefore present a different radiographic density also the detail contrast is reduced by a veil of fog. Slightly separated, though identical structures, may present different radiographic appearances in the same image because of the difference in contrast caused by different object-film distances. The effect in degree would be present regardless of the kilovoltage employed.

When Part is Distant From Film

An important situation in which the amount of secondary radiation reaching the film is reduced occurs when the body part is distant from the film. The intensity of the secondary radiation emitted by the body part is diminished by the operation of the inverse square law under these circumstances, and fogging of the image is thereby lessened. When attempts are made to control secondary radiation fog by long object-film distances, it must be remembered that sharpness of definition is adversely influenced and considerable enlargement of the image takes place. Unsharpness, however, may be somewhat controlled by using a very small focal spot and a longer FFD. For routine radiography, however, the method is not to be recommended.

SUMMARY

Fog can be controlled by (1) limitation of the amount of tissue irradiated, (2) the use of correct exposures, and (3) the use of cones and/or grids. Kilovoltage can then be employed as the factor for influencing contrast. An unrestricted beam of x-rays always causes a larger amount of secondary radiation to be emitted by the tissues than a beam confined by a cone or diaphragm. As may be expected, any method of limiting the amount of secondary radiation produces radiographic images of better diagnostic quality. When a cone or grid is not used, kilovoltage then becomes the only remaining factor in the control of secondary radiation. With a knowledge of how secondary radiation fog affects the over-all density of the image and hence the quality of the radiograph, a balance of exposure factors and accessory apparatus can lead to the selection of an exposure procedure that will be best suited to each body part examined.

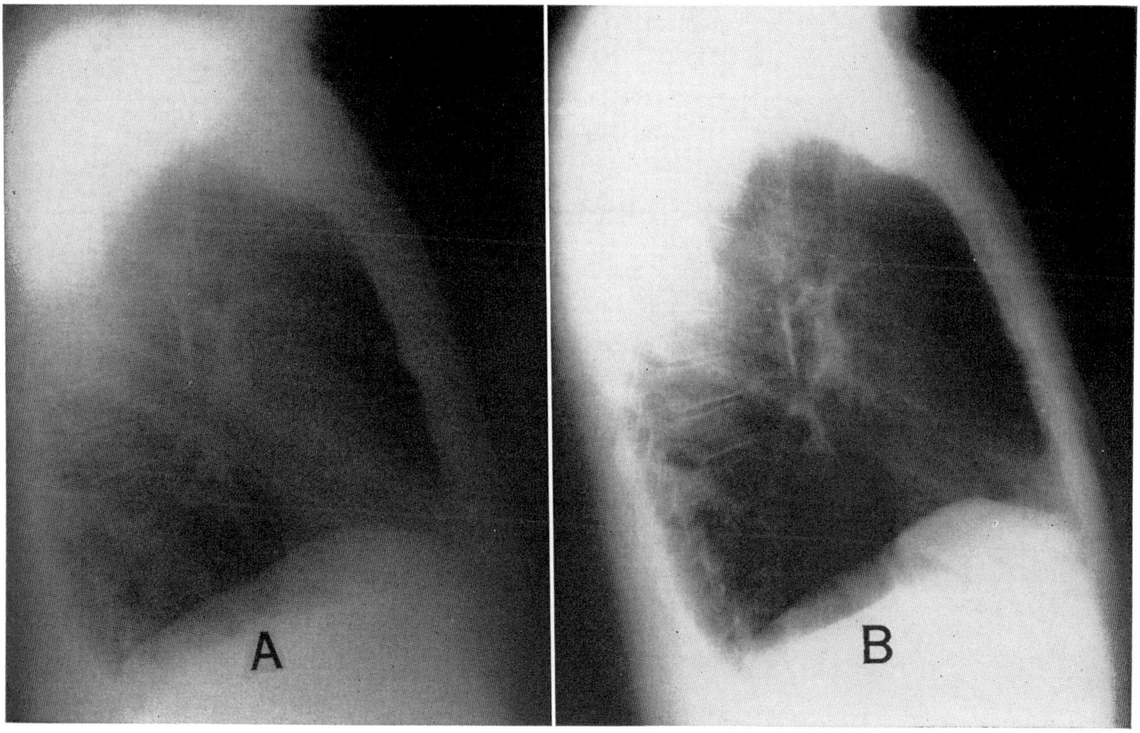

Figure 83. Two lateral screen radiographs of a 34-cm. chest.

Chapter 11

Function of Milliampere-Seconds

THE MILLIAMPERE-SECONDS factor, indicated by the symbol MaS, directly influences radiographic density when all other factors are constant. It is the product of the *milliamperage* (Ma) and the duration of the exposure time in *seconds* (S). Either factor of *Ma* or *S* may be changed at will to conform to required radiographic exposures as long as their product—*MaS*—remains the same. This fact holds true on all *direct* x-ray exposures. However, intensifying screen exposures may show some loss in radiographic density when they are exceedingly long because of failure of the *reciprocity law*. In practice, the *Ma* factor is seldom changed for a given projection and may usually be considered as a constant. The time of exposure, however, can be readily changed and should constitute the variable in the *MaS* factor. For ease in general compuation and expression, the *MaS* factor may be employed for a given projection rather than citing its components.

RULE-OF-THUMB FOR DENSITY CHANGES

It requires at least a 35 per cent increase in MaS to produce a significant increase in density. To produce a worthwhile increase or decrease in density, a rule-of-thumb can be employed to effect density changes in an orderly and easy manner. When the *KvP* and processing are constant, serious underexposures should be corrected by doubling the initial *MaS* value, to change density; in cases of serious overexposures, the MaS should be halved. If further alteration in density is necessary, a change of 50 per cent either way from the last MaS employed should produce the desired density, or one so close, that a slight adjustment of the MaS value will provide a satisfactory final density. In other words, changes in *MaS* to compensate over or underexposure are facilitated arithmetically by indicating the *original MaS* value as *X*. *Halving* the *MaS* would be indicated by ½X; *doubling* the *MaS* would be indicated by 2X. Greater refinement can be effected by smaller changes in *MaS* to produce a more satisfactory density once the *basic MaS* value is established. These changes would be indicated by ¾X or 1½X. (At times, these values would only be approximations due to timer, or *Ma* station limitations.)

RECIPROCITY LAW

An important concept advanced by Bunsen and Roscoe in 1875 states that the reaction of a photographic emulsion to light is equal to the product of the intensity of the light and the duration of exposure. This is known as the reciprocity law. The phenomenon occurs in radiography only when intensifying screens are used, because exposure of the film under these circumstances is chiefly caused by the fluorescent light emitted by the screens and very little by x-rays. Failure of this law may be observed when the radiographic density is greater upon short exposure with a large quantity of fluorescent light than that produced by a long exposure and a small amount of fluorescent light even though the total quantity of x-radiation exposing the film remains the same, i.e., MaS. Fortunately, it is not necessary to be concerned about this effect in routine work, for today it is seldom encountered because it has been largely compensated by the characteristics of the x-ray film emulsion. Therefore, the *MaS* value may be considered reliable for use as an exposure factor in general radiography. For example, approximately the same radiographic density will be obtained whether 50 *Ma* is used for 1/10 second or 10 *Ma* for 5/10 second—both conditions entail the use of 5 *MaS*.

TABLES OF MaS VALUES

Tables VI and VII make possible rapid determination of *MaS* values when the time of exposure and the milliamperage are known. Table VI lists the common fractional exposures and the number of impulses employed for short exposures. Table VII lists exposure times of longer duration. The *Ma* values in each table are identical. To use the tables, find the exposure to be employed in the left-hand vertical column; then, in the horizontal row at the bottom of the table, find the *Ma* value to be used. The required *MaS* value is found at the point where these two columns meet in the body of the table.

Example 1. An exposure of 1/30 second was employed in a given projection at 100 *Ma*. What is the *MaS* value?

Solution. Find 1/30 second in the left-hand vertical column of Table VI; then, locate 100 in the horizontal row at the bottom of the table. Follow the horizontal line at the 1/30 level to the right until it meets the vertical volumn headed by 100 *Ma*. The *MaS* value common to both columns is found at this point, and the answer is 3.33.

Example 2. An exposure of 2¾ seconds was given in a specific projection at 30 *Ma*. What *MaS* was employed?

Solution. Locate 2¾ seconds in the left-hand vertical column of Table VII; then, locate the value 30 in the horizontal row at the bottom of the table. Follow the horizontal line at the 2¾ level to the right until it meets the vertical column headed by 30 *Ma*. The *MaS* value common to both columns is found at this point, and the answer is 82.5.

DECIMAL EQUIVALENTS OF FRACTIONAL EXPOSURES

In computing MaS values, it is often convenient to use the decimal equivalent of the exposure time fraction. Table VIII lists decimal equivalents of commonly employed exposure fractions. It will be recalled that in any fraction, the number above the line is called the *numerator* and the number below the line, the *denominator*. For example, in the fraction 3/20, the number 3, above the line, is the numerator and the number 20, below the line, is the denominator. Table VIII is arranged so that the numerators of fractions are listed horizontally, at the top of the table; and

TABLE VI

MAS VALUES DERIVED BY MULTIPLYING SPECIFIC MA AND TIME VALUES FROM 1/60 TO 1/4 SECOND

Impulses	*Time (Seconds)*	*Milliampere Seconds*											
2	1/60	.16	.25	.33	.41	.5	.83	1.66	2.5	3.33	5.	6.66	8.33
3	1/40	.25	.37	.5	.62	.75	1.25	2.5	3.75	5.	7.5	10.	12.5
4	1/30	.33	.5	.66	.83	1.	1.66	3.33	5.	6.66	10.	13.33	16.66
5	1/24	.41	.62	.83	1.04	1.25	2.08	4.12	6.25	8.33	12.5	16.66	20.83
6	1/20	.5	.75	1.	1.25	1.5	2.5	5.	7.5	10.	15.	20.	25.
7		.58	.87	1.16	1.56	1.75	2.91	5.83	8.75	11.66	17.5	23.33	29.16
8	1/15	.66	1.	1.33	1.66	2.	3.33	6.66	10.	13.33	20.	26.66	33.33
9	3/40	.75	1.12	1.5	1.87	2.25	3.75	7.5	11.25	15.	22.5	30.	37.5
10	1/12	.83	1.25	1.66	2.08	2.5	4.16	8.33	12.5	16.66	25.	33.33	41.66
11		.91	1.37	1.83	2.27	2.75	4.58	9.16	13.75	18.33	27.5	36.66	45.83
12	1/10	1.	1.5	2.	2.5	3.	5.	10.	15.	20.	30.	40.	50.
13		1.08	1.62	2.16	2.77	3.25	5.41	10.83	16.25	21.66	32.5	43.33	54.16
14		1.16	1.75	2.33	2.91	3.5	5.83	11.66	17.5	23.33	35.	46.66	58.33
15		1.25	1.87	2.5	3.12	3.75	6.25	12.5	18.75	25.	37.5	50.	62.5
16	2/15	1.33	2.	2.66	3.33	4.	6.66	13.33	20.	26.66	40.	53.33	66.66
17		1.41	2.12	2.83	3.54	4.25	7.08	14.16	21.25	28.33	42.4	56.66	70.83
18	3/20	1.5	2.25	3.	3.75	4.5	7.5	15.	22.5	30.	45.	60.	75.
19		1.58	2.37	3.16	3.95	4.75	7.91	15.83	23.75	31.66	47.5	63.33	79.16
20		1.66	2.5	3.33	4.16	5.	8.33	16.66	25.	33.33	50.	66.66	83.33
21		1.75	2.62	3.5	4.37	5.25	8.75	17.5	26.25	35.	52.5	70.	87.5
22		1.83	2.75	3.66	4.58	5.5	9.16	18.33	27.5	36.66	55.	73.33	91.66
23		1.91	2.87	3.83	4.79	5.75	9.58	19.16	28.75	38.33	57.5	76.66	95.83
24	1/5	2.	3.	4.	5.	6.	10.	20.	30.	40.	60.	80.	100.
25		2.08	3.12	4.16	5.20	6.25	10.41	20.83	31.25	41.66	62.5	83.33	104.16
26		2.16	3.25	4.33	5.41	6.5	10.83	21.66	32.5	43.33	65.	86.66	108.33
27		2.25	3.37	4.5	5.62	6.75	11.25	22.5	33.75	45.	67.5	90.	112.5
28		2.33	3.5	4.66	5.83	7.	11.66	23.33	35.	46.66	70.	93.33	116.66
29		2.41	3.62	4.83	6.04	7.25	12.08	24.16	36.25	48.33	72.5	96.66	120.83
30	1/4	2.5	3.75	5.	6.25	7.5	12.5	25.	37.5	50.	75.	100.	125.
Milliamperes		**10**	**15**	**20**	**25**	**30**	**50**	**100**	**150**	**200**	**300**	**400**	**500**

Milliampere Seconds

the denominators are listed vertically, in the columns to the left and the right. The body of the table contains the decimal equivalents of various combinations of numerators and denominators.

Example. To determine the decimal equivalent of the fraction 3/10, find the numerator 3 in the horizontal row at the top of the table. Then, find the denominator 10 in the left-hand *vertical* column; now, follow the horizontal row of decimals on line 10 until it meets the vertical column containing the numerator 3. At the intersection of these columns, the decimal equivalent of the fraction 3/10 is indicated as 0.3. The Ma may be multipled by this decimal to obtain the MaS value.

TABLE VII

MAS VALUES DERIVED BY MULTIPLYING SPECIFIC MA AND TIME VALUES FROM 1/10 TO 4 SECONDS

Time (Seconds)	*Milliampere Seconds*								
1/10	1.	1.5	2.	2.5	3.	5.	10.	15.	20.
2/10	2.	3.	4.	5.	6.	10.	20.	30.	40.
1/4	2.5	3.75	5.	6.25	7.5	12.5	25.	37.5	50.
3/10	3.	4.5	6.	7.5	9.	15.	30.	45.	60.
4/10	4.	6.	8.	10.	12.	20.	40.	60.	80.
5/10	5.	7.5	10.	12.5	15.	25.	50.	75.	100.
6/10	6.	9.	12.	15.	18.	30.	60.	90	120.
7/10	7.	10.5	14.	17.5	21.	35.	70.	150.	140.
3/4	7.5	11.25	15.	18.75	22.25	37.5	75.	112.5	150.
8/10	8.	12.	16.	20.	24.	40.	80.	120.	160.
9/10	9.	13.5	18.	22.5	27.	45.	90.	135.	180.
1	10.	15.	20.	25.	30.	50.	100.	150.	200.
1¼	12.5	18.75	25.	31.25	37.5	62.5	125.	187.5	250.
1½	15.	22.5	30.	37.5	45.	75.	150.	225.	300.
1¾	17.5	26.25	35.	43.75	52.5	87.5	175.	262.5	350.
2	20.	30.	40.	50.	60.	100.	200.	300.	400.
2¼	22.5	33.75	45.	56.25	67.5	112.5	225.	337.5	450.
2½	25.	37.5	50.	62.5	75.	125.	250.	375.	500.
2¾	27.5	41.25	55.	68.75	82.5	137.5	275.	412.5	550.
3	30.	45.	60.	75.	90.	150.	300.	450.	600.
3¼	32.5	48.75	65.	81.25	97.5	162.5	325.	487.5	650.
3½	35.	52.5	70.	87.5	105.	175.	350.	525.	700.
3¾	37.5	56.25	75.	93.75	112.5	187.5	375.	562.5	750.
4	40.	60.	80.	100.	120.	200.	400.	600.	800.
Milliamperes	**10**	**15**	**20**	**25**	**30**	**50**	**100**	**150**	**200**

Milliampere Seconds

TABLE VIII

TABLE FOR DETERMINATION OF DECIMAL EQUIVALENTS OF FRACTIONAL EXPOSURE TIMES

Denominators	*Decimal Equivalents of Fractional Exposures* — *Numerators*												Denominators
	1	**2**	**3**	**4**	**5**	**6**	**7**	**8**	**9**	**10**	**11**	**12**	
2	0.5	1.	1.5	2.	2.5	3.	3.5	4.	4.5	5.	5.5	6.	**2**
3	.333	.666	1.	1.33	1.666	2.	2.33	2.66	3.	3.33	3.66	4.	**3**
4	.25	.5	.75	1.	1.25	1.5	1.75	2.	2.25	2.5	2.75	3.	**4**
5	.2	.4	.6	.8	1.	1.2	1.4	1.6	1.8	2.	2.2	2.4	**5**
6	.167	.333	.5	.667	.835	1.	1.167	1.333	1.5	1.667	1.833	2	**6**
7	.143	.286	.429	.572	.715	.858	1.	1.143	1.286	1.429	1.57	1.7	**7**
8	.125	.25	.375	.5	.625	.75	.875	1.	1.125	1.25	1.375	1.5	**8**
9	.111	.222	.333	.444	.555	.666	.777	.888	1.	1.111	1.222	1.333	**9**
10	.1	.2	.3	.4	.5	.6	.7	.8	.9	1.	1.1	1.2	**10**
11	.09	.18	.27	.363	.455	.545	.636	.727	.818	.090	1.	1.09	**11**
12	.083	.167	.25	.333	.415	.5	.583	.667	.75	.833	.917	1.	**12**
15	.067	.134	.2	.267	.333	.4	.467	.533	.6	.667	.733	.8	**15**
20	.05	.1	.15	.2	.25	.3	.35	.4	.45	.5	.55	.6	**20**
24	.042	.083	.125	.167	.208	.25	.292	.333	.375	.416	.458	.5	**24**
30	.033	.067	.1	.133	.167	.2	.233	.267	.3	.333	.367	.4	**30**
40	.025	.05	.075	.1	.125	.15	.175	.2	.225	.25	.275	.3	**40**
60	.017	.033	.05	.067	.083	.1	.117	.133	.15	.167	.183	.2	**60**
120	.008	.017	.025	.033	.042	.05	.058	.067	.075	.083	.092	.1	**120**

ARITHMETICAL RELATIONS

RELATION NO. 5—Ma AND TIME

Rule. The Ma required for a given radiographic density is inversely proportional to the time of exposure when remaining factors are constant. This rule may be expressed by the following formula:

$$\frac{\text{(A) Original Ma}}{\text{(B) New Ma}} = \frac{\text{(F) New Time}}{\text{(E) Original Time}}$$

Example 1. Assume that 10 Ma (A) and an exposure time (E) of 0.5 sec. was employed in making a radiograph. It is desired to decrease the exposure time (F) to 0.05 sec. What milliamperage (B) would be needed to assure comparable radiographic densities?

Solution. A, E, and F are known and B is unknown.

$$B = \frac{AE}{F}$$

$$B = \frac{10 \text{ x } 0.5}{0.05} = \frac{5}{.05} = 100 \text{ Ma. Answer.}$$

Example 2. Assume that 10 Ma (A) and

an exposure time (E) of 0.5 sec. was employed in making a radiograph. It is desired to increase the milliamperage (B) to 100. What time of exposure (F) would be needed to obtain comparable radiographic densities?

Solution. A, E, B are known and F is unknown.

$$F = \frac{AE}{B}$$

$$F = \frac{10 \times .5}{100} = \frac{5}{100} = 1/20 \text{ sec. Answer.}$$

EXPOSURE EXPERIMENTS

EXPERIMENT NO. 12—TIME-DENSITY RELATION

Purpose. To demonstrate the relation between exposure time and radiographic density when all other factors are constant.

Theory. When all other factors but time are constant, the quantity of x-rays emitted by the x-ray tube increases in direct proportion to the time of exposure. Thus, the quantity of x-rays applied in 1 second is approximately doubled when the exposure is 2 seconds, etc. Since radiographic density is influenced by this action, increasing the time increases the density and vice versa.

Procedure No. 1

1. Two series, Figure 84, A and B, of three exposures each are to be made *without* an object on the film using the following materials and exposure factors for each series.

Materials	Film:	Screen-type, 8 x 10-inch	
	Exposure holder:	8 x 10-inch	
	Cone:	To cover exposure area	
Constant Factors	Development:	5 min. 68° F.	
	KvP:	35 (Series A)	
	KvP:	50 (Series B)	
	Ma:	10	
	FFD:	36 inches	
	Filter:	1 mm. aluminum	
Variable Factors	Exposure No.	Time	MaS
	1	2/10 sec.	2
	2	4/10 sec.	4
	3	8/10 sec.	8

2. Place the mask on the exposure holder containing a film. Place a small lead sheet over the No. 2 and No. 3 exposure holes and

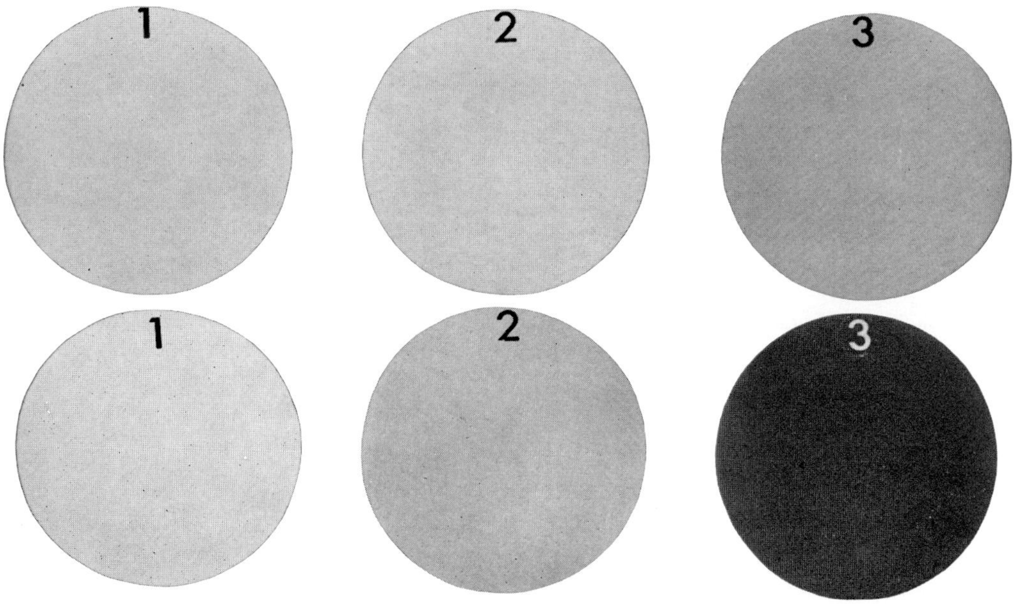

Figure 84. Demonstration of the effect of exposure time on radiographic density when no absorber is employed. (*Top*) Series A, using 35 KvP. (*Bottom*) Series B, using 50 KvP.

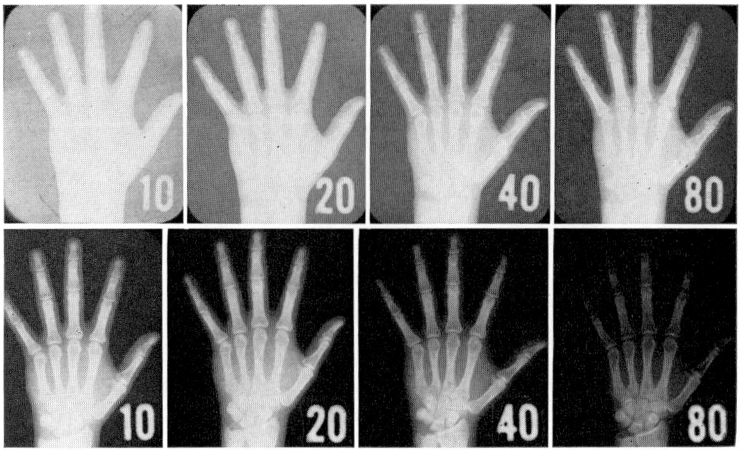

Figure 85. Demonstration of the effect of exposure time on radiographic density when an absorber (hand) is used. (*Top*) Series A, using 35 KvP. (*Bottom*) Series B, using 50 KvP. The respective MaS values are inscribed on each radiograph.

expose No. 1. Then, cover No. 1 and No. 3 and expose No. 2, etc., until all exposures in both series are completed. Process films.

Comment

a. Series A. The radiographs, (Figure 84 *Top*) made using 35 KvP and with all factors constant except the exposure time, demonstrate that as the exposure time increases, radiographic density increases. Although each exposure is progressively doubled for exposures 1, 2, and 3, the respective densities are not markedly changed when 35 KvP is employed.

b. Series B. The radiographs, (Figure 84 *Bottom*) using 50 KvP and with all factors constant except the exposure time, demonstrate that as the respective times used for exposures 2 and 3 are doubled, a more decided change in density occurs. The shorter wave lengths of x-radiation emitted with 50 KvP produce a greater exposure effect.

c. This experiment demonstrates that when low kilovoltages are employed, larger MaS increments must be used for gaining density than when a higher KvP is employed. In both series A and B, however, it may be observed that radiographic density increases with the exposure time when all other factors are constant.

Procedure No. 2

1. The time-density relation can also be demonstrated by making two series of posteroanterior radiographs of the hand, (Figure 85) employing 35 and 50 KvP. Series A is made with 35 KvP and all other factors are constant except exposure time, which is increased in accordance with the rule of thumb for changing density. Series B is made with 50 KvP and all other factors are constant except exposure time, which is increased in the same manner as in Series A. The following materials and factors are employed.

Materials	Film:	Screen-type, 8 x 10-inch	
	Exposure holder:	8 x 10-inch	
	Cone:	To cover exposure area	
Constant Factors	Development:	5 min. 68° F.	
	KvP:	35 (Series A)	
	KvP:	50 (Series B)	
	Ma:	100	
	FFD:	36 inches	
	Filter:	1 mm. aluminum	
Variable Factors	Exposure No.	Time	MaS
	1	1/10 sec.	10
	2	2/10 sec.	20
	3	4/10 sec.	40
	4	8/10 sec.	80

Comment. With all factors constant except time, the two series of radiographs demonstrate the progressive increase in density that results when the exposure time is increased as was related in Procedure No. 1.

a. Series A. In this series (Figure 85 *Top*) the densities do not materially increase as the time of exposure increases, because the intensity of the radiation is relatively small, i.e., 35 KvP. Prolonged and impractical exposures would, therefore, be necessary to produce radiographic densities that might be satisfactory.

b. Series B. When an optimum kilovoltage of 50 is employed for this projection of the hand, (Figure 85, *Bottom*) a greater intensity of radiation is provided and any desired density may be obtained simply by increasing or decreasing the time of exposure. The most satisfactory density is provided by 40 MaS.

EXPERIMENT NO. 13—Ma-DENSITY RELATION

Purpose. To demonstrate the relation between milliamperage and radiographic density when all other factors are constant.

Theory. When all other factors except milliamperage are constant, radiographic density increases in direct proportion to the milliamperage and vice versa.

Procedure No. 1

1. A series of three exposures made ***without*** an object on the film using the following materials and exposure factors demonstrates the influence of Ma on radiographic density when all other factors are constant.

Materials	Film:	Screen-type, 8 x 10-inch	
	Exposure holder:	8 x 10-inch	
	Cone:	To cover exposure area	
Constant	Development:	5 min. 68° F.	
Factors	KvP:	50	
	Time:	2/10 sec.	
	FFD:	36 inches	
	Filter:	1 mm. aluminum	
Variable	Exposure No.	Ma	MaS
Factors	1	10	2
	2	50	10
	3	100	20

2. Place the mask on the exposure holder containing a film. Place a small lead sheet over the No. 2 and No. 3 exposure holes and expose No. 1. Then, cover No. 1 and No. 3 and expose No. 2, etc., until all exposures are completed. Process film.

Comment. These radiographs, (Figure 86 *Top*) demonstrate that, as the Ma increases

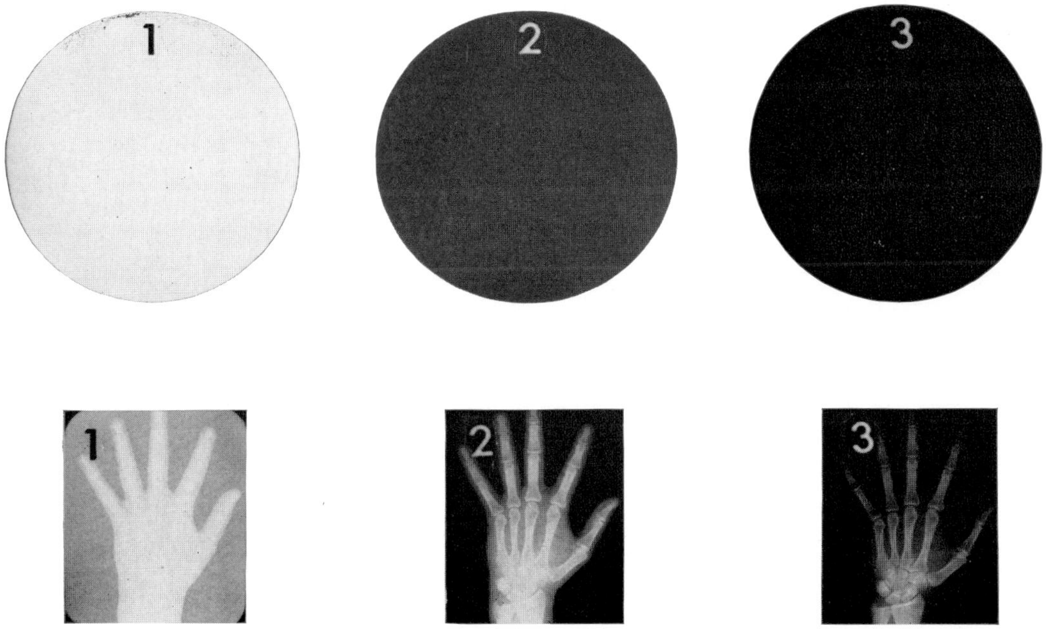

Figure 86. Demonstration of influence of Ma on radiographic density. (*Top*) Without absorber. (*Bottom*) with absorber (hand). The respective exposures are indicated by numerals on the images.

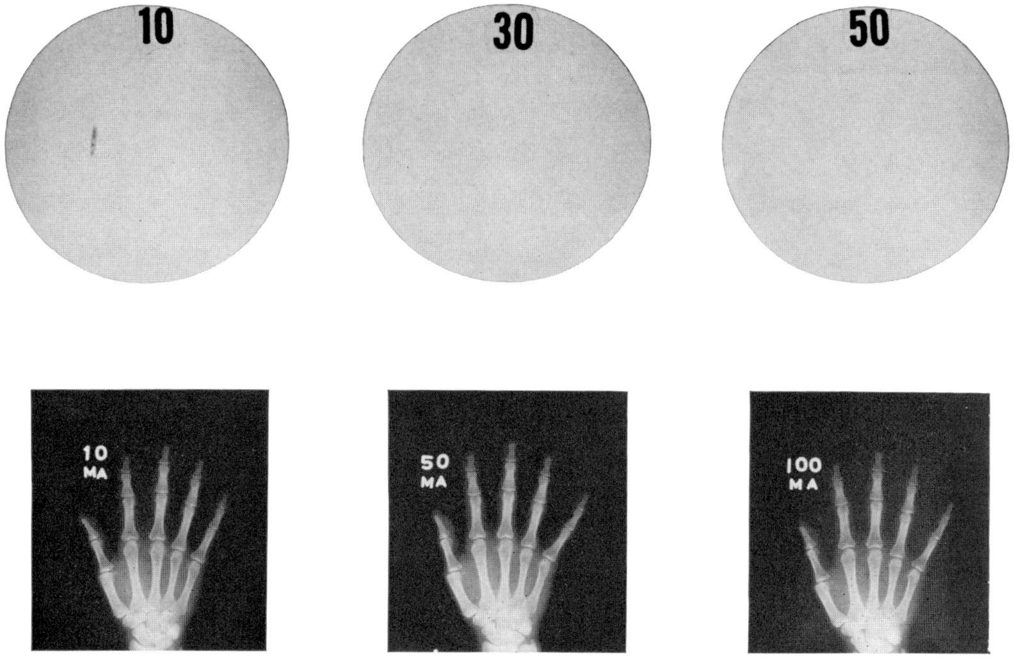

Figure 87. Demonstration of the influence of Ma and time on radiographic density when all other factors are constant. (*Top*) Without absorber; (*bottom*) with absorber (hand). Ma values are inscribed on each image.

with all other factors constant, the radiographic density increases. Compare the densities of exposures No. 1 and No. 3. Note that the greater density exhibited by No. 3 was the result of the application of 10 times the Ma of No. 1.

Procedure No. 2

1. The Ma-density relation may be demonstrated by three posteroanterior radiographs of the hand wherein the following materials and exposure factors were employed. All factors but Ma are constant:

Materials	Film:	Screen-type, 8 x 10-inch	
	Exposure holder:	8 x 10-inch	
	Cone:	To cover exposure area	
Constant	Development:	5 min. 68° F.	
Factors	KvP:	50	
	Time:	½ sec.	
	FFD:	36 inches	
	Filter:	1 mm. aluminum	
Variable	Exposure No.	Ma	MaS
Factors	1	10	5
	2	50	25
	3	100	50

Comment. The radiographs of the hand, (Figure 86 *Bottom*) demonstrate that as the milliamperage increases, the radiographic density increases. The radiographic effect is similar to the influence of time on density. Compare exposures No. 1 and No. 3 and note that the latter has greater density because ten times the milliamperage of No. 1 was employed.

EXPERIMENT NO. 14—Ma-TIME DENSITY RELATION

Purpose. To demonstrate the interrelation of milliamperage and exposure time with respect to radiographic density when all other factors are constant.

Theory. The milliamperage required for a given radiographic density is inversely proportional to the exposure time when all other factors are constant.

Procedure No. 1

1. A series of three exposures made *without* an object on the exposure holder, using

the following materials and exposure factors, demonstrates the interrelationship of Ma and time when all other factors are constant.

Materials	Film:	Screen-type, 8 x 10-inch	
	Exposure holder:	8 x 10-inch	
	Cone:	To cover exposure area	
Constant	Development:	5 min. 68° F.	
Factors	KvP:	50	
	FFD:	36 inches	
	Filter:	1 mm. aluminum	
	MaS:	4	
Variable	Exposure No.	Ma	Time
Factors	1	10	4/10 sec.
	2	30	2/15 sec.
	3	50	1/12 sec. (approx.)

2. Place the mask on the exposure holder containing a film. Place a small lead sheet over the No. 2 and No. 3 exposure holes and expose No. 1. Then, cover No. 1 and No. 3 and expose No. 2, etc., until all exposures are completed. Process film.

Comment. This experiment (Figure 87 *Top*) demonstrates (1) that as the Ma is changed, radiographic densities are equalized when the exposure time is adjusted in accordance with the increase or decrease in Ma and, (2) that as the exposure time is changed, densities are equalized when the Ma is adjusted.

Procedure No. 2

1. The MaS-density relation is demonstrated by three posteroanterior radiographs of the hand, the following materials and exposure factors being employed.

Materials	Film:	Screen-type, 8 x 10-inch	
	Exposure holder:	8 x 10-inch	
	Cone:	To cover exposure area	
Constant	Development:	5 min. 68° F.	
Factors	KvP:	50	
	FFD:	36 inches	
	Filter:	1 mm. aluminum	
	MaS:	50	
Variable	Exposure No.	Ma	Time
Factors	1	10	5 sec.
	2	50	1 sec.
	3	100	1/2 sec.

Comment. The radiographs (Figure 87 *Bottom*) demonstrate that as the milliamperage is increased and all other factors but time are constant, the latter may be reduced to equalize radiographic densities. Since milliamperage and time directly influence density, in actual practice the Ma is usually established as a constant and the exposure time as a variable. The greater ease with which small changes in time can be made with modern timers suggests this procedure. Modern apparatus is usually calibrated with present Ma stations, and it is difficult to convert to manual control operation and accurately select all milliampere readings from the meters.

SUMMARY

The influence of Ma and time of exposure in relation to radiographic density is summarized as follows:

MILLIAMPERAGE-DENSITY RELATION

When all exposure factors but milliamperage are constant, radiographic density increases as the Ma increases and vice versa.

TIME-DENSITY RELATION

When all other factors but time of exposure remain constant, radiographic density increases as the time is increased and vice versa.

Ma-TIME RELATION

When Ma is changed, time must be changed to maintain the same density.

MaS-DENSITY RELATION

The MaS factor is the product of Ma and time (in seconds) and should be employed as the factor of density control.

Chapter 12

Additional Density Factors

I. Influence of "Heel Effect"

MANY TECHNICIANS have occasionally been puzzled by radiographic density differences which could not always be attributed to the incorrect use of exposure factors. For example, an anteroposterior radiograph of a thoracic spine would show overexposure in the upper thoracic area and underexposure in the lower thoracic area, Figure 90. This regional lack of density balance is often caused by improper alignment of the long axis of the x-ray tube to the body part so that the "heel" effect of the anode was manifested in its worst form. This inherent characteristic of all x-ray tubes—the "heel" effect—may be employed to advantage in a limited manner to balance radiographic densities in the image.

WHAT "HEEL" EFFECT IS

The "heel" effect is a variation in x-ray intensity output along the longitudinal tube axis (depending upon the angle of x-ray emission from the focal spot). The intensity diminishes fairly rapidly from the central ray toward the *anode* side of the x-ray beam; on the *cathode* side of the beam, the intensity increases over that of the central ray and then slightly diminishes.

Using average or short focus-film distances (25 to 30 inches) and large film areas, its effect is most advantageous, particularly where decided differences in tissue densities require the balancing of radiographic densities to avoid over- and underexposures within the same image. The "heel" effect is more apparent when using rotating anode tubes because the angle of the anode face is more acute than it is in stationary anode tubes, Figure 31.

DISTRIBUTION OF X-RAY INTENSITY OVER FILM AREA

The approximate percentage of x-ray intensity emitted by a tube at various angles of emission may be determined directly from photographic measurements of the radiographic blackening of an x-ray film. For radiographic purposes, this procedure is adequate and gives an indication of the approximate percentage of intensity variation to be expected when the x-ray beam falls on specific areas of different sizes of

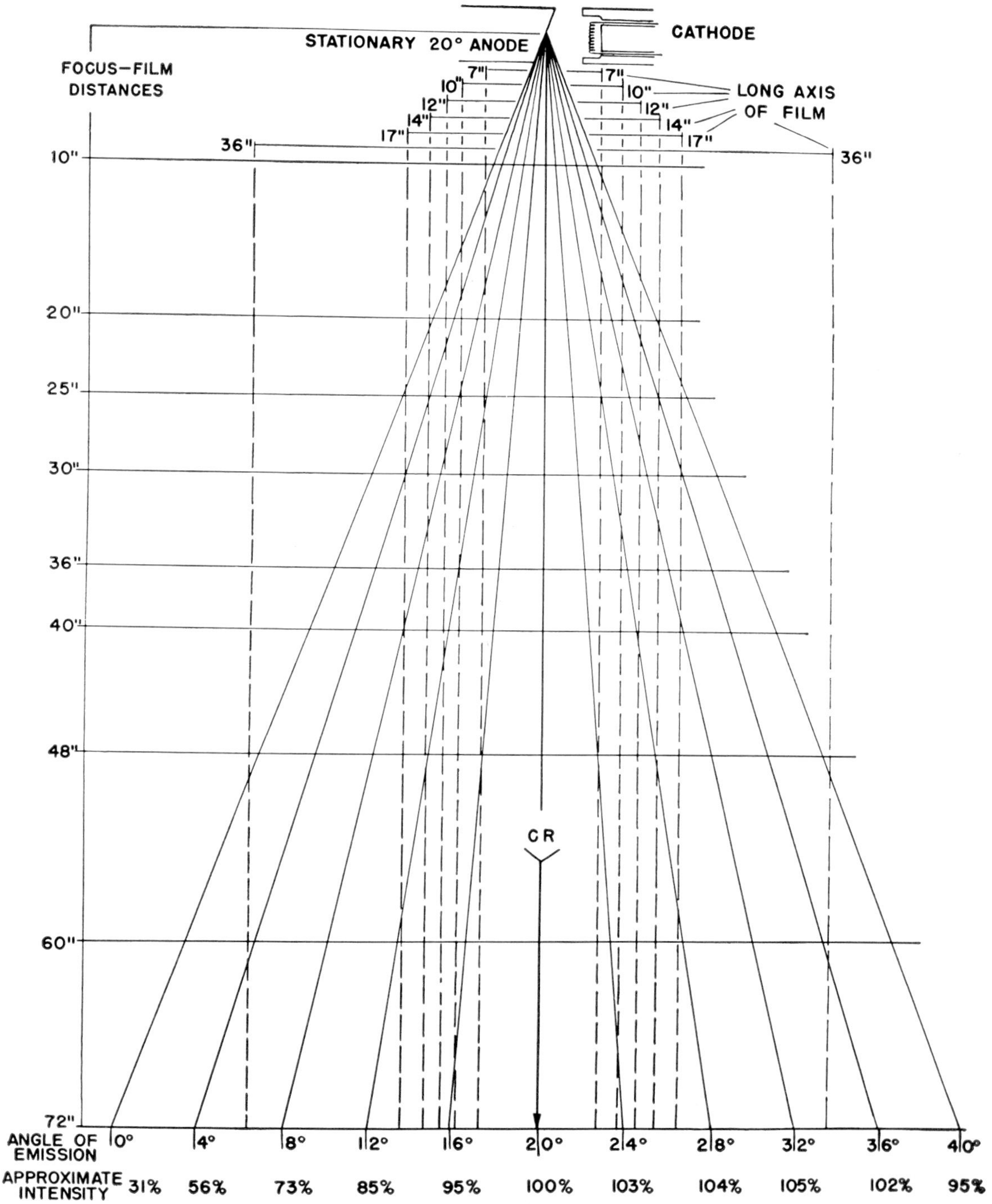

Figure 88. Graphic illustration of the mean values of radiographic density measurements over the x-ray beam at different focus-film distances obtained from many intensities emitted by various x-ray tubes.

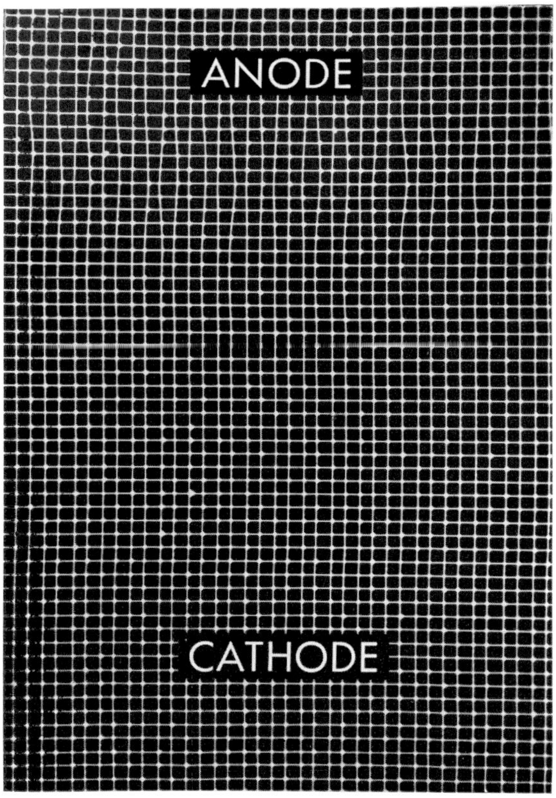

Figure 89. Radiographic illustration of the differences in intensity manifested by differences in radiographic density when heel effect is utilized.

x-ray films at various focus-film distances.

The mean values of radiographic density measurements obtained from many intensities emitted by various x-ray tubes are graphically shown in Figure 88. This diagram shows radii emanating from the target face, drawn at 4° intervals from 0° to 40° and intercepting horizontal lines representing various focus-film distances. At the termination of the radii at the bottom of the chart, the mean intensity values in percentages are indicated. For convenience, the intensity at the central ray (CR) is assumed to be 100 per cent. To the left, or anode side of the central ray, the intensities diminish in value, while those to the right or cathode side, increase moderately and then decrease slightly.

A radiographic illustration of the differences in intensity is shown in Figure 89. A wire mesh was placed on a 14 x 17-inch film. The long axis of the tube was aligned on the center film axis, and the anode portion of the beam was directed toward the top edge of the film. An exposure at a focus-film distance of 20 inches caused the upper portion of the image of the mesh to have less density than the bottom portion where the cathode portion of the beam exposed the film.

INTENSITY-FILM AREA RELATION

Consulting Figure 88, the vertical dotted lines beginning just below the diagram of the cathode and terminating at the 72-inch focus-film distance line, indicate various film lengths. Focus-film distances are shown as solid horizontal lines. The respective intensity values created by the radiation emitted at various angles of x-ray emission at various focus-film distances is shown at the bottom. For example, on the 48-inch focus-film distance line the outermost pair of vertical lines representing the 36-inch length of film passes outside the limits of the x-ray beam. In order to make use of the entire range of intensities on this length of film, it would be necessary to employ a focus-film distance of 49 inches. All intensity radii would intercept at this distance; consequently, if an exposure were made, the entire range of intensities would be expected to become evident, let us say, on a radiograph of an entire spine. Since the minimal intensity in the anode portion of the beam, approximately 31 per cent, is emitted in advance to the angle indicated as 0°, it is obvious that the portion of the spine having the least tissue density (the neck) should be exposed by this portion of the beam, and the heavier portion (the lumbar vertebrae) should be exposed by the cathode portion of the beam.

When radiographs on large film are made at relatively short focus-film distances, the percentage distribution of x-ray intensity delivered to a particular size of film at a known focus-film distance should be known. This knowledge will aid in correct alignment of the tube and part to the film at the most favorable focus-film distance. Radiographic densities cannot be balanced if only the intensity of the central ray is considered.

Example 1. An example of the "heel" effect is demonstrated by a radiograph, Figure 90, *Left,* of the thoracic vertebrae in which the cathode portion of the beam was directed cephalically. Note the high density in the upper thoracic region and the insufficient density in the lower thoracic vertebrae. By correctly applying the "heel" effect, a radiograph, Figure 90, *Right,* was obtained in which all the densities were properly balanced in the image because the anode portion of the beam was directed cephalically. Note that the densities are less in the upper thoracic region and greater in the lower thoracic area.

Example 2. To demonstrate the influence of the focus-film distance on the "heel" effect, a series of anteroposterior radiographs of the humerus, Figure 91, A-D, were made. Radiograph A was made with an FFD of 20 inches and the anode portion of the x-ray beam was directed cephalically. Note the underexposure of the upper portion of the humerus and the overexposure of the distal end. The intensity of the radiation passing to the heavier end of the humerus was insufficient and that portion of the beam passing to the thinner distal end overexposed the area. Radiograph B was made with the same exposure factors after the tube axis was rotated 180°. It may be seen that all densities have been approximately equalized. Radiograph C was made with a 40-inch FFD and the anode portion of the beam was directed cephalically.

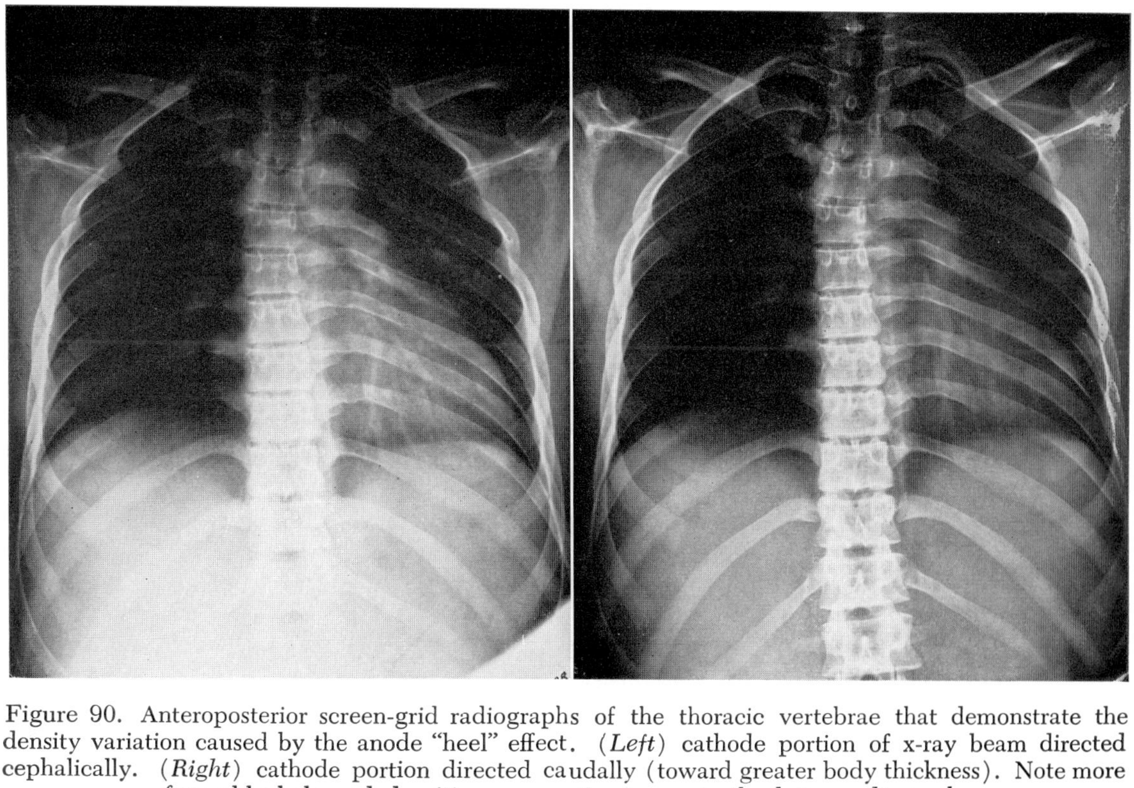

Figure 90. Anteroposterior screen-grid radiographs of the thoracic vertebrae that demonstrate the density variation caused by the anode "heel" effect. (*Left*) cathode portion of x-ray beam directed cephalically. (*Right*) cathode portion directed caudally (toward greater body thickness). Note more favorably balanced densities over entire image in the latter radiograph.

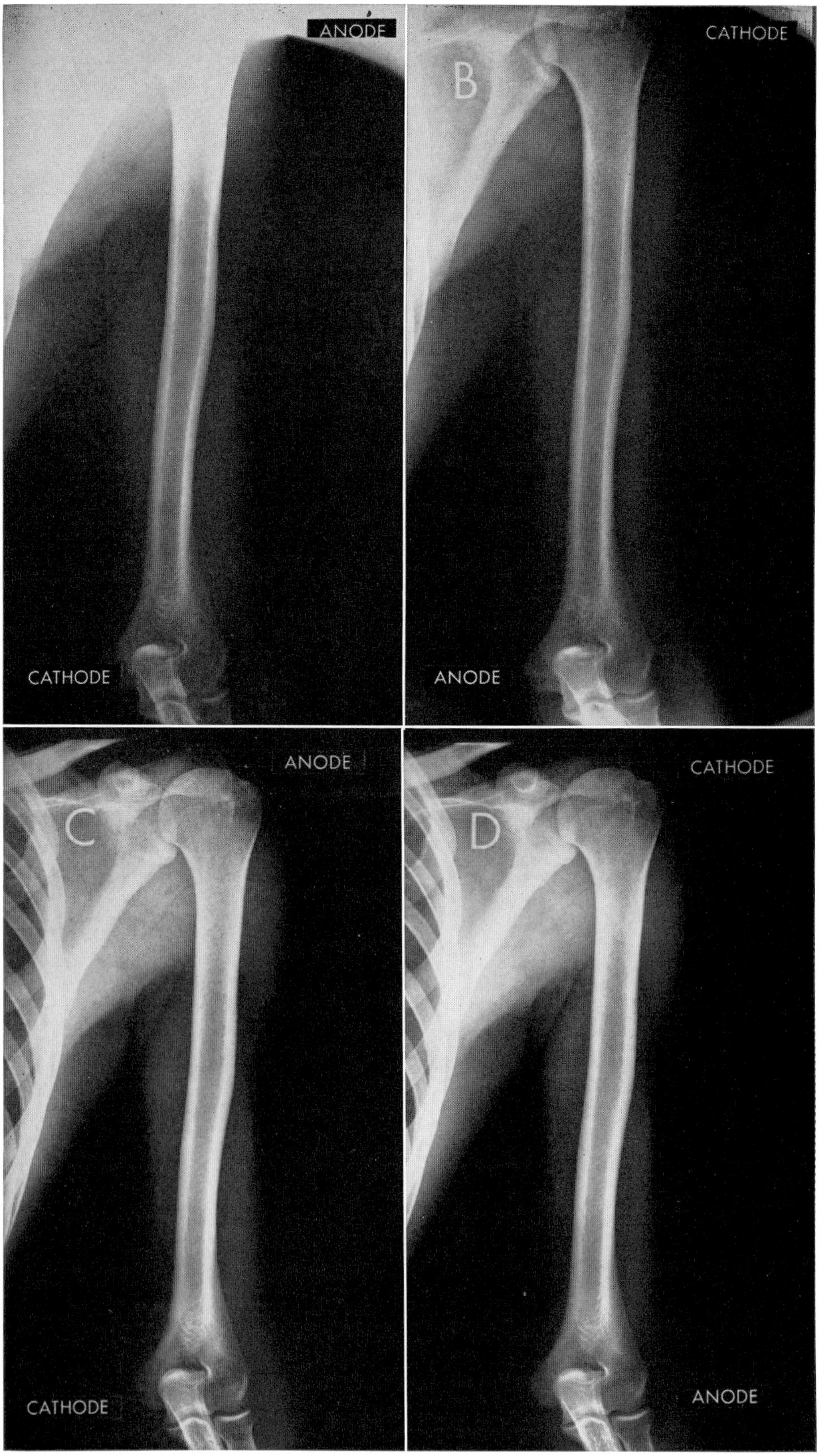

Figure 91. Series of radiographs of the humerus that demonstrate the "heel" effect with change in focus-film distance.

Note that, because the center portion of the beam only was employed, there was little variation in intensity and all areas have a fairly uniform density. Yet, radiograph D, also made with a 40-inch FFD after the tube axis was rotated 180° shows no improvement over the densities depicted in radiograph C. This example demonstrates that as the focus-film distance increases, the "heel" effect diminishes.

Example 3. An anteroposterior radiograph of an abnormal pelvis, Figure 92, A, was made with the long axis of the tube coincidental with the short axis of a 14 x 17-inch film at a 30-inch FFD. This example demonstrates an underexposure of the left side of the image produced by the anode portion of the beam. When the exposure was increased to provide perhaps a satisfactory image of the underexposed area, Figure 92, B, the contralateral side became overexposed. The underexposed left side was caused by the greater tissue density of normal structures, whereas the abnormal side possessed less tissue density because of disuse and was therefore overexposed by the cathode portion of the beam. The proper course would have been to direct the anode portion of the beam toward the abnormal side.

Rule. When body parts of unequal thickness or tissue density are to be recorded the following rule should be observed.

Align the long axis of the x-ray tube with the long center axis of the part and film, and direct the cathode portion of the x-ray beam toward the anatomic area of greatest tissue density or thickness.

It should be observed that the "heel" effect diminishes with an increase in the focus-film distance and with the use of

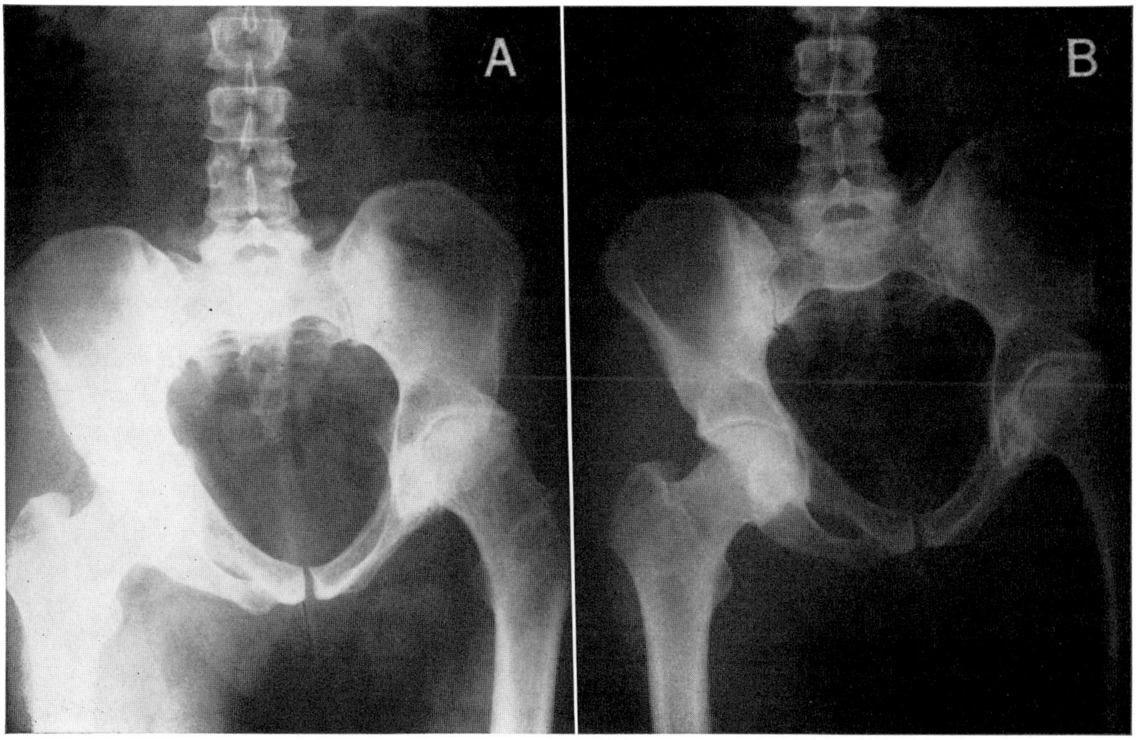

Figure 92. Series of anteroposterior screen-grid radiographs of the pelvis that demonstrate the "heel" effect when the tube axis is directed translaterally with the anode portion of the beam projected toward the left hip shown as an underexposed area in A.

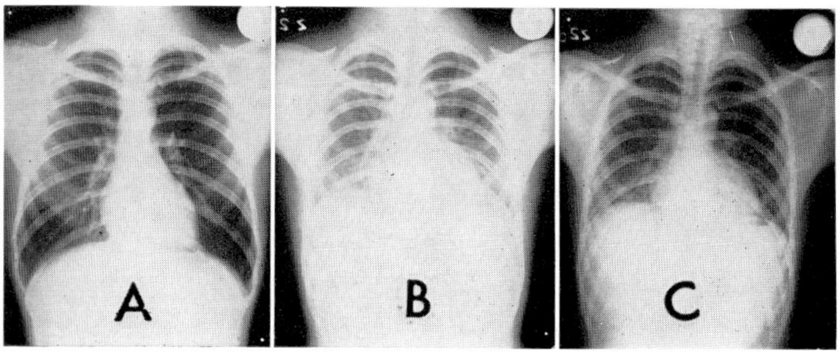

Figure 93. Posteroanterior chest screen radiographs. Radiograph A, made upon inspiration; B and C, upon expiration. Factors: 80 KvP, 72-inch FFD, average speed screens. Radiographs A and B, 2.5 MaS; C, 3.3 MaS.

small-size films since the more uniform intensities of radiation exist in the neighborhood of the central ray. Its greatest effect is observed when the focus-film distance is relatively short, when a large film is employed and the body part is unequal in thickness or tissue density.

II. Influence of Respiration

In radiography of the thorax, the influence of the phase of respiration on the over-all image density should be recognized. The great permeability of air-containing tissues to x-rays is well known and generally offers no great exposure problem. However, when the patient is not correctly instructed as to the phase of respiration in which the radiograph is to be made, confusing results are often obtained.

EFFECT OF DENSITY

For an initial posteroanterior radiograph of the lungs, the exposure should be made when the patient suspends respiration upon full inspiration. If the same exposure is made at expiration or partial expiration, the resulting consolidation of pulmonary tissue will cause underexposure and a loss in radiographic density. Hence, when an exposure of the lungs is to be made at the expiratory phase, an approximate MaS increase of one-third is necessary to approximate the original density.

Example 1. These conditions may be illustrated by three posteroanterior radiographs of the chest, Figure 93. Radiograph A was exposed at the inspiratory phase and radiograph B, at the expiratory phase; the exposure factors being identical. Note that a definite loss of over-all image density occurred in radiograph B. Radiograph C was then made using an approximate increase of one-third in MaS to equal the density shown in radiograph A. Note the change in position of the heart silhouette between radiographs A and C.

Example 2. To demonstrate the appearance of the image obtained in both respiratory phases in lateral radiography of the chest, two radiographs were made, Figure 94. Radiograph A was made at inspiration; radiograph B, made on expiration, was exposed with approximately a one-third increase in the MaS so as to compensate for the increase in density of the consolidated pulmonary tissues.

Example 3. In lateral radiography of the thoracic vertebrae, the high contrast influence of the air-filled lungs frequently prevents satisfactory recording of the spine. The high densities may be avoided by permitting the patient to breathe during a rather long exposure time at low Ma. The thorax is immobilized and the air-bearing pulmonary tissues move continuously during the exposure and blur themselves to such an extent that sharp details of the immobile vertebrae are clearly rendered, Figure 95.

EFFECT ON HEART MEASUREMENTS

It is most important to recognize that the cardiac silhouette changes position in each respiratory phase and the cardiac measurements will vary. Exposure should, therefore, occur at the commonly accepted respiratory phase (inspiration) to obtain comparable cardiac measurements. (When special apparatus is available, the exposure can be made in any cardiac cycle.)

Example. The influence of expiration on the cardiac contour is illustrated in Figure 96. Radiograph A was made at full inspiration; radiograph B, at expiration. Note the differences in shape between the car-

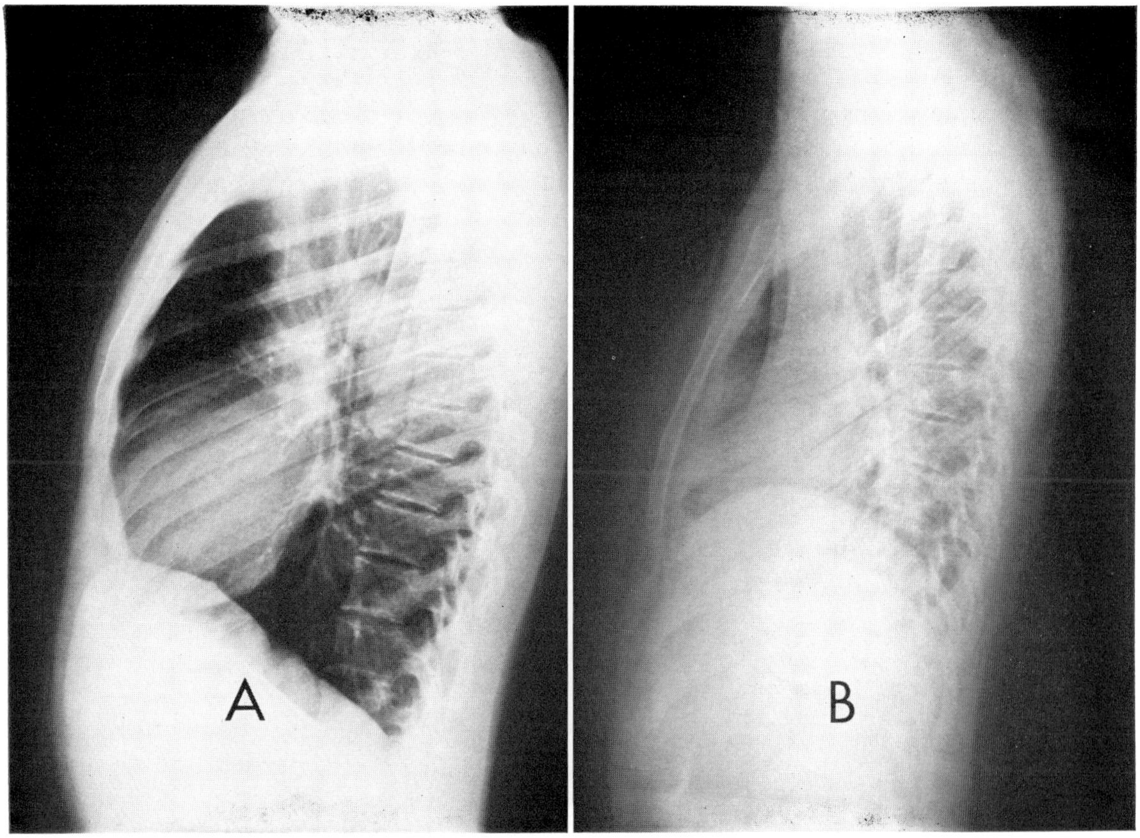

Figure 94. Lateral chest screen radiographs demonstrating influence of respiration on density. A, made at inspiration; B, at expiration. Factors: 85 KvP, 72-inch FFD; average speed screens. Radiograph A, 10 MaS; B, 13.3 MaS.

diac images as well as the changes in the cardiac measurements.

Rule. In radiography of the chest, the MaS value always should be adjusted to the respiratory phase in which the exposure is to be made. The MaS should be increased approximately one-third when exposure occurs at the expiratory phase if pulmonary densities are to be equalized.

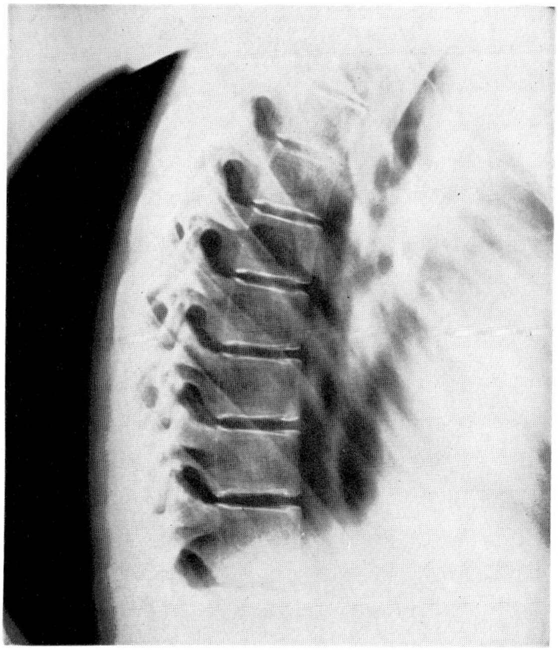

Figure 95. Lateral screen-grid radiograph of the thoracic vertebrae to demonstrate the value of immobilizing the thorax and permitting breathing during the exposure to blur out the unwanted pulmonary details and reveal the required structures.

III. Compensating Filtration

There are occasions when it is difficult to balance densities in radiography of large and irregular anatomical areas by making use of kilovoltage or the "heel" effect. However, by selective absorption of various portions of the x-ray beam *before* it traverses the subject, balanced densities may be secured.

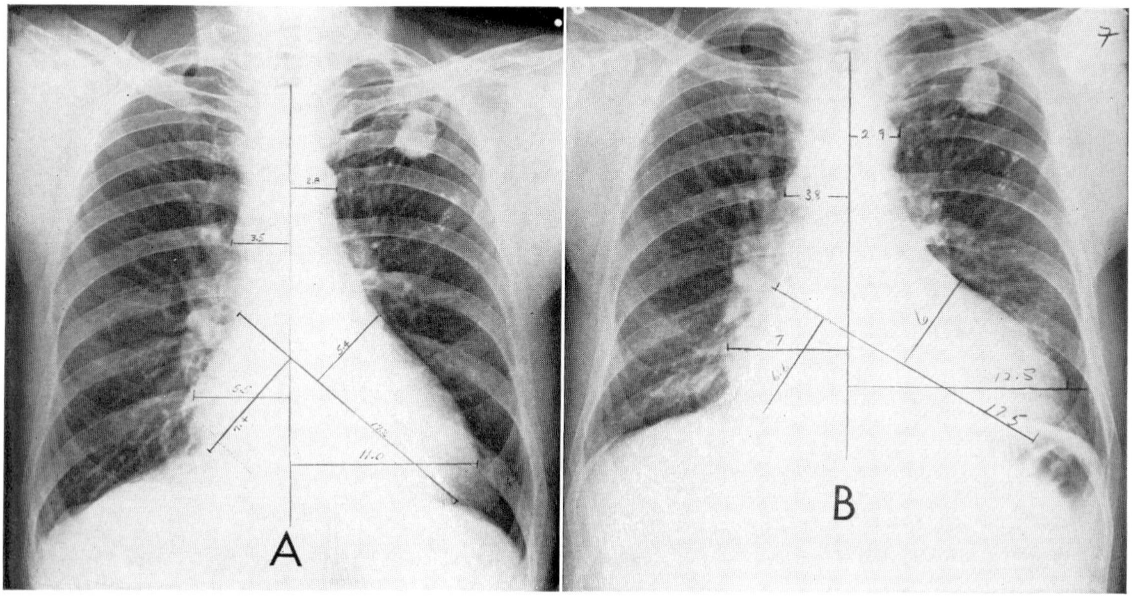

Figure 96. Posteroanterior chest screen radiographs exhibiting the change in cardiac dimensions upon respiration. Radiograph A made upon full inspiration; B, upon partial expiration.

Absorption of the beam can be effected by placing an absorbing medium such as barium impregnated clay or graduated aluminum in the filter channel. The material is so shaped that the beam must pass through the larger amounts of absorbing material when directed toward the thinner anatomical portions. The material should be thin or omitted for that portion of the beam passing toward the heavier parts.

In radiography of the entire spine on a 14 x 36-inch film, a normal image would exhibit high density in those portions representing the thinner tissue areas. The upper segment of the vertebral column would be overexposed because the expo-

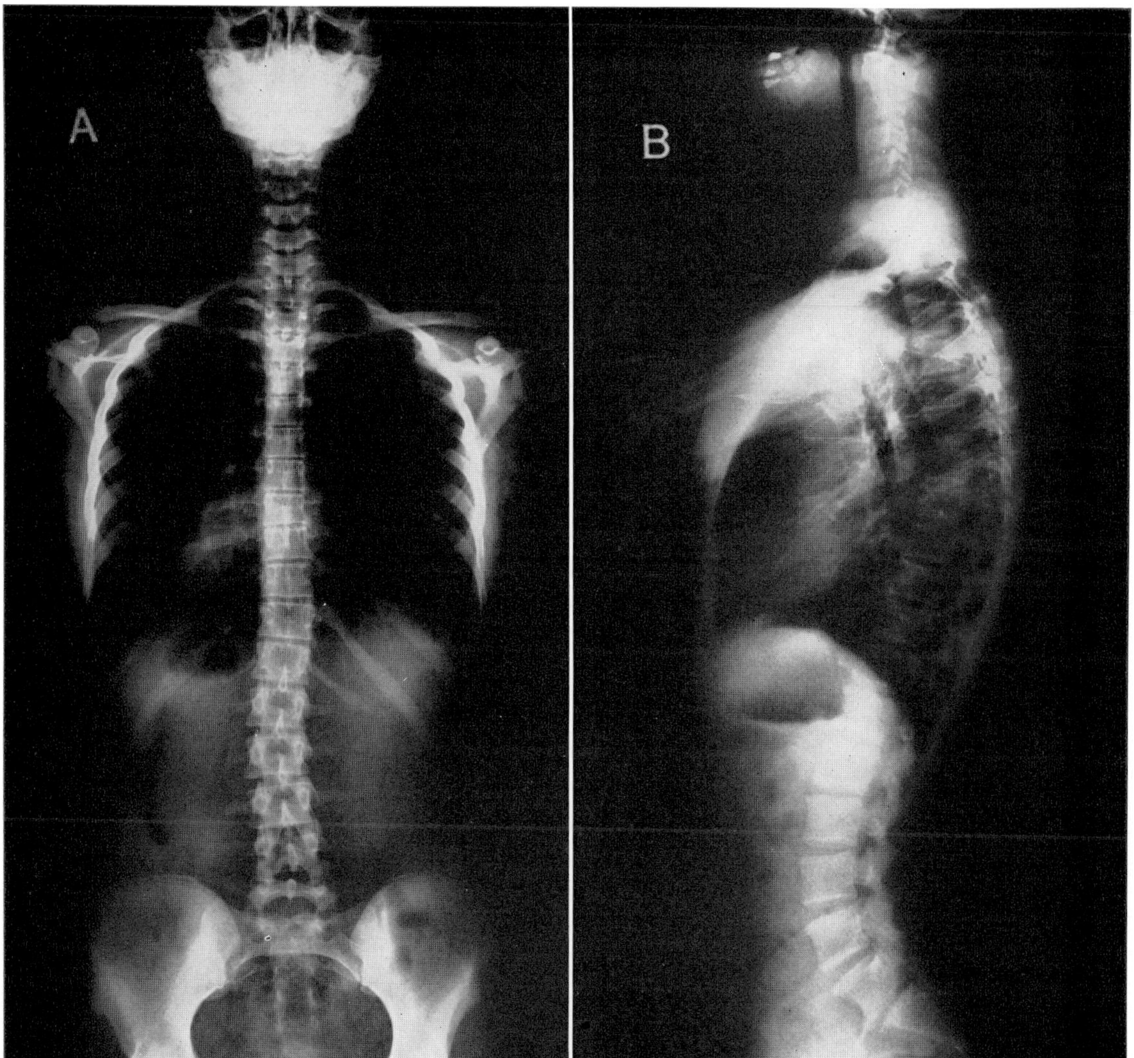

Figure 97. Anteroposterior (A) and lateral (B) screen-grid radiographs of entire spine exposed with compensating filtration. Note balanced densities.

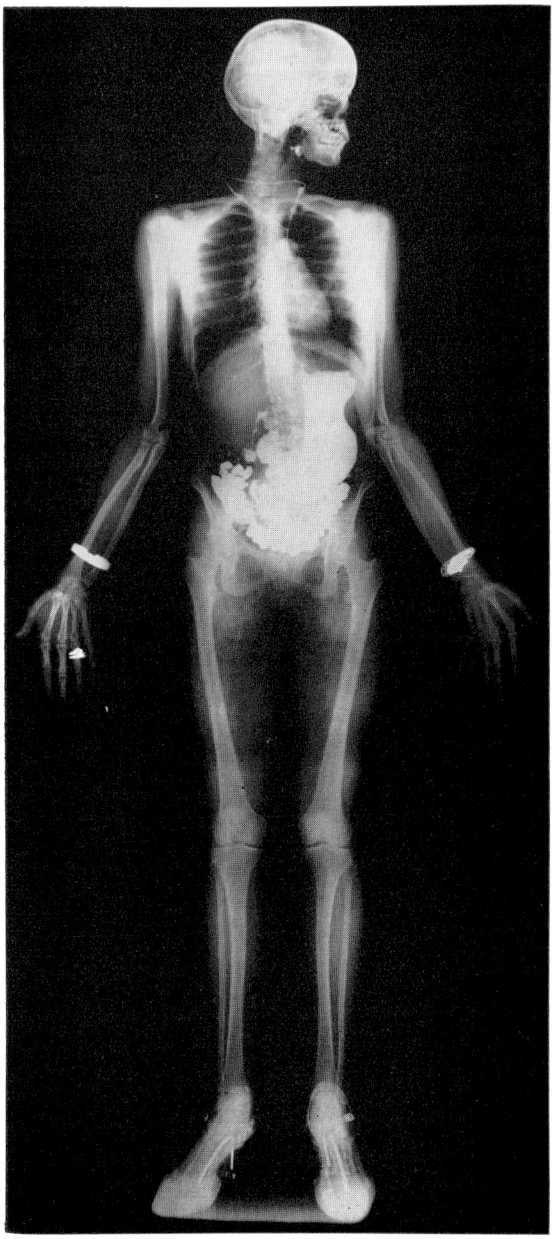

Figure 98. Entire body radiograph of a living girl made with a compensating filter. The stomach and intestinal tract was filled with a barium sulfate meal for their delineation.

sure would necessarily be adjusted to suit the heavier or lumbosacral portion of the spine. This condition would still arise on occasion because the anode portion of the beam would ordinarily be directed toward the thinner area—the cervical vertebrae. Despite this arrangement, however, overexposure of the cervical area often would occur. By constructing a suitable compensating filter of barium impregnated clay, anteroposterior and lateral views of the entire vertebral column that exhibit balanced radiographic densities may be secured, Figure 97.

Radiography of chests wherein extensive consolidations or thoracoplastys are present, shielding the normal pulmonary area with a compensating filter, permits using an exposure that is more appropriate for the diseased area or the one wherein surgery was employed without overexposing the contralateral side.

Compensating filters are also used to advantage in placental studies and orthopedic radiography. Herein, however, employment of the higher kilovoltages and the heel effect are of great assistance.

In radiography of the entire living body, a compensating filter can be made to produce radiographs as shown in Figures 1 and 98 wherein all densities are equalized to produce balanced images.

Chapter 13

Geometry of Image Formation

THE FORMATION of the radiographic image is dependent upon geometric conditions associated with its projection. Actually, the image is composed of various details that are renditions of the anatomical structures through which the x-ray beam passed. These details are defined by various degrees of sharpness and shape, depending upon the geometric conditions existing at the time of exposure. *Radiographic detail* constitutes the recorded image. *Definition* is the term employed to describe the sharpness with which the detail is recorded. Radiographic details are never points in the image but are minute areas of black metallic silver. Since many of these facts also apply to light, their understanding may be facilitated by comparing the characteristics of light and of x-rays with respect to the recording of an image.

SHADOW FORMATION BY LIGHT

To demonstrate shadow formation by light, Figure 99, a source of light (LS), an opaque object (OB) to be projected by the light, and a recording card (RC) are needed. The plane of the object should be parallel to the plane of the recording card.

POINT LIGHT SOURCE

Assume that light from a point source (LS) falls on the recording card (RC), A, and the object (OB) is interposed between LS and RC. A shadow (S) of the object will be formed, the edges of which are sharply defined. The shadow naturally is larger than the size of the object. The degree of enlargement will vary according to the distance of the object from RC and from LS. When the object is moved nearer the light source, the margins of the shadow are still sharply defined but the shadow is larger, B. When the object is placed at the same distance from the recording card, as shown in diagram B, but the distance from the light source is increased, the size of the shadow is reduced, C. In all examples, the periphery of the shadow is sharply delineated because a *point* source of light was employed; the size of the shadow, however, varied with the distance between the object and the recording card as well as between the object and the light source.

AREA LIGHT SOURCE

Assume another situation wherein the light source is a small area, Figure 99, D, instead of a point. The relation of the

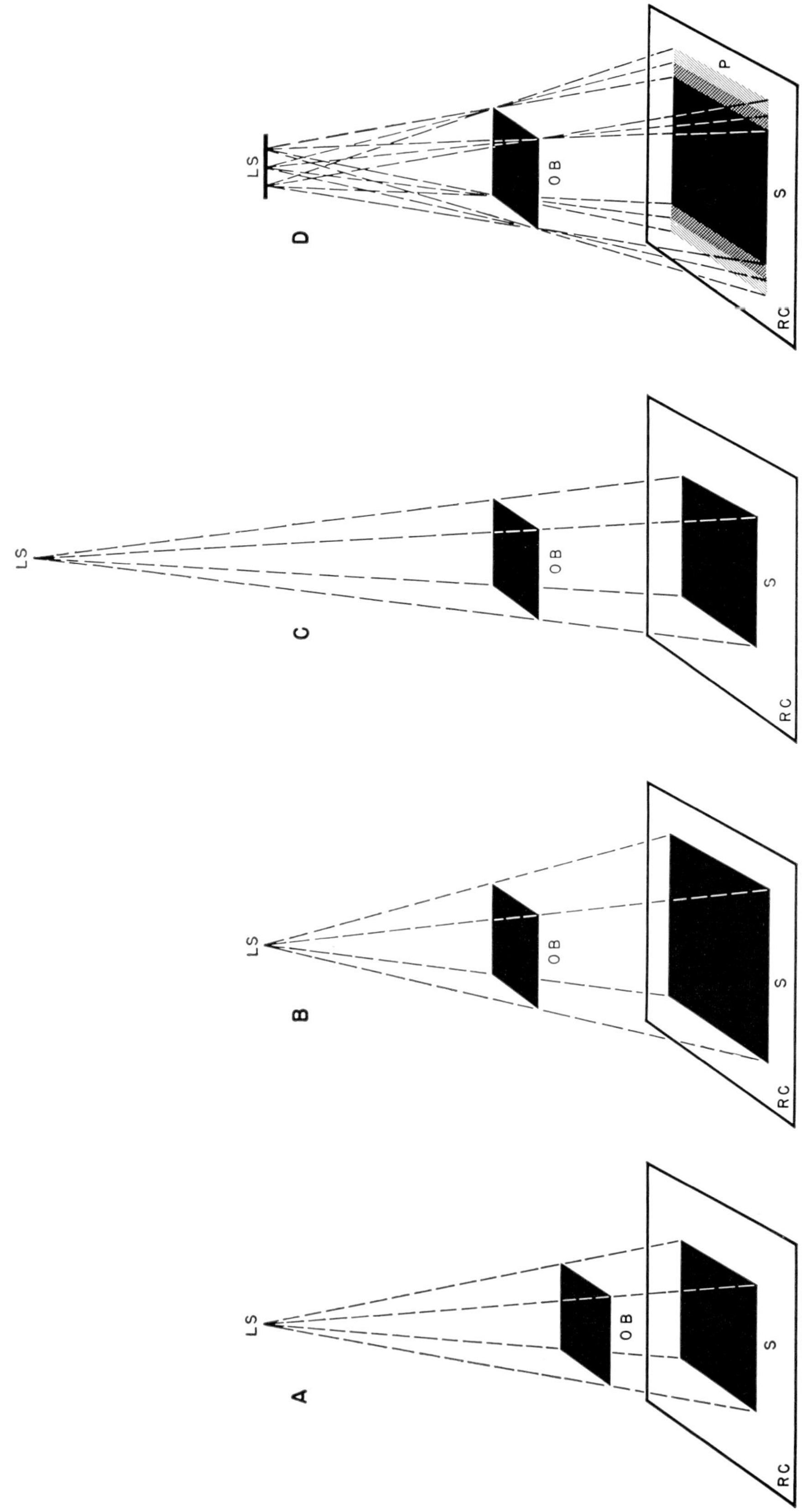

Figure 99. Diagrams illustrating shadow formation by light.

object to the recording card is the same as shown in diagram B. Many points of light emanate from this source and many light beams strike the object and each, in turn, produces its shadow of the object on the recording card. The result of these combined shadows is to diffuse the margins of the image so that it is not sharply defined. The shadows produced in diagrams A, B, and C are known as umbras and their margins sharply defined. In diagram D, an umbra is present, but the margins are not sharp. The area of unsharpness is known as the *penumbra (P)*, D. Some improvement in definition may be secured if the object is placed nearer to the recording card or if the light source is moved farther away.

Comment. From the above it, may be observed that the following apparent conditions must be fulfilled when an enlarged though sharp shadow of the object is to be produced by means of light—

1. The source of the light must be small.
2. The source of the light should be at a sufficient distance to avoid objectionable enlargement.
3. The recording card should be as close to the object as possible so as to avoid a great degree of enlargement.
4. The light should be directed perpendicularly to the recording card.
5. The plane of the object and the plane of the recording card should be parallel.

X-RAY "SHADOW" A MISNOMER

To avoid misunderstanding, it is necessary at this point to explain what light shadows are as compared to x-ray "shadows." A shadow may be defined as a mass of darkness or shade produced on a recording surface by an object that intercepts a beam of light; details of the object are not present in the shadow. Actually, it is a silhouette.

DISSIMILARITY OF SHADOW AND IMAGE

The physical laws responsible for the formation of a shadow by visible light are identical to those that serve to make an x-ray image, but there is no similarity between a shadow and an x-ray image beyond this point. The shadow caused by light and the image produced by x-rays are very dissimilar in appearance. There is some resemblance, however, between an image produced by a lens and that produced by an x-ray beam, but the means for producing either are entirely dissimilar. The laws governing the formation of a light shadow such as size and shape of light source and its distance from the object and recording surface, have a definite influence on the size, shape, and peripheral sharpness of the shadow. This situation is comparable to the production of an x-ray image using such factors as an x-ray focal spot, focus-and-object-film distances, etc.

It must be pointed out that in a true shadow no details are visible since the object is opaque to the passage of light. A shadow only has outline. On the contrary, abundant details are found within an x-ray image because most objects can be *penetrated* by x-rays.

RADIOGRAPH VERSUS SKIAGRAPH

When Röntgen discovered the x-rays, the low power of his apparatus produced only weak x-ray images on the fluorescent screen of objects placed in the x-ray beam. These images were little better than shadows, but some details were discernible. Early enthusiastic investigators, however, called x-ray images "shadows" and coined the word *skiagraph* (shadow picture) comparable to the presently accepted term of *radiograph.* The tendency to call x-ray images "shadows" has persisted through the years. A careful analysis of how a radiograph is produced should convince one that the word "shadow" is a misnomer when it is applied to an x-ray image, whether it occurs on the radiograph or on the fluoroscopic screen. An x-ray "shadow" is more accurately termed *radiographic image* or *fluoroscopic image* depending upon the manner in which the images are produced.

GEOMETRIC CHARACTERISTICS

Every radiographic image represents a projection on a two-dimensional surface of a number of body details disposed in a three-dimensional medium. A spatial situation of this character produces distortions that are a departure from the actual situation and variations from the true shapes and sizes of the object occur. Consequently, the projection of the x-ray beam should be such that these image-degrading effects be reduced to a minimum.

The source of the x-ray beam is at the target in the x-ray tube and it cannot be a point—it must be a small area. In practice, the size of the area varies with the electrical capacity of the tube. It may be 1 or 2 millimeters or as large as 4 millimeters. The radiographic image cannot ever be geometrically sharp because it consists of a large number of minute specks of silver located on *both* sides of the film base. The borders of the image are really broken up into a number of microscopic specks which our eyes are not capable of seeing individually and which may seem to consist of diffused lines of configuration. The sharpness of detail is directly influenced by the width of the marginal diffusion.

REDUCTION OF UNSHARPNESS

Measures may be taken to reduce detail unsharpness to a minimum value by observing the following recommendations. The size and shape of an image of an object placed in the path of an x-ray beam depend upon the object-film distance, which should be as short as possible. The focal spot should be as small as possible depending upon the choice of the current and kilovoltage to be used, and it should be as remote from the x-ray film as is practical. The film should be placed as near the object as possible and the central ray should be perpendicular to the plane surface of the film except where diagnostic requirements necessitate an oblique projection.

The effects produced when various changes are made in the above factors are diagrammatically represented in Figure 100. In diagram A, an object (OB) was placed so that the object-film distance (OFD) was long; a large focal spot (FS) was employed. The penumbra (P) as projected on the film was wide, indicating excessive image unsharpness that was also influenced by the relatively short focus-film distance (FFD). The situation represents the worst sort of geometric relationship between the image and the object.

In diagram B, the same conditions prevailed as in A, with the exception that a smaller focal spot was used. The narrower penumbra indicates that less unsharpness was obtained. In diagram C, a long focus-film distance was employed with other conditions remaining as in A. The increased focus-film distance narrowed the penumbra, but not to the same extent as in B, where a smaller focal spot was employed. In diagram D, the same conditions

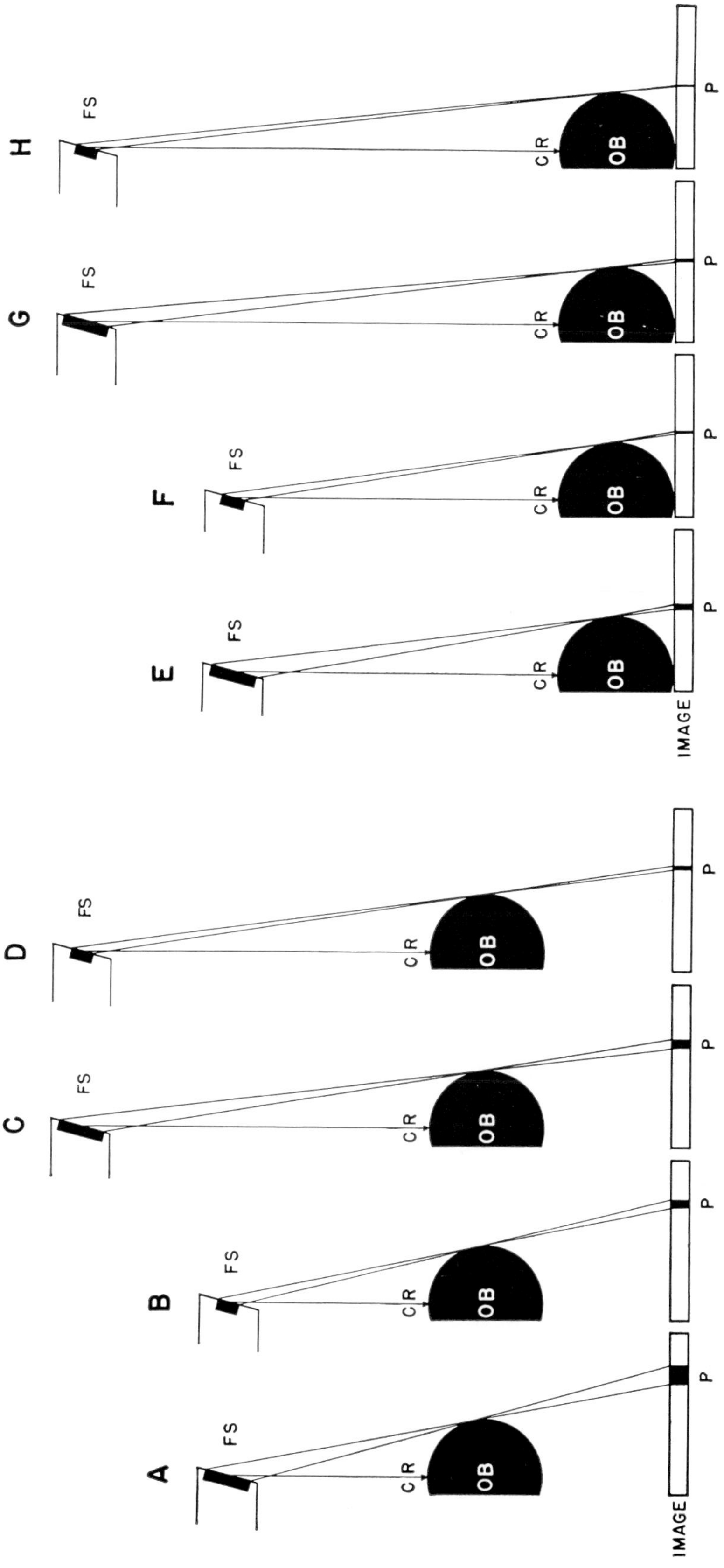

Figure 100. Diagrams illustrating situations affecting image sharpness.

prevailed as in C, with the exception that a small focal spot was used. The very narrow penumbra indicates a decrease in unsharpness due to the use of a smaller focal spot. This condition should prevail when an appreciable object-film distance exists.

Diagram E shows the object close to the film; an average focus-film distance and a large focal spot were used. A fair degree of sharpness was achieved, although a smaller focal spot as shown in diagram F, slightly improved the sharpness. From diagrams E and F, it is obvious that when the object is close to the film, the size of the focal spot has a smaller effect upon image sharpness. A large focal spot at a long focus-film distance with the object close to the film as shown in diagram G, produced a very narrow penumbra. By employing a smaller focal spot under the same conditions as in G, the maximum sharpness was obtained as shown in diagram H. Of all the situations depicted in diagrams A to H, the image sharpness is at its maximum in H.

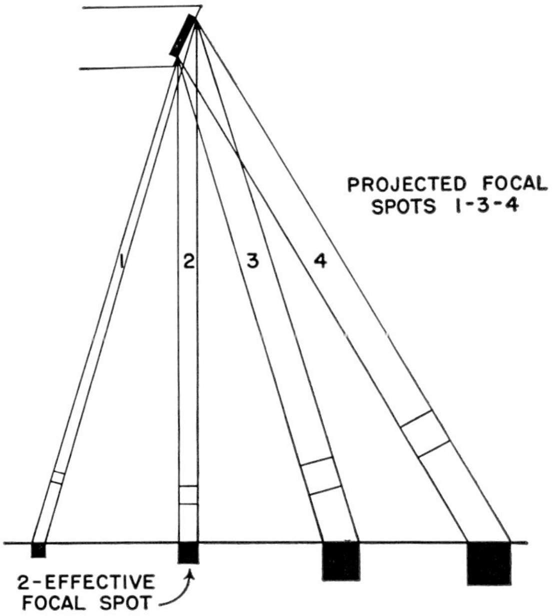

Figure 101. Diagram illustrating how the size of the focal spot varies with the angle at which it is projected from the target.

TYPES OF DEFINITION

Definition may be divided into three types: (1) geometrical unsharpness, which is influenced by the focal spot, object-film distance, or focus-film distance; (2) motion unsharpness, which may be voluntary or involuntary on the part of the patient, or caused by vibration of the apparatus; and (3) screen unsharpness, which is influenced by the character of the screens and screen-film contact. In considering unsharpness, it is well to realize that all these factors contribute to the total resultant unsharpness. The correction of some factors may induce unsharpness by some other factor. For example, if a radiograph was made without screens to ensure image sharpness, patient movement may cause blurring if a long exposure time is employed. It is necessary, therefore, that the various influences which these factors have upon unsharpness in the image should be considered.

GEOMETRICAL UNSHARPNESS

Geometrical unsharpness is influenced by all factors of projection that alter the size, shape, and location of images of structures traversed by the x-rays.

Influence of Focal Spot

The focal spot of the x-ray tube is comparable to the light source employed in shadow formation, as previously described. The influence of the focal spot on definition is confined to image sharpness. With all other factors constant, the smaller the focal spot, the sharper the definition. A large focal spot, although capable of withstanding high electrical energies, does not produce the sharpness of detail that is characteristic of tubes with a small focal spot, though relatively much lower energies are employed in the latter. In some instances, a long focus-film distance will aid in showing sharper detail when employing a large focal spot, but it is generally considered advantageous to use, whenever possible, a smaller focal spot with smaller tube capacities or a rotating anode tube. The relative unsharpness produced by a larger focal spot is not so significant when the object is close to the film.

Projected Focal Spot

From the diagram, Figure 101, it may be seen that the size of the projected focal spot varies with the angle at which it is projected from the target. When the projected focal spot is nearly perpendicular to the face of the target, it is large (4). As the angle decreases toward the central ray, the projected focal spot becomes smaller. The focal spot as projected at the central ray (2) is characteristic of the rated or effective focus of the tube. As the projected focal spot moves anode-wise from the central ray, it becomes smaller (1) until it reaches the limits of the anode side of the beam. Actually, at routine focus-film distances, the differences in sharpness of definition are minimal and are difficult to determine visually.

INFLUENCE OF OBJECT-FILM DISTANCE

When the object is at some distance from the film as shown in diagram, Figure 66, D, the sharpness is not as great as it is in Figure 66, A, wherein the object is shown next to the film. The larger the object-film distance, the greater the unsharpness. The use of grids requires an increase in object-film distance, but the gain in contrast offsets the small amount of image unsharpness introduced. The effect of object-film distance may be also demonstrated by the example shown in Figure 66.

Example. The series of four posteroanterior radiographs of a hand, Figure 66, was made in which all factors were constant except the object-film distance. Radiograph A was made with the hand on the film; B, the object-film distance was 2 inches; C, 6 inches; and D, 8 inches. Note that as the object-film distance increased, the size of the hand also increased.

INFLUENCE OF FOCUS-FILM DISTANCE

When a body part is placed on a film, image unsharpness is minimal, and its degree is directly attributable to the pro-

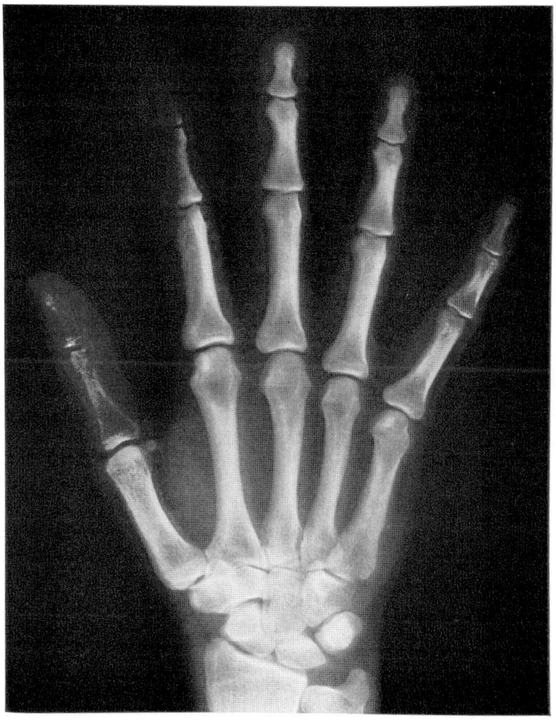

Figure 102. Posteroanterior direct-exposure radiograph of the hand which exhibits movement that occurred during the exposure.

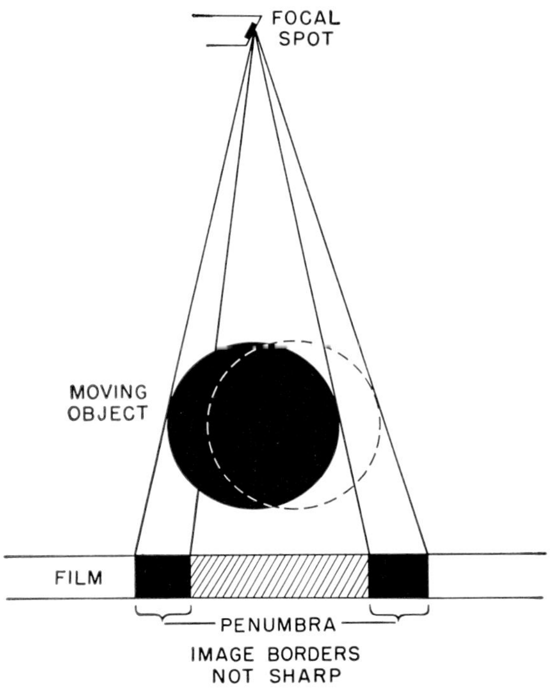

Figure 103. Diagram illustrating the influence of motion in producing image unsharpness.

jected focal spot and the focus-film distance. When a short focus-film distance is employed, the unsharpness increases. The image of the plane of that portion of the body part next to the film is always sharper than the image of the plane farthest away.

The degree of unsharpness depends upon the size of the focal spot and the focus-film distance. At maximum focus-film distance definition is improved and the image is also more nearly the actual size of the body part. In all situations sharpness is improved as the focus-film distance is increased. However, it is impractical to extend the focus-film distance to the point where the unsharpness is much less than that due to the intensifying screens. Also, the greater the focus-film distance, the greater the probability of introducing motion unsharpness because of the need for longer exposures. When a body part cannot be placed close to the film, the focus-film distance should be increased beyond that normally employed. A good beginning would be to double the normal value.

MOTION UNSHARPNESS

Motion of a body part being examined directly influences sharpness of image definition. Motion may be voluntary on the part of the patient, or may be involuntary. The only means for controlling the effects of motion are—(1) patient cooperation, (2) immobilization of the part being examined, and (3) short exposures.

Voluntary Motion

Voluntary motion may take several forms. The noncooperative child who needs restraint is common. The patient who does not understand the manner in which he is to cooperate is usually the fearful one, Figure 102. A satisfactory explanation of the procedure usually suffices to create confidence. When in doubt, immobilize the part and use short exposures.

Involuntary Motion

Involuntary motion is normally associated with the physiologic activity of the body tissues. Respiration produces movement of the thorax and its contents so that short exposures are mandatory, Figure 104. The normal adult respiratory rate is 16 to 18 respirations per minute; in some pulmonary or cardiac lesions, the rate may be greater; in the newborn, it may be 30 to 40 per minute. Respiration also influences in some degree the viscera adjacent to the diaphragms.

Movement of the heart and great vessels is an important factor in radiography of the chest. The pulsation of the arterial system in all parts of the body at the rate of about 5 to 8 meters per second creates various degrees of movement in the tissues they supply.

Esophageal peristalsis begins about 1 second after the initial swallowing act. The rate of travel is not the same at all levels. In the first 7 to 8 centimeters of its course, the rate is rapid (1 second); in the next 7 centimeters, the rate is 1 to 2 seconds; and in the lower segment, the rate is about 3 seconds. Solid or semisolid food takes between 6 and 7 seconds to pass from the mouth to the stomach. When liquids are ingested, the rate is relatively more rapid. Movement of the gastrointestinal tract requires proper use of exposure time to avoid unsharpness in the image. Motion of the stomach exhibits great individual variations. In some stomachs, the peristaltic wave travels rapidly and lasts 10 to 15 seconds. In others, the wave may occupy as much as 30 seconds to move from its origin to the pyloris. The slower waves, however, are more common. Peristalsis in the small intestine is about 10 centimeters per second; the colonic rate is very slow.

The gallbladder exhibits rhythmic contractions that may last 5 to 30 minutes. Contractions also occur in the common bile duct.

In the urinary tract, peristaltic waves begin at the kidney and extend to the urinary bladder at the rate of 20 to 30 millimeters per second or 3 to 6 contractions per minute.

Effect of Motion on Image

The influence of motion in producing image unsharpness is diagrammatically shown in Figure 103. In this illustration, the object moved during the exposure resulting in unsharpness in the margins of the image. A typical radiographic example of patient movement is shown in radiographs of the chest, Figure 104. Note the blurring of all image details in radiograph A while radiograph B shows no movement.

Immobilization

Immobilization is imperative in radiography, for differential diagnoses depend upon the visualization of sharp, undistorted images. Movement should be practically eliminated during the exposure in order to avoid blurring of details in the image.

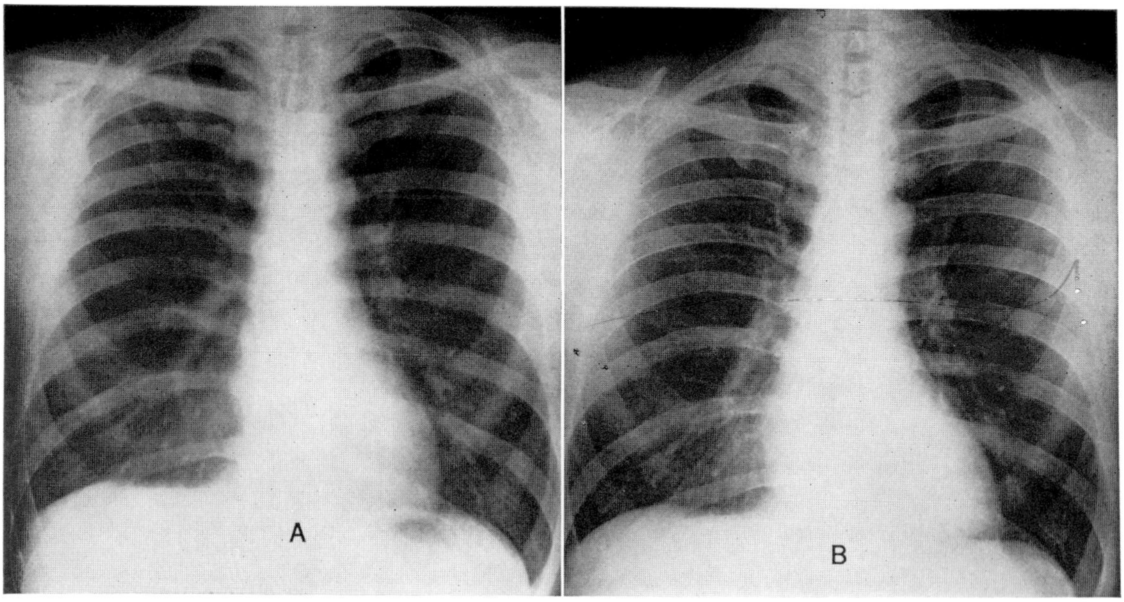

Figure 104. Posteroanterior radiographs of the chest demonstrating pulmonary movement (A); and, (B) at full inspiration, without movement of the pulmonary structures.

Composing the Patient

The responsibility of keeping the part immobile is the job of the technician, not the patient, for movement may occur consciously or unconsciously. Respiration and body tremor are physical conditions that are important enough to warrant close attention. To some patients, the mere fact it is necessary to lie on a table for an x-ray examination is perturbing. Some may show signs of trembling. A few words of assurance will help to restore peace of mind. Too much cannot be left to the patient in the matter of keeping still during the exposure because most patients are not familiar with the requirements for making a radiograph. Frequently, they are nervous and afraid; so it is the job of the technician to put the patient at ease—so that he will be comfortable, mentally and physically. When the patient is passive and relaxed as a result of his comfort, he will be most co-operative. The technician's task does not end there, however, for much of his success is dependent upon the closeness and the firmness with which the part is juxtaposed to the filmholder and the method of immobilization used. Even with the short exposures now possible, immobilization is necessary. There is no usable exposure so short as to fail to record uncontrollable or involuntary tremor of the area under examination. Proper immobilization assures comparison of symmetrical parts, for it also serves to prevent involuntary rotation of the part. The tube carriage always should be locked in position, because its vibration is a common cause for blurred radiographs.

Immobilization Methods

There are a number of good methods for immobilizing the body part: sandbags, compression bands, cones, and special clamps, etc. Many of these devices for immobilization are found in the modern laboratory. An important aspect of immobilization is compression of tissues, particularly in the abdomen. By displacing some of the tissues, less secondary radiation is produced and better definition attained because of the improvement in contrast.

An Advantage of Motion

Tissues in motion can in some instances serve diagnostic purposes, because their movement can be made to blur out undesirable details of superimposed structures. This can be effectively accomplished in lateral radiography of the thoracic vertebrae, Figure 95, and the sternum.

SCREEN UNSHARPNESS

The influence of x-ray intensifying screens on the radiographic image will be discussed in Chapter 14. It will be shown that, when screens are employed in radiography, unsharpness is introduced, the degree of unsharpness depending upon the size of the crystals incorporated in the screen upon the thickness of the fluorescent layer, and upon the film-screen contact. Since the level of unsharpness is usually acceptable provided film-screen contact is good and does not materially influence the diagnostic features of the image, screens have become an indispensable means for shortening the exposure.

MAGNIFICATION

Magnification in the radiographic image is a normal occurrence. The degree of enlargement is a function of the focus-film and object-film distance. When the object is close to the film, enlargement is minimal. When the center of the part is traversed by the central ray, normal magnification occurs. Whether the FFD is great or small, the image will always be magnified when a large OFD exists. The use of a long FFD in these situations serves only slightly to increase the sharpness of definition and decrease the image size. Therefore, the film should always be placed as near the object as possible even though some distortion of the image may occasionally result.

EFFECTS OF MAGNIFICATION

The following example will illustrate the effects of simple magnification when the FFD or the FFD and the OFD are varied.

Example. Two series of lateral radiographs of a dry skull, Figure 105, were made in which the focus-film distance was varied as indicated on the radiographs. The dry skull was placed directly on the exposure holder. Radiographs A-D, Top: A, FFD 20 inches; B, FFD 30 inches; C, FFD 40 inches; and D, FFD 72 inches. Note that as the FFD was increased, the images became smaller. Radiographs E-H, Bottom: the various focus-film distances were the same as in Figure 105, Top, but the OFD was increased to 4 inches in each case. Note the decrease in enlargement as the FFD was increased. The least enlargement is shown in each group at an FFD of 72 inches. In reality, FFD distances beyond 48 inches do not contribute materially to reduce magnification and improve definition.

WHEN THE FOCAL SPOT IS GREATER THAN THE OBJECT

Occasionally, an opaque object in the tissues may have a diameter *less* than that of the tube focal spot. If there is sufficient magnification achieved by a reasonable OFD and a short FFD, the object may be visualized as a diffuse grey area. This condition is diagrammatically represented, Figure 106, in which a small object (OB) at an extended object-film distance is shown projected by a larger focal spot (B). If details composed the object, all image details would be blurred and indis-

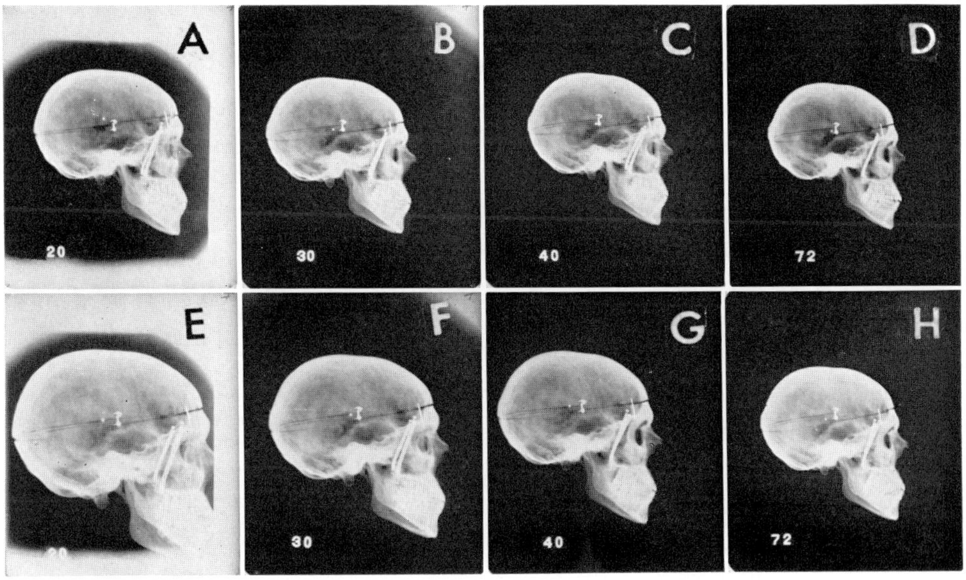

Figure 105. Series of lateral direct-exposure radiographs of a dried skull illustrating the influence of FFD and OFD with respect to magnification of the image. (*Top*) Influence of FFD (A-D); OFD none. (*Bottom*) Influence of OFD (4 inches) and FFD (E-H). The FFD is inscribed on each radiograph.

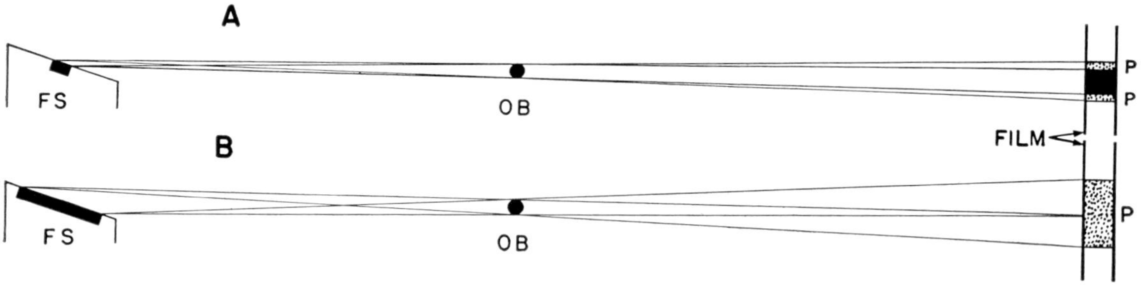

Figure 106. Diagram illustrating the effects of magnification when the focal spot is greater than the object.

tinguishable, having only the gross shape of the object. If secondary radiation undercut the object the blurred details would be superimposed by fog, and any suggestion of image might then be entirely eliminated. In A, the object is shown projected by a focal spot *smaller* than the diameter of the object. The image would then contain details with small blurred margins.

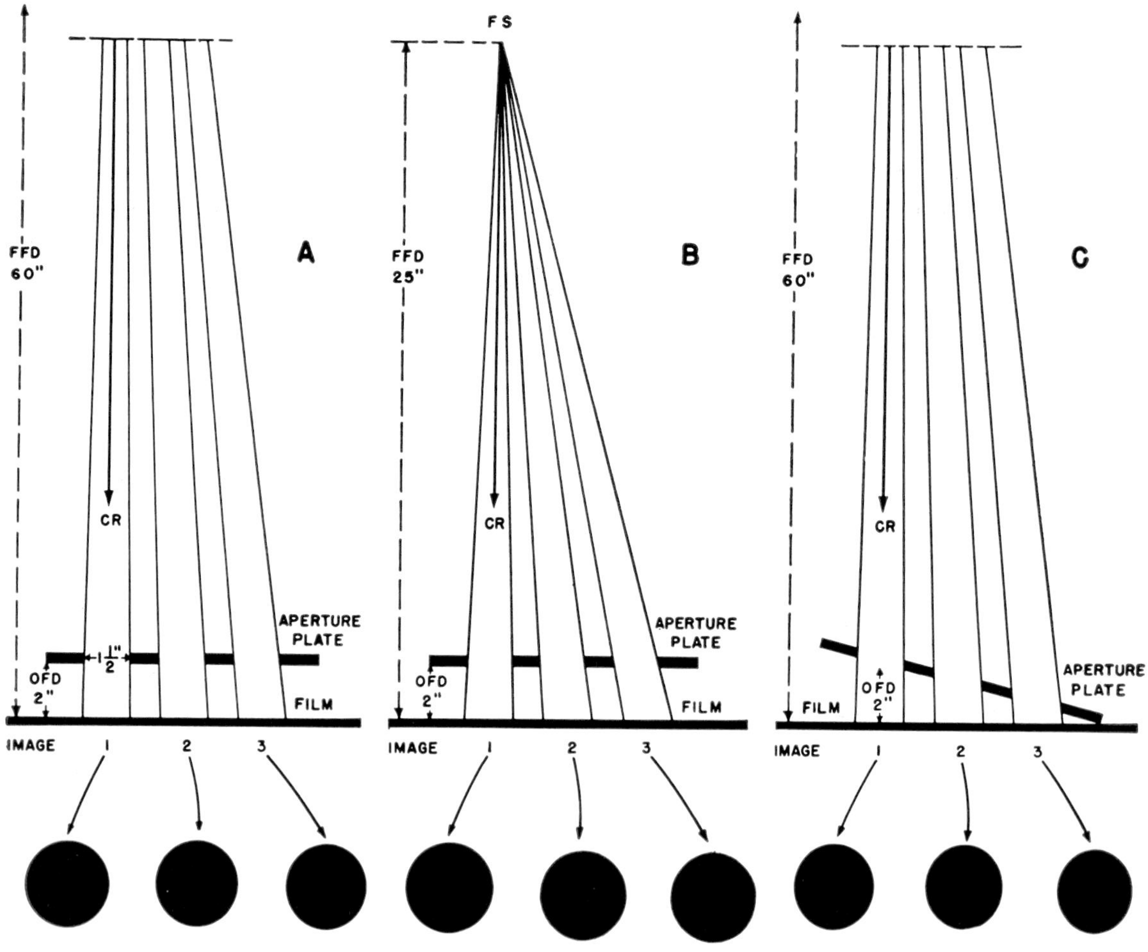

Figure 107. A series of diagrams demonstrating the effects of distortion.

DEGREE OF MAGNIFICATION

The percent magnification of an object at any focus-film distance (FFD) and object-film distance (OFD) can readily be determined by the following formula:

$$\frac{\text{FFD}}{\text{FFD} - \text{OFD}} - 1 \times 100\% = \text{Per Cent Magnification.}$$

Example. Determine the percent magnification of an object situated 5 inches from the film (OFD) when employing an FFD of 48 inches.

$$\frac{48}{48 - 5} - 1 \times 100\% = 11.5\% \text{ Answer.}$$

DISTORTION

Distortion in a radiographic image is a variation from the true size and shape of a body part. Body parts are not always symmetrical since the body is an irregularly shaped object. All parts cannot be over the center of the film, nor can all tissue planes be parallel with the film. Some distortion will always be present because some portions will be projected obliquely and their details distorted more than those in the center of the film.

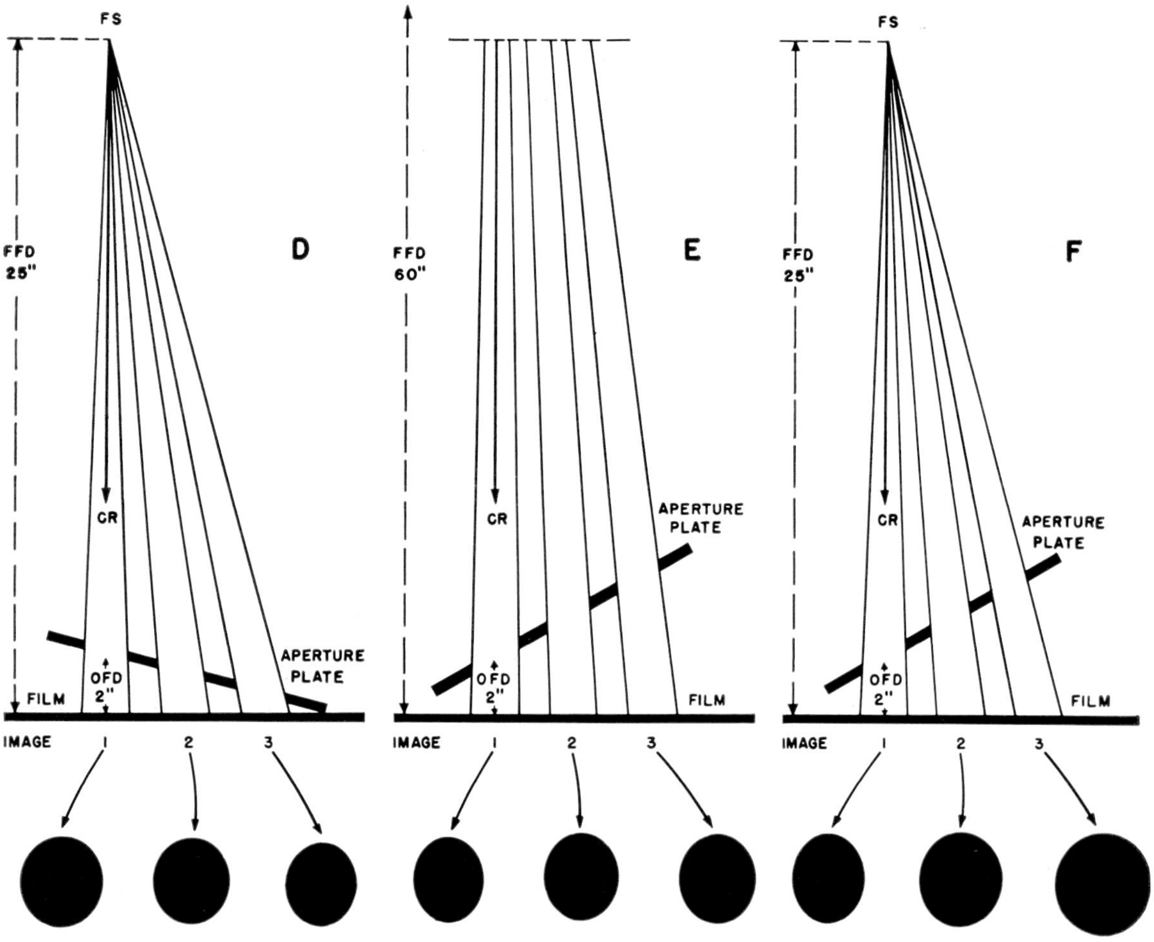

Figure 107. (*Continued. See legend on opposite page.*)

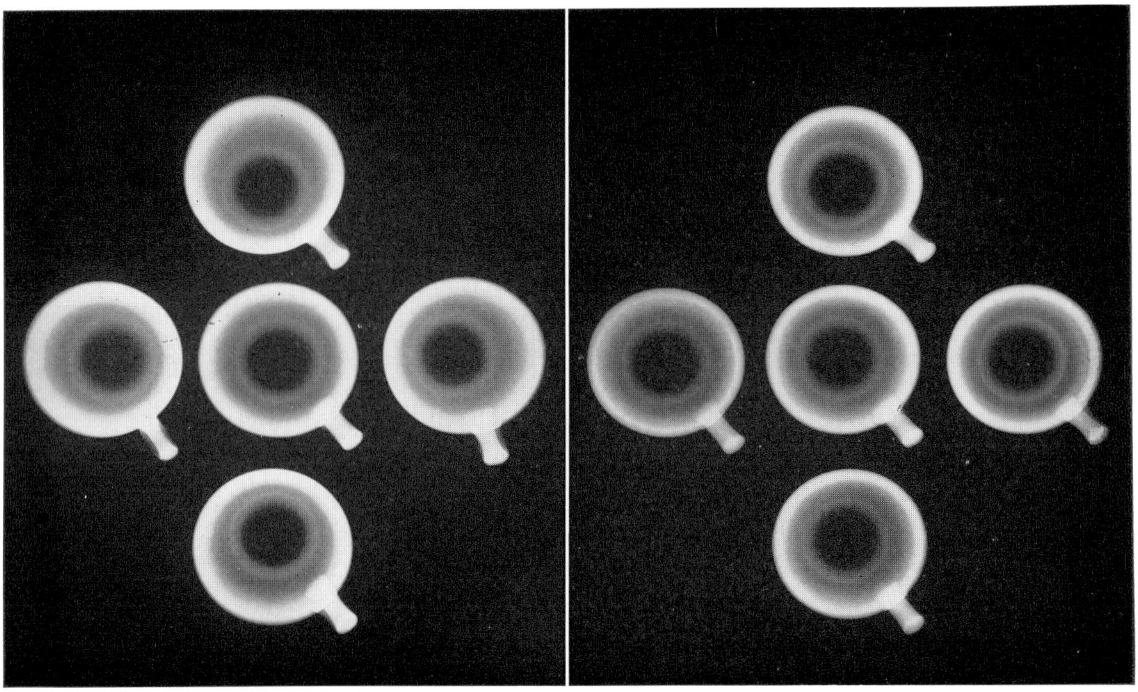

Figure 108. Radiographs of cups (china) to demonstrate the effect of FFD on image distortion. (*Left*) FFD 30 inches; (*right*) FFD 72 inches.

DEMONSTRATION OF DISTORTION

To demonstrate the effects of distortion, a series of radiographs of apertures, Figure 107, in a lead plate was made. The aperture plate is shown in Figure 28. Only the center row of three holes was exposed. From left to right, the holes were numbered 1, 2, and 3. The focus-film distances were alternated so that in diagrams A, C, and E, the focus-film distance was 60 inches. An object-film distance of 2 inches was used. In diagrams B, D, and F, the focus-film distance was 25 inches. In all diagrams, the central ray passed through the center of hole No. 1, and divergent portions of the x-ray beam passed through holes No. 2 and No. 3. Diagrams of the various positions assumed by the aperture plate with respect to the focal spot and film are shown in Figure 107. Below the diagrams are the radiographic images which were obtained under each set of conditions.

Diagram A. All radiographic images exhibit simple magnification because the 60-inch focus-film distance permits projection of approximately parallel x-rays.

Diagram B. Since the focus-film distance was shortened to 25 inches, simple magnification of the images resulted, although it is greater than that shown in diagram A. Some oblique radiation partially altered the shape of the No. 3 image.

Diagram C. In this situation, the aperture plate was tipped so that the right-hand edge rested on the film. The center of hole No. 1 was supported 2 inches from the film; the focus-film distance was 60 inches. Besides simple magnification of all images, the horizontal image axis is foreshortened and distortion of the original shape occurs.

Diagram D. When the focus-film distance is reduced to 25 inches, greater magnification and distortion are shown. In both diagrams C and D, image No. 1 in each diagram shows less distortion, because it is produced by the central portion of the beam containing the central ray.

Diagram E. In this diagram, the aperture plate was inclined in a reverse direction to that shown in diagram D and at a greater angle to the film plane. The center of hole No. 1 is supported 2 inches above the film. A focus-film distance of 60 inches was employed. Magnification of the images in their vertical axes is shown in Nos. 1 to 3 but foreshortening of the horizontal image axes occurs, thereby producing distortion.

Diagram F. The focus-film distance was reduced to 25 inches in this diagram and the size and shape of image No. 1 is about the same as that shown in diagram E. However, because of the great angle at which holes No. 2 and No. 3 are inclined, considerable distortion and magnification occurs in image No. 2; No. 3 image assumes a more spherical form although greatly magnified.

Comment. From diagrams A and B, it may be assumed that when body parts are in one plane parallel to the film, the shape of the parts remain substantially unaltered but the size of the image is increased. In diagrams C and D, it was shown that when the central ray passes through the center of the part, very little distortion takes place in that area. However, the shape of parts lying in the fringe of the area is distorted as well as enlarged. Diagrams E and F illustrate the point that when body parts are grossly misaligned and lie in the fringe area of the x-ray beam, the images become grossly distorted. It is most important that the size and shape of the image of various anatomical structures be comparable to

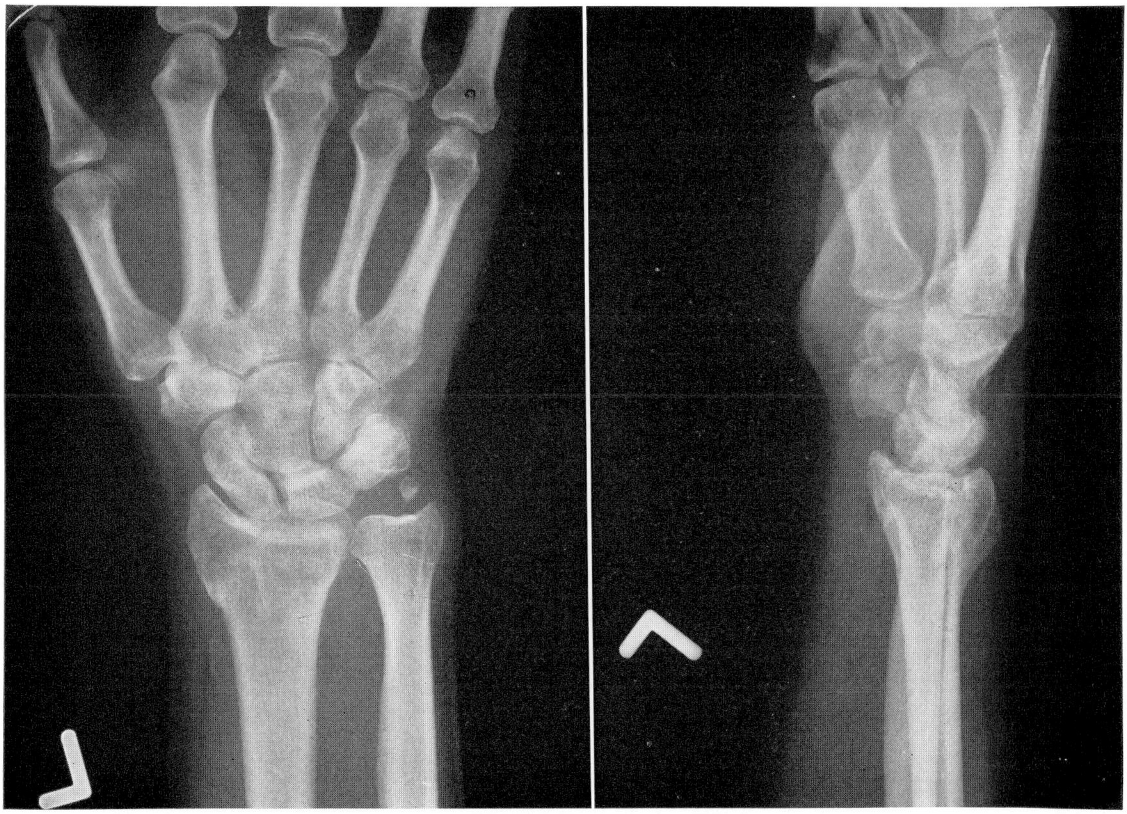

Figure 109. Posteroanterior and lateral direct-exposure radiographs of the wrist that demonstrate anatomical relationships after fracture.

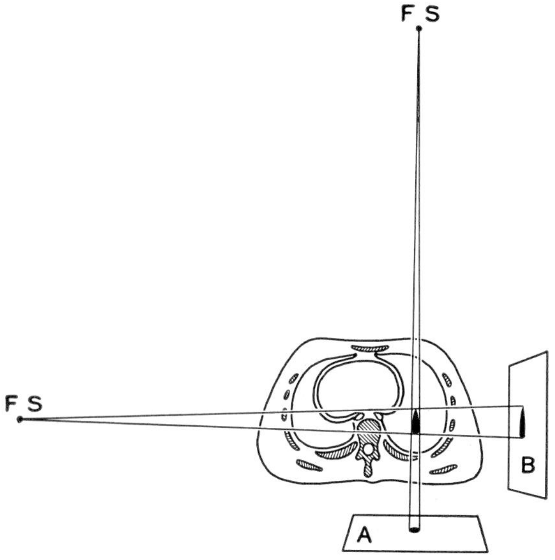

Figure 110. Two diagrams illustrating the need for projections from two positions to determine nature of foreign body.

the original. There are occasions in which body parts are deliberately distorted to obtain more diagnostic information, as in posteroanterior radiography of the sinuses. In the main, however, the central ray should be perpendicular to the plane of the film and the major planes of the object.

Example. An example of distortion is shown in radiographs, Figure 108, of a number of coffee cups. In each radiograph, the center cup was placed directly under the central ray and four other cups arranged around the center cup to be recorded on the film by divergent rays in the primary beam. The radiograph (Left) was made at an FFD of 30 inches. Note that the center cup shows little evidence of distortion. However, the images of all outer four cups show unmistakable evidence of distortion. When the FFD was increased to 72 inches and another radiograph (Right) was made, the center cup is shown free of distortion and a *lesser* amount of distortion is evidenced in the outer four cups indicating that fewer divergent rays were employed in exposing the cups. Therefore, reduction in the amount of image distortion can be effected by increasing the FFD.

POSITIONING

The diagnostic radiograph is dependent upon proper posing of the patient before exposure. This is facilitated by the use of standard projections. Such projections produce images that reveal the maximum amount of diagnostic information with a minimum of distortion. An accurate idea of the anatomic arrangement of the internal structures with relation to some external landmark aids materially in posing the patient. A convenient method is to visualize the part as though it were transparent, so that the usual structures which appear on the radiograph may be identified in relation to an external landmark. The relation of the central ray to the part to be examined, and to the film, must be carefully considered in each projection. Imperfect centering of the part on the film and alignment of the tube to the part are probably the most common causes of image distortion. The requirements of radiography are such that slight differences in position do not necessarily rule out the diagnostic value of the radiograph. A certain degree of latitude in routine may be permissible, because the radiologist ordinarily can make satisfactory adjustment by reason of his experience and knowledge. However, in order to secure reliable diagnostic results, it is best to conform to a procedure which is precise and accurate.

To derive the maximum information concerning the size and shape of body parts and foreign objects in relation to their position in the body, projections should be made from different directions. The need for multiple views is clearly demonstrated in Figures 109-111.

In routine radiography, two views, each at right angles to the other, are made as shown in Figure 109, wherein postero-anterior and lateral views of the wrist are illustrated.

To determine the nature of a foreign body, two views are also necessary, Figure 110. In this diagram an anteroposterior radiograph would show a foreign body as a circular object (image A). Another, when viewed at right angles to the original projection (image B) would show by its shape that the foreign body was a bullet.

The radiographs of a dried femur, Figure 111, further demonstrate the value of two opposing projections. In radiograph A, a portion of the image appears abnormal. When viewed at right angles, it may be seen in radiograph B that the ends of the bone are not united but are quite distant to each other, yet their ends were projected so that their images were superimposed.

SUMMARY

The ultimate in image sharpness is not absolutely necessary, because visualization of most images is facilitated by appropriate contrast. However, to attain the best in geometric projection of body parts, the following recommendations should be observed.

1. As small a focal spot as possible should be employed, consistent with the safety limits of the electrical load on the x-ray tube.
2. The focus-film distance should be as long as possible within practical working limits.
3. The object-film distance should be minimal.
4. The central ray should pass through the center of the part and perpendicular to its major planes and that of the film.
5. Movement of the patient should be controlled by immobilization and short exposures.
6. Intensifying screens should be in good contact with the film.
7. The patient should be correctly posed.

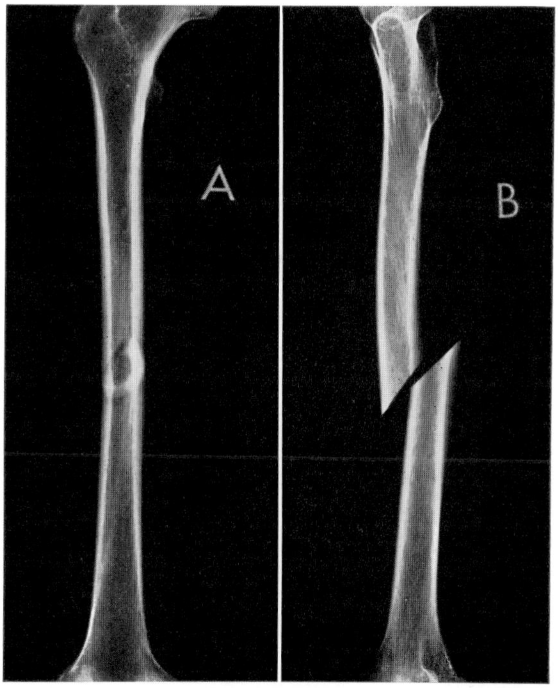

Figure 111. Two radiographs of a dried femur, one made with anteroposterior (A) and lateral (B) projections to determine true relationships of the fracture.

Chapter 14

X-Ray Intensifying Screens

X-RAY INTENSIFYING screens are radiographically indispensable. Although they introduce some measure of detail unsharpness in the image, their value in radically shortening exposures and reducing motion unsharpness is of prime importance. Less than 1 per cent of the x-rays striking an x-ray film is absorbed by the emulsion to expose it; the balance fails to perform any useful radiographic work. The absorption of the x-rays by the emulsion primarily governs the formation of the latent image. It is obvious, therefore, that a means for fully utilizing this small percentage of energy, without complicating the technical procedure, is desirable. This may be accomplished by the use of x-ray intensifying screens that serve to increase the effect of the x-radiation on the sensitized emulsion by means of fluorescence, thereby reducing the exposure. Certain chemicals have the ability to absorb x-rays and instantaneously emit light. This property is called *fluorescence.*

HISTORICAL

Fluorescence was first systematically studied by Sir George Gabriel Stokes of Cambridge, England, in 1852. He showed that a large number of solid bodies and solutions possess the power of absorbing light of various wave lengths and then transforming and emitting them in such a manner that an increase in the wave length occurs. For example, a solution of quinine sulphate was found to absorb ultraviolet rays and then emit them as visible blue rays. Also, an alcoholic solution of chlorophyl would absorb yellow rays and emit red light; the principle being that the emitted ray is of greater wave length, hence lower in the spectrum than the absorbed or exciting ray. As might naturally be expected—and which later proved to be true in Röntgen's discovery—the extremely short wave length of the rays above the visible violet of the spectrum caused them to be absorbed by most fluorescent bodies and to be emitted as rays of longer wave length so that they became visible. Stokes applied this principle in other experiments by employing a sheet of paper coated with a paint made from pulverized crystals of barium platinocyanide —another fluorescent chemical. There were a number of other investigations conducted with fluorescent materials from this time up to discovery of the x-rays, but little knowledge was added to the discoveries made by Stokes.

FLUORESCENCE

At the time of his discovery, Röntgen was searching for light rays beyond the visible spectrum, and the nature of the experiment which he was making at the time with low-pressure discharge tubes in a darkened room led him to cover the tube completely with black paper. When the tube was excited, he noticed that a barium platinocyanide fluorescent screen lying on a table a few feet away glowed brightly. The covered discharge tube precluded any possibility of the effect being due to ordinary or ultraviolet light, and he reasoned that there must be some strange radiation emanating from the tube. Objects that were interposed between the energized tube and the screen caused images to appear. Since this strange light caused the screen to fluoresce, it became possible to photograph and record the images. Röntgen then made those first radiographs, which have become very familiar to us.

Development of Fluorescent Chemicals

Röntgen's discovery of x-rays by means of the fluorescent screen served as a new means to further intensive research in the study of fluorescent compounds. In fact, subsequent experimental work with x-rays and various fluorescent crystals finally led Becquerel to the discovery that uranium or its compounds constantly emitted radiations which were very similar to x-rays in that they penetrated opaque objects, ionized gases, and also caused fluorescence. Thus was acquired the knowledge of the phenomenon of radioactivity which ultimately led to the isolation of a new element—radium—by the Curies.

To understand more fully the development of the fluoroscopic and intensifying screen, some knowledge relative to the modern conception of fluorescent compounds is necessary.

Edison's Work

In the period, January to March, 1896, Thomas Alva Edison ambitiously tested some 8,500 different materials in his efforts to build a new incandescent lamp. Finally, from among 1,800 which fluoresced, he discovered that the fluorescence of calcium tungstate crystals has approximately six times more intensity than barium platinocyanide. He then recommended the use of this salt for x-ray fluoroscopic screens in March of 1896. Edison prepared his calcium tungstate screens by mixing the crystals with collodion and spreading a thick layer upon paper; later, cardboard was employed, and on occasion, thin sheets of aluminum.

FIRST USE OF INTENSIFYING SCREENS

At the time of the discovery of x-rays, Professor Michael Pupin of Columbia Uni-

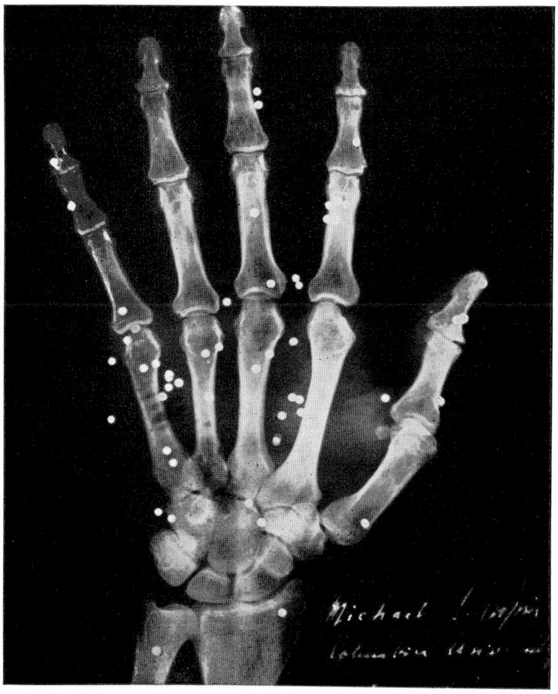

Figure 112. First radiograph of the hand made (1896) by Professor Michael Pupin with a fluorescent screen to enhance the x-ray exposure.

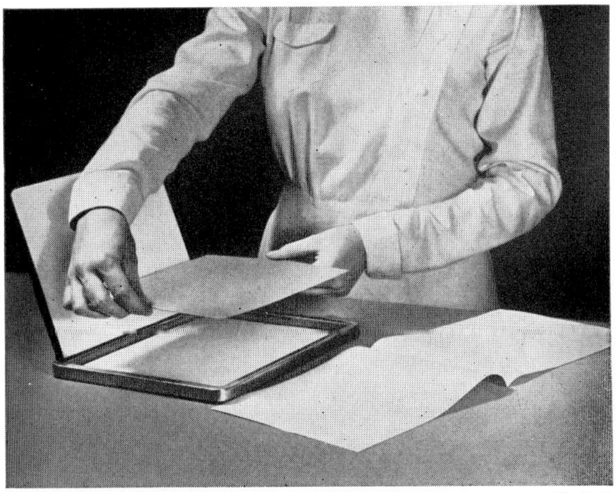

Kodak

Figure 113. Photograph of an x-ray cassette containing two intensifying screens into which an x-ray film is being correctly placed.

versity had been keenly interested in the work conducted in Germany on discharge-tube phenomena; consequently he was one of the few persons in 1896 who had any equipment adequate to produce x-rays. Pupin immediately began to study these rays and accomplished a tremendous amount of experimental work. In addition, a large number of patients were sent to him for examination by the local physicians. The exposures necessary for him to employ were very long and he made every effort to increase the efficiency of his apparatus so that he could shorten the exposure. This he accomplished in February of 1896 by sandwiching together a photographic plate and a fluorescent screen that Thomas Edison had sent to him. He then made an exposure of a hand in a few seconds that formerly had required an hour's exposure. A large number of buckshot were revealed in the image, Figure 112. Subsequent improvement in fluorescing power of the fluoroscopic screen by Edison, and its application to radiography by Pupin, meant much to radiology, for it made possible shorter exposures and consequently increased the life of those fragile, unstable x-ray tubes then in use.

SCREEN CHARACTERISTICS

The compound that is most commonly employed today in intensifying screens is the crystalline salt, calcium tungstate, because of its effectiveness as a fluorescent agent and its general advantages in manufacture and use. It is finely powdered, mixed with a suitable binder, and coated in a thin, smooth layer on a special cardboard or plastic support to form the screen. The fluorescence of calcium tungstate crystals is confined to the violet and near-ultraviolet region of the spectrum, and x-ray film is most sensitive to this type of light.

MODE OF USE

When intensifying screens are employed, the double-coated x-ray film is placed between the active faces of the two screens, Figure 113, which absorb the x-ray energy and then fluoresce. When the film is exposed to x-rays, it receives not alone an x-ray exposure but also a photographic one from the fluorescent light of both screens. This combined action serves to produce the required radiographic density. Almost the entire effect of the x-radiation on the film is caused by the fluorescent light of the screens and relatively short exposures become practicable.

TYPES OF SCREENS

The three types of screens most widely employed in radiography are of three speeds: (1) *slow;* (2) *average-speed,* and (3) *fast.* The slow type is used where sharpness of definition is of first importance at some expense to exposure time. The average-speed screens are valuable where good definition is obtained with shorter exposure. The fast screens are designed for situations wherein shortness of exposure is of prime importance at some sacrifice in image sharpness.

Crystal Size Versus Speed

The size of the calcium tungstate crystals in a screen and the thickness of the fluorescent layer determine its speed and the sharpness of definition. *Small* crystals in thin layers are employed in slow screens to attain maximum sharpness in definition. The average-speed screen possessing slightly larger crystals provides an image with intermediate sharpness in definition. The fast screens provide for maximum practical speed that modern screens possess. Large crystals are used in these screens and some sharpness of detail is sacrificed to effect a gain in speed. When employing the higher kilovoltages, the slow and average-speed screens provide excellent detail sharpness and the exposure times are well within the range of capabilities of all apparatus. The effect of screen-crystal size on sharpness of definition is diagrammatically shown in Figure 114. In this diagram, a large crystal is shown (A) being activated by x-rays and the fluorescence is brilliant and extensive. Although more of the silver emulsion is exposed, some sharpness of definition is lost because the fluorescence extends across detail boundaries. In B, the fluorescence of the small crystal is less, but the sharpness in definition is improved.

The light emission of screens is widely influenced by change in x-ray wave length. As the wave length decreases, emission increases, i.e., as kilovoltage increases, intensity of fluorescence increases. The speed of screens as compared to film speed varies between 1:20 and 1:30, depending upon the crystal size of the fluorescent salt. Screen speed varies in small degree from one screen of given speed to another. It is contingent upon the care given the screen and its manufacture. It cannot be expected to possess a constant speed because exposure conditions dictate its performance. With kilovoltages around 50, the speed factor is low; whereas at 80 to 90 KvP, it is high. The average-speed screen in the 65 KvP region is about 5 KvP faster than the slow type. Fast screens are 5 KvP faster than the average-speed screen in this region.

Screen Thickness

Modern intensifying screens are made in two thicknesses: (1) The front screen is thin so that the x-rays can more readily pass through it. The front screen, there-

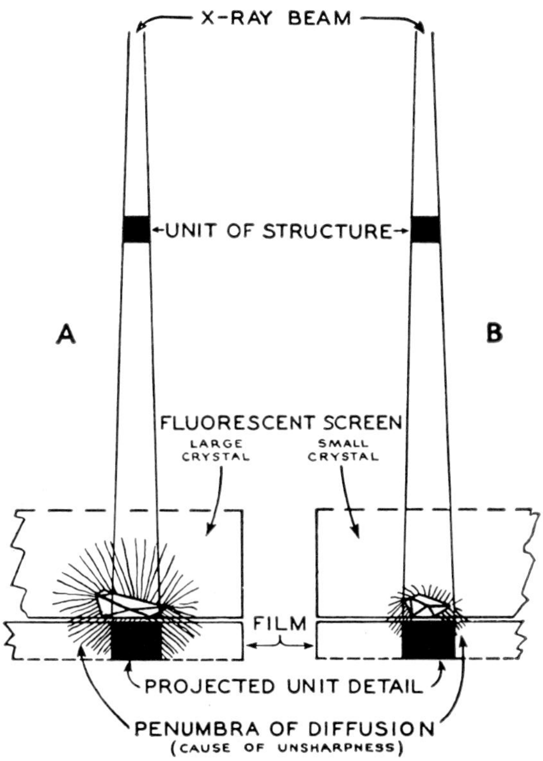

Figure 114. Diagrams illustrating the radiographic effect on image sharpness: A, using screens with large crystals, lessens image sharpness; B, using screens with small crystals, increases image sharpness.

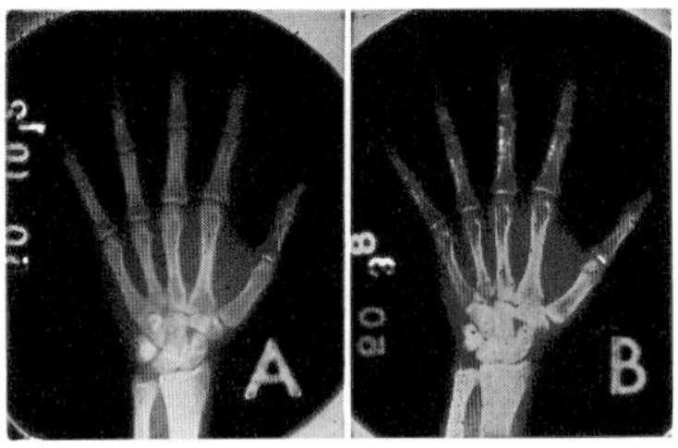

Figure 115. Radiographs of the hand to show lower contrast obtained upon direct exposure (A) and higher contrast when screens are used (B), when employing screen-type film and 50 KvP.

fore, emits less fluorescent light because fewer crystals absorb only a small amount of radiation. (2) The back screen is about twice the thickness of the front screen so that a larger percentage of radiation can be absorbed resulting in a larger amount of fluorescent light. In general, the thicker the screen, the greater the speed and the poorer the definition.

Screen Contrast

Screen radiography produces higher contrast in the image than can be attained by direct exposure when using the same kilovoltage. The higher contrast is a characteristic response of the emulsion to the fluorescent screen light. Also, the front screen tends to absorb some of the longer wave length secondary radiation emitted by the patient, thereby reducing the level of fog on the image. However, the contrast scale may readily be lengthened by increasing the kilovoltage, which also tends to increase the speed of the screen-film combination. By the use of the higher contrast and shorter exposures, there is less opportunity for details of low contrast being "blurred away" by motion unsharpness; for example, the kidney contours may be easily blurred into the background densities when a patient breathes. A comparison between contrasts produced on direct exposure (A) and on screen exposure (B) employing 50 KvP is shown in Figure 115.

Screen Lag

As previously mentioned, the property of fluorescence in a substance is its ability to emit radiation of one quality when stimulated by radiation of another quality. A common example is the luminous paint employed on instrument dials to render them visible in darkness. Such paints are excited by tiny quantities of radioactive material included in a paint mixture consisting usually of zinc sulfide or a sulfide of some other metal. *Phosphorescence,* however, is another phenomenon comparable to fluorescence. In a fluorescent material, the glow of light only takes place as long as the substance is excited by radiation. In a phosphorescent chemical, the glow continues for an appreciable period *after* the exciting radiation is cut off. A typical example is the action of x-rays on an intensifying screen showing screen lag or afterglow. In such an example, the glow of light continues after the x-rays are turned off. When screen lag is present, the technician cannot reload his cassette immediately for an image made by the previous exposure would be recorded on a fresh unexposed film. The second radiograph might contain two images if the afterglow from the first exposure was sufficiently strong in intensity. It is possible for an afterglow to remain for months after exposure if the screen is of poor quality. Fortunately, the rigid production controls employed in the manufacture of modern screens precludes the use of fluorescent chemicals that exhibit phosphorescence. In good-quality screens, the intensity of fluorescence must rapidly reach its peak as the x-rays strike the crystals and should cease immediately upon termination of the exposure.

A test for persistent screen phosphorescence (test for screen lag) may be made by exposing the lower lumbar vertebral area laterally with 85 KvP and an appropriate MaS value at an FFD of 36 inches. The exposed film is removed from the cassette and replaced by another film. The second film is left in the cassette for 10 to 15 minutes, and then processed. If no image is produced, the problem of phosphorescence does not exist with respect to the screens tested.

Influence of Temperature

The fluorescent property of screens excited by x-rays decreases as the temperature increases. At 95° F. screens emit less fluorescent light than at 70° F. One might assume that this fact is important radiographically. Actually, it is not, for the x-ray sensitivity of the x-ray film used with screens increases with the temperature. Since film and screens are used in combination at a given temperature, the screen effect balances the film effect and there is no need to observe the differences from a practical radiographic standpoint.

SCREENS VERSUS UNSHARPNESS

Loss in image sharpness always ensues when screens are employed, because the fluorescent light diffuses across image boundaries within the body of the screen itself. No matter how fine a crystal is used in screens, its fineness does not compare with that of the film emulsion crystals. Any radiograph made with screens cannot compare favorably as to detail sharpness with a radiograph made without screens. However, when screens are not used, patient movement may occur during the longer exposure times required whether the part is immobilized or not. However, the amount of unsharpness that may accrue for this reason is so insignificant that it should not deter one from doing radiography of the smaller parts of the body without screens. Screens should always be employed whenever there is a possibility of movement, and the exposure time should be as small as possible.

SCREEN-FILM CONTACT

Close contact between the active surfaces of the screens and the emulsion surfaces of the film is essential so that sharpness of detail will not be impaired. Poor or uneven contact allows the fluorescent light to spread and produce blurring of the image. For that reason each pair of screens is placed in a rigid holder (cassette) so that they will be in direct contact with the film. The effect of poor screen-film contact is shown in Figure 116. The fluorescent light spreads in all directions in the space between the film and the screens resulting in image unsharpness.

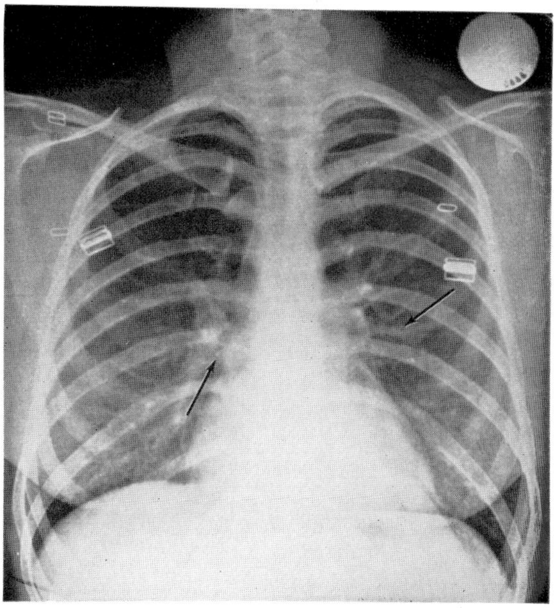

Figure 116. Radiograph of chest made with a cassette that provided poor screen-film contact resulting in image unsharpness.

CARE OF SCREENS

As screens influence the quality of the radiograph, their proper care is important. The fluorescent light emitted by intensifying screens obeys the laws of light, and any foreign matter on a screen will absorb light during the exposure and cause objectionable marks in the radiograph. Consequently, bits of paper, lint, and dust should be carefully removed and dirt and stains should never be allowed to remain on the surfaces of the screens. To avoid scratches and finger marks, the active surfaces should not be touched or handled except in washing. Cassettes may be stored in the processing room, but they should be kept at a safe distance from chemicals and all other possible sources of contamination or damage. Developer stains cannot be removed from screens. Therefore, as a safeguard, handle cassettes on the "dry side" of the processing room. They should be kept closed when not in use.

SUMMARY

Calcium tungstate screens were first developed by Thomas Alva Edison (1896). The first radiograph made with fluorescent screens was produced by Professor Michael Pupin in February, 1896.

The advantages of x-ray intensifying screens in radiography are:

1. They provide means for short exposures.
2. They make possible the use of small focal-spot tubes.
3. They reduce possibility of motion unsharpness.
4. They increase contrast.
5. Density increases more rapidly with screen exposures than with direct exposures.

The disadvantages of screens in radiography are:

1. They increase image unsharpness.
2. The image of the screen-crystal pattern is more noticeable as the kilovoltage is increased.

Chapter 15

Standardization of Exposure

THE FUNDAMENTALS of exposure are easy to understand and there seems to be no reason why they should be made complicated. It must be realized that the radiologist is not so much interested in the occasional "beautiful" radiograph—or poor one—as he is with *uniform* radiographic quality. Such uniformity from day to day and year to year can only be achieved through complete control and standardization of exposure and processing procedures. The *appearance* of the radiographic images should always be fairly consistent. The busy radiologist should not be obliged to interpret radiographs made with a particular projection in which the image of a body part is seldom twice alike. The apparatus, x-ray tube, x-ray film, and processing chemicals have been scientifically designed so that radiographic standardization may be more readily employed to produce radiographs from which the radiologist can make competent interpretations.

The common lack of unanimity on the subject of radiographic exposure is aptly demonstrated by the numerous recipes advanced in the form of complicated exposure tables. The lack of a systematic and workable exposure method becomes readily apparent when it is necessary to train a student in radiographic exposure.

Standardized projections of an anatomic part portray the structures always in the same manner. It has been demonstrated repeatedly that an essential point in the radiographic diagnosis often appears in an inconspicuous portion of the image. Therefore, a systematic analysis and evaluation of the *entire* image should always be made. This requires that the entire image should be diagnostically informative and that translucent silver deposits representative of the anatomic structures always be produced.

RADIOGRAPHIC QUALITY

Radiographic quality should be evaluated along realistic lines rather than upon the emotional response of the individual observer to the image. Quality results when sound judgment is employed in the selection of the exposure factors and in the manner in which the exposed x-ray film is processed. Also, there should exist a balance in compromise between the exposure factors employed, the clinical situation as it is presented to the technician, and the objective of the examination—the diagnosis. When a radiologist views a good radiograph, he is not particularly interested in how it was produced. But, if the quality is not what he should reasonably expect, then the *practical* reasons for failure should be recognized and investigated.

CRITERIA

The following criteria for attaining satisfactory radiographic quality may serve as a guide to better radiography.

1. All image densities should be *translucent* when viewed before a conventional x-ray illuminator.
2. All portions of the image should have silver deposit. Areas devoid of silver deposit are diagnostically useless. Excessive silver deposits should be avoided for they obscure detail and also are diagnostically useless.
3. The part examined should be fully penetrated.
4. The *basic MaS* factor should be selected so as to provide the best over-all radiographic density for the patient whose measurement is within the *average* thickness range.
5. Contrast should be such that differentiation between densities or details can be readily made.
6. Image details should not be obscured by secondary radiation or chemical fog.
7. Maximum sharpness and true shape of the image should be consistent with the clinical needs of the examination.

Image Should Represent Anatomic Situation

In making his interpretation, the radiologist must be confident that the radiographic image represents the true anatomic situation. His knowledge of the normal appearance of anatomic structures in the image and his visual acuity in noting deviations from the normal are the tools which he uses in making his interpretation. But he needs translucent *silver* on the film to do it. Images that merely depict the size, shape, or outline of the desired object are not satisfactory. The image must be composed of a multitude of gray tones that make for differentiation of detail. However, there is a limit to the number of tones necessary to produce a good image, because differentiation between densities becomes extremely difficult when the contrast scale is unduly lengthened.

Contrast Extremes

The extremes of the contrast scale in a radiograph — opacity and transparency — cannot reveal all the details of a radiographic image. It is necessary to have a large number of intermediate tones or shades of gray in the middle of the scale for this purpose. In other words, there should be a good balance of densities to satisfy diagnostic requirements. Unfortunately, many technicians have not been trained to recognize the importance of the gray tones in an image, but they are attracted toward the brilliant images in which the heavier silver deposits are more distinctive. It is only through the recognition of the value of long-scale contrast for a given image or projection that faults or errors in the application of exposure factors can be corrected.

Contrast and Sharpness

Image contrast and sharpness are the basic factors in detail visibility. It is desirable to record with sufficient contrast slight variations in radiographic density of all details within the part examined and to show small differences over a wide range of tissue thicknesses in the same exposure. If *all* radiographic densities are *translucent,* there is, then, image representation of all tissue details because all elements within the part have been penetrated. It is most necessary that the scale of existing contrast not be shortened beyond the point where essential detail, when viewed before an x-ray illuminator, begins to be lost to the eye in the higher and lower densities of the radiograph; it is preferable to stop short of this limit so as to have sufficient latitude to allow for unavoidable density deviations that may occur because of unusual or unpredictable tissue absorption. As a rule, improvements in detail visibility of some body parts can be effected by increasing the contrast within limits. However, certain restrictions as to over-all detail visibility are imposed. On occasion, small areas of image detail are rendered brightly visible because the exposure factors may be optimum for the region. However, adjacent areas may be devoid of sufficient silver to produce a satisfactory over-all image because the radiation did not penetrate all the tissues. Except for special cases, it is best to be satisfied with a lower image contrast and assured penetration that will reveal details in the over-all image. The greater number of densities provided by long-scale contrast makes possible the visualization of a larger number of tissue components.

VALUE OF TOTAL IMPRESSION

Our eyes cannot always distinguish image details by contrast or sharpness alone. In reality, it is the *total* impression of the product of these two factors that makes this possible. Two radiographs of the chest may be made, Figure 117, one (A) with long-wave length x-rays (50 KvP), the other (B) with short-wave length x-rays (80 KvP). Owing to the shorter exposure time for radiograph B, it

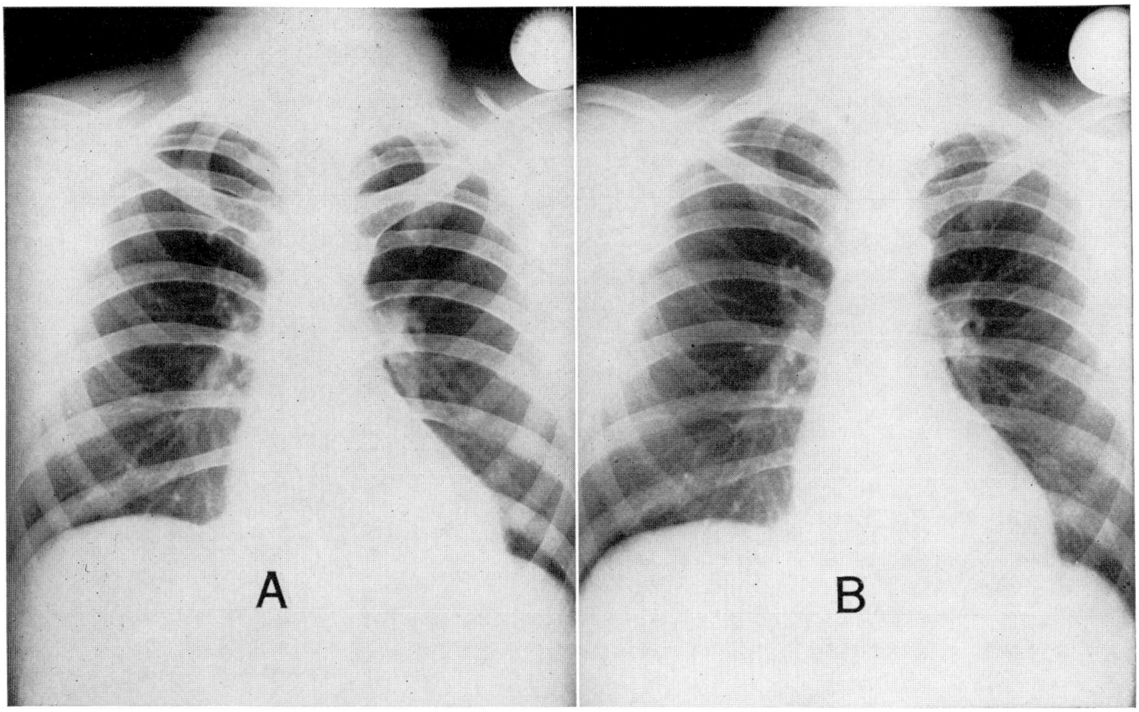

Figure 117. Posteroanterior chest screen radiographs: Radiograph A made with 50 KvP and radiograph B, with 80 KvP. Factors: A, 20 MaS, 72-inch FFD; B, 3.3 MaS, 72-inch FFD. Note wide differences in contrast between radiographs.

will be sharper than radiograph A and will possess a wider range of densities. It may happen, however, that the high contrast of radiograph A may create the impression of greater sharpness because of the exaggerated density values. This optical peculiarity is usually submerged when all radiographs are made carefully, since the evaluation of an x-ray image is dependent upon the distinctness of all the recognizable detail and not on the contrast alone or the sharpness alone. In the examination of unsatisfactory radiographs, these two qualities must be carefully evaluated. Generally, it is easier to correct unsatisfactory image sharpness by greater contrast, rather than the opposite; but one should not go too far in this direction. In many laboratories, unfortunately, sharpness is often neglected in striving for higher radiographic contrast with resultant lack of tissue penetration.

VIEWING RADIOGRAPHS

A radiograph is only as good as its illumination. The manner in which radiographs are viewed is as important to the technician as it is to the radiologist. Radiographs are made with translucent densities of varying tone value and details only become visible when they are transilluminated by light of conventional color and intensity.

THE ILLUMINATOR

The modern illuminator is designed for viewing radiographs up to 14 x 17 inches in size and consists of two fluorescent tubes suitably mounted in a reflecting box and behind opal diffusing glass. The quality and quantity of light transmitted through the radiograph by the illuminator determines the diagnostic worth of the image. The technician should provide a standard level of density that is translucent when the radiograph is viewed on the illuminator. The radiologist should view the radiographs on an illuminator that provides comparable color and intensity. To maintain the same quality and intensity of light, the illuminator should be cleaned regularly and old fluorescent tubes should be replaced.

To obtain the best transmission of illuminator light through a radiograph, all light that might pass *around* the radiograph should be blocked out. For example, when an 8 x 10-inch or a 10 x 12-inch radiograph is viewed on a 14 x 17-inch illuminator, a mask should be used with an aperture cut to suit the size of the film being viewed. If this is not done, the density of the radiograph appears greater than it actually is. In fact, it may appear fogged. The phenomenon may be demonstrated by a simple experiment, Figure 118. Two gray squares are shown: the square at the left is surrounded by a black mask and the other at the right is located in a white field. The gray square on the right looks darker than the one on the left, yet both squares have identical reflectances that may be verified by placing a black mask around the square on the right. The former situation simulates the conditions existing when a radiograph is masked on the illuminator; the latter represents the conditions existing when a mask is not used. The extraneous light causes the pupils of the eyes to contract so that it is more difficult for the eye to accommodate to the light that passes through the radiographic image.

LEVEL OF ROOM ILLUMINATION

When radiographs are being read, the level of general illumination in the viewing room should be sufficiently low so that extraneous light is not reflected from the surfaces of the radiographs, thus lessening the brightness of image details.

EVOLVING THE EXPOSURE SYSTEM

The foregoing chapters have described in detail the functions of x-ray exposure factors. From this material may be summarized essential features that can serve as a basis for formulating a standardized exposure system. The ideal should establish all factors as constants with the exception of one to be employed as a variable. Hence, kilovoltage should be regarded as the factor of penetration, exposure latitude and radiographic contrast; milliampere-seconds as the factor of radiographic density; and the focus-film and object-film distances as geometric factors influencing image sharpness, shape, and size. Thus, standardization of radiography resolves itself into four phases.

1. Standardization of Exposure Factors. The reduction of all exposure factors in a given projection to constants with the exception of one variable (MaS).

2. Standardization of Radiography. Standardization of radiography requires its division into three major classes:

a. *Direct*-exposure technics.
b. *Screen*-exposure technics.
c. *Screen-grid* exposure technics.

3. Standarization of Projections. A standard method for posing the patient and projection of the central ray for a given projection.

4. Standardization of the Processing Procedure. The reduction of time and temperature values to constants so that changes in radiographic density can more properly be attributed to exposure.

OPTIMUM KILOVOLTAGE TECHNIC

The bulk of modern radiography is "production-line" effort. A standardized system for selecting and applying exposure factors therefore becomes a necessity. Such a system, however, must produce consistently good radiographic quality. The optimum kilovoltage technic satisfies these requirements. This technic was evolved to eliminate many complexities in the application of exposure factors and reduce them to simplicities. Specifically, it is based upon standardization of the processing procedure and the reduction of exposure factors to constants with the exception of one variable. The technic is based on the following general principles. By trial, a fixed or optimum kilovoltage is established for an average tissue thickness range and for a given projection. Once it has been found that the kiolovoltage selected produces the most desirable amount of penetration and contrast for the given human part, irrespective of size, it is established as a constant. A basic MaS value is then decided upon that will produce the required amount of radiographic density within the average range. When a patient is classified as outside the average thickness range—smaller or larger—the basic MaS value is halved or doubled, respectively. This is the initial operation, since further refinement in the MaS may, on occasion, be necessary and desirable. All other factors, including processing, are constants.

TECHNIC

In working out an optimum kilovoltage technic, each projection must be considered individually. It must be understood that for a given thickness of a particular body part, the wave length of the x-rays employed to penetrate the tissues must be adequate or, in other words, *optimum*. The amount and kind of tissue—the relation of bone to soft tissue—and its penetrability by x-radiation must be evaluated.

TABLE IX

TABLE LISTING AVERAGE THICKNESS RANGES FOR VARIOUS PROJECTIONS AND THE FREQUENCY WITH WHICH THE ADULT PATIENT DIMENSIONS FALL INTO EACH AVERAGE RANGE

Region	*Average Thickness Adult—Cms.*			*Per Cent Frequency*
	AP	*PA*	*LAT*	
Thumb, fingers, toes	1.5–4			99
Hand	3–5			99
			7–10	93
Wrist	3–6			99
			5–8	98
Forearm	6–8			94
			7–9	92
Elbow	6–8			96
			7–9	87
Arm	7–10			95
			7–10	94
Shoulder	12–16			79
Clavicle		13–17		82
Foot	6–8			92
			7–9	91
Ankle	8–10			86
			6–9	96
Leg	10–12			85
			9–11	89
Knee	10–13			92
			9–12	92
Thigh	14–17			77
			13–16	76
Hip	17–21			76
Cervical C1-3	12–14			77
Vertebrae C4-7	11–14			98
C1-7			10–13	90
Thoracic	20–24			76
Vertebrae			28–32	81
Lumbar	18–22			69
Vertebrae			27–32	77
Pelvis	19–23			78
Skull		18–21		96
			14–17	88
Sinuses Frontal		18–21		97
Maxillary		18–22		88
			13–17	96
Mandible			10–12	82
		20–25		82
Chest	OBL		27–32	84
	24–30			83

Measurement of the part must be made along the course traversed through the tissues by the central ray, and the average range of measurements verified by checking many individuals. On the basis of this information, a kilovoltage is selected that will thoroughly penetrate the part, irrespective of size, and produce a satisfactory contrast. Once established as optimum for the projection, it should not be changed unless the conditions under which the KvP was established are changed.

With the KvP fixed, a basic MaS or density value must be established for the average thickness range of the part. In deriving MaS values for thicknesses outside the average range or for variations in the physiologic or pathologic state of the tissues, the rule of thumb for density changes by MaS is employed. The focus-film distance need seldom be changed and may, in most cases, be considered a constant.

When the wave length is optimum, a lower MaS value is usually more adequate for the exposure than that habitually employed for the same purpose with the lower kilovoltages. Less MaS, of course, permits a greater number of radiographs to be made in a given projection before the limit of radiation safety is reached. The over-all radiographic density produced by this method is uniform from case to case—a point of considerable diagnostic value because any differences from the normal density may then be attributed to abnormal changes within the tissues. Duplication of results is easy to attain in follow-up cases. The technic may be employed with any type of rectified or self-rectified apparatus. Whatever the type of generator, the only variable factor to adjust is the MaS; all other factors are constant.

Role of Thickness Ranges

Average thickness ranges are actually guides for establishing basic MaS values for various projections since approximately 85 per cent of all patients fall within these ranges. However, thickness ranges have been established for a number of projection shown in Table IX. The approximate frequency in percentage with which these thicknesses appear is also listed.

Rules for Application

The successful operation of the optimum kilovoltage technic is dependent upon a rigid acceptance and application of the following facts, which should be reviewed at this point. When all other exposure factors remain constant, the functions of the factors listed below operate in the manner described.

1. *Focus-film distance (FFD).*
   a. Influences the *sharpness* and *magnification* of the radiographic image.
   b. Influences radiographic *density.*
2. *Kilovoltage (KvP).*
   a. Regulates *wave length* of radiation.
   b. Determines degree of *penetration* of tissues.
   c. Influences production of *secondary radiation fog.*
   d. Regulates scale of radiographic *contrast.*
   e. Determines degree of exposure *latitude.*
   f. Influences radiographic *density.*
3. *Milliampere-seconds (MaS).*
   a. Regulates the *quantity* of x-radiation emitted by the x-ray tube.
   b. Regulates *radiographic density,* i.e., amount of black metallic silver deposited on the x-ray film.

SELECTION OF FACTORS

The selection of factors that influence the image should be based upon consideration of all aspects that might have an eventual effect on radiographic quality.

FOCAL SPOT

The focal spot should always be selected so that the maximum image sharpness is obtained assuming that the exposure factors to be used conform to the rated capacity of the x-ray tube.

CONES

Cones should be employed for all projections. Their size (diameter) should be such as to exactly cover the size of the film employed at a given focus-film distance. There are occasions when the cone size should conform to the size of the anatomical area being examined. For example, a certain cone might be suitable to cover an 8 x 10-inch film, but it would be inadequate for delineating a very small area, such as the mastoid process. A smaller cone, therefore, would need to be employed.

GRIDS

Stationary or moving grids are used in examining the heavier tissue parts. The technician should be familiar with grid ratios as well as the focus-film distances that can be used with the various grids. The higher the grid ratio, the greater the care that must be exercised in selecting the focus-film distance and in centering the tube to the grid and part to avoid "grid cutoff." For best results, conventional moving grids of 8 to 1 ratio should be used when employing optimum kilovoltages. The stationary grid of the Lysholm type is also a very useful accessory in many situations where it is impractical to employ a moving grid.

FOCUS-FILM DISTANCE

The focus-film distance should be chosen to produce the most realistic geometric image pattern with satisfactory sharpness of definition. Once the focus-film distance is selected for a specific projection, it should be established as a constant. The number of focus-film distances should be maintained at a minimum. If the distance must be changed for a given projection, the MaS can be adjusted so that the resulting radiographic density is approximately equal to the density obtained with the original focus-film distance by applying the MaS-FFD law (Table I).

KILOVOLTAGE

The variety of effects that may be produced on the radiographic image by kilovoltage makes it an important and influential exposure factor. Consequently, it should be closely controlled and established as a constant for a given projection. When a kilovoltage provides an acceptable contrast scale in a given projection of a normal part, that kilovoltage should be fixed. Thereafter, the images produced by a given projection will present the same relative scale of contrast.

The Optimum Kilovoltage

When an x-ray beam is capable of penetrating all segments of interest of a specific body part irrespective of its thickness, the wave length of the x-rays is said to be *optimum*. Since the higher kilovoltages assure more complete penetration of tissues, they provide a wider range of densities, hence, greater exposure latitude, shorter exposures, and less heating of the x-ray tube. The kilovoltage selected should provide radiation that is transmitted through the part. This is the only radiation that is useful in making a radiograph; the radiation that is absorbed by the patient is useless radiographically. In practice, an excess of kilovoltage is often used to "make sure" that the part is fully penetrated. This is unnecessary since in every projection there is a limit to the amount of kilovoltage that can be employed and still maintain good radiographic quality. Invariably, such overexposure results in attempts to "sight" develop the film at the final expense of quality. In either case, the excess of secondary radiation fog will degrade image contrast.

When an optimum kilovoltage is to be selected for projection of a body part, the part must be considered as an entity. The thickness and density of the tissue, the proportionate relation of bone to soft tissue in the normal adult and its relative absorption properties must be evaluated. Once an optimum kilovoltage is established as a constant for each projection, it is remarkable how few kilovoltages are needed to adequately radiograph the many parts of the body. Also, using kilovoltage as a constant to establish contrast places the burden of providing sufficient silver in the image for diagnostic purposes upon the MaS. The use of optimum kilovoltages has the advantage of making a group of exposure factors relatively insensitive to the absorption values of different tissue components. Employing the principles advocated in these pages, kilovoltages for other projections may be easily made.

Illustrated in Figures 127-129 are groups of unretouched radiographs in which, for the respective projections, the exposure factors were identical since the thicknesses of the parts in each case were within the average range. Note the uniformity in density and contrast manifested in each group.

Change in Kilovoltage

Once the kilovoltage has been established as a constant for a given projection, it is not changed so long as the conditions upon which it was established remain the same. When these conditions are changed, then the kilovoltage may require change (Tables III and IV); but after the change is made, the kilovoltage then becomes a constant for the new projection.

SELECTION OF BASIC MaS

The MaS factor is the most reliable factor for regulating the *amount* of over-all silver (density) in the image. There should be a satisfactory range of densities for interpretations of all portions of the image. The MaS can become a constant within certain limitations for a given projection. A *basic* MaS value can be established for any average thickness range of a part, provided it is established for an adult person.

Thickness Only a Guide

The thickness of any part serves only as a guide which the technician can use to expose the normal part and in determining what MaS will compensate for abnormal tissue changes. Obviously, if the part is normal and is in the average thickness range, the basic MaS can be employed. Knowledge of the structural makeup of the area is necessary when the kilovoltage has been fixed as a constant for the projection. The part should also be judged from a physiologic and pathologic standpoint as to whether it is reasonably normal. As previously mentioned, the normal thickness range need not be accurately determined in radiography by the experienced technician. All that is needed is a visual classification of the part as small, average, or large. For the *small* part, the basic MaS value is halved; for the *average* part, the basic MaS value is employed; and for the *large* part, the basic MaS value is doubled. By means of these modifications, the radiographic density obtained will be approximately correct. If not, a slight increase or decrease in the MaS value in exposing a second film should provide the most desirable density. However, it will be found that a "remake" is seldom required.

The first requirement in establishing a basic MaS is that the correct *quality* of radiation is selected for a given projection. The *quantity* of radiation then must be determined by making three initial radiographs of a part, *the thickness of which is approximately at the middle of the average thickness range* (see Table IX). In determining exposure factors for a given projection, the first radiograph should be made with the kilovoltage listed as optimum for the part (Tables XI-XV), and with an MaS value estimated to be correct. This value may be considered as X. The second radiograph is made with an MaS that is twice in value to that used for the first radiograph. This is 2X. The third radiograph is made with one-half the original MaS or ½X. All other factors are constant. The three radiographs are viewed on the illuminator and the density that is most appropriate for the part is chosen. Sometimes when using the above method, it may be found that none of the densities are exactly correct. However, one of the radiographs perhaps contains a density close to the one desired, so that another radiograph made with an appropriate change in the MaS will provide the required radiographic density and a more correct basic MaS value. The final MaS value is then used on several patients whose measurements fall within the average thickness range.

If the density level is satisfactory for measurements at the center and at the extremes of the range, this MaS value should be established as basic and employed for all patients measuring in the average range. Once the correct MaS is determined, it then becomes the basic value to be employed for all thicknesses in the aver-

TABLE X

LIST OF PHYSICAL CHARACTERISTICS OF THE PATIENTS WHOSE RADIOGRAPHS APPEAR IN FIGURE 119

Radio-graph	*Thick-ness (CM)*	*Sex*	*Age (Years)*	*Height (Inches)*	*Weight (Lbs.)*
A	17	F	20	65	105
B	18	F	24	63	110
C	19	F	29	60	101
D	20	F	22	63	107
E	21	M	61	67	135
F	22	F	21	58	132
G	23	F	24	60	123
H	24	M	60	68	165
I	25	M	34	63	130
J	26	M	60	67	173
K	27	M	55	67	199
L	28	M	36	70	206
M	29	M	60	69	193

age thickness range established for the projection. Departures from the basic MaS value should only be made when the influence of disease or trauma alters the absorption characteristics of the part, or when the speed characteristics of the x-ray film or screens change.

Example 1. In posteroanterior adult chest screen radiography, the average thickness range may be considered to be 20 to 25 centimeters. As shown in Table IX, this range of measurements represents those of about 82 per cent of patients. A basic MaS of 3.3 or 5, whichever is more suitable to the apparatus, may be employed when an optimum kilovoltage of 80 is used at a film-focus distance of 72 inches and with average-speed screens. In this projection the basic MaS (X) should be established for a normal healthy adult measuring 23 cm. (the middle thickness in the range). When the patient's measurement exceeds 25 centimeters, the MaS is doubled (2X), and when it is less than 20 centimeters, the MaS is halved, (½X). Projections that have relatively little variation from the average thickness range, such as a posteroanterior view of the chest, require refinement in application of the MaS values to those thicknesses in excess of or less than the average. These values are respectively 1½X MaS and ¾X MaS. To apply the rule of thumb would not provide good radiographic quality of these borderline thicknesses. A typical example of a standardized posteroanterior technic is shown in the unretouched radiographs, Figure 119. It is interesting to statistically evaluate in Table X the physical characteristics of the patients whose radiographs are shown in Figure 119.

Radiation that completely penetrates the part and produces a consistently uniform density and contrast is most important in applying a standardized technic. It becomes readily apparent that the characteristics of height, weight, or sex cannot *per se* be employed to determine the x-ray absorbing properties of the tissues being exposed.

Thickness Greater than Average

When a chest measurement is slightly greater than average, the only change that need be made in the factors is in the MaS. The increased thickness of the 26- and 27-centimeter chest only requires *more* radiation of the quality as produced with 80 KvP on chests within the average range. The kilovoltage is held constant since it has been predetermined that 80 KvP provides the necessary quality of radiation to penetrate any size adult chest within a reasonable range in the posteroanterior direction.

When a basic MaS (X) is given to a 26-centimeter chest, the radiographic density may be too low. When the MaS is raised to 2X, the density may be too great, largely because of secondary radiation fog. Consequently, a value should be employed which is one-half the difference between 2X and X, or 1½X. The density produced will then be comparable to that provided by X MaS on a 23-centimeter chest. The original contrast is maintained because the presence of secondary radiation fog has been maintained at an acceptable level. If the same procedure is followed for a 27-centimeter chest, a similar result will be obtained. Chests with a thickness of 28, 29, and 30 centimeters can be exposed with 2X MaS because the increase in thickness requires only an increase in MaS and not necessarily in KvP. It should be noted, however, that due to the gradual accumulations of secondary radiation fog, chests with thicknesses greater than 26 centimeters and greater will exhibit lower contrast. Chests exceeding 30 centimeters in thickness require an increase not only in MaS but also in kilovoltage to provide adequate penetration. The kilovoltage, therefore, should be raised to 100 to increase penetration and secondary radiation fog can be eliminated by the use of a stationary parallel grid—Lysholm type. Consequently, a new group of conditions must be set up just as if another projection is to be standardized, and a new basic MaS should be established to assure proper density. The same focus-film distance and screens should be employed.

Smaller Thicknesses

If the basic MaS is used for a 15-, 16-, or 17-centimeter chest, the density would be excessive. A satisfactory result can be obtained, however, by exposing with ½X MaS. To balance the densities for the 18- and 19-centimeter chests, ¾X MaS may be used. For chests that are in the range of 10 to 14 centimeters, ¼X MaS may be employed. For infants (less than 10 centimeters) ¼X MaS may be employed, but the kilovoltage should be reduced from 80 to 70 to provide the increase in contrast that may be needed for the chests of these young subjects. However, 80 KvP can still be employed with ⅛X MaS, if desired.

Figure 118. Demonstration of the effects of the transmission of light through and around a radiograph: (*Left*) square surrounded by a black mask; (*Right*) square located in a white field.

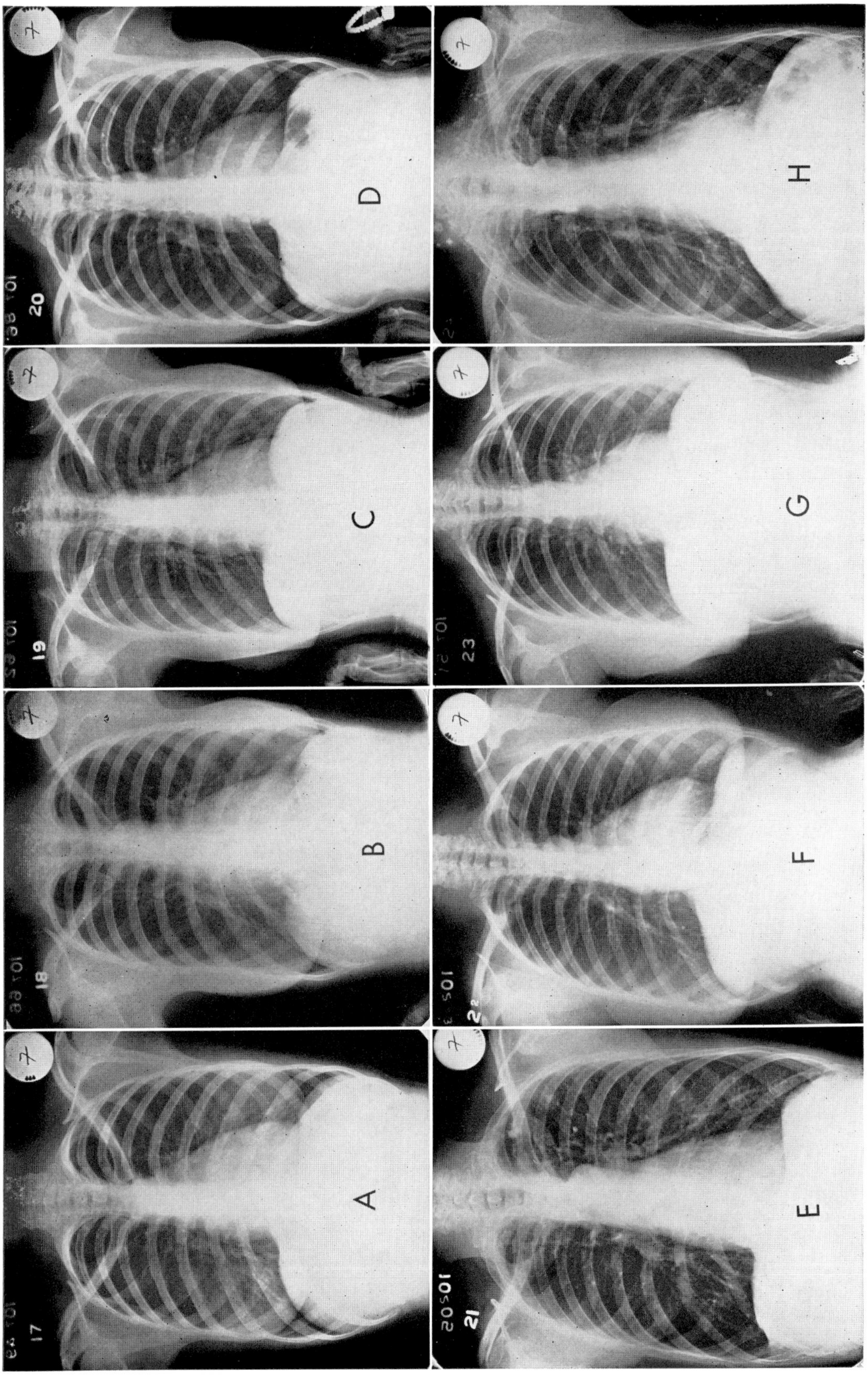

Figure 119. (*See legend on opposite page.*)

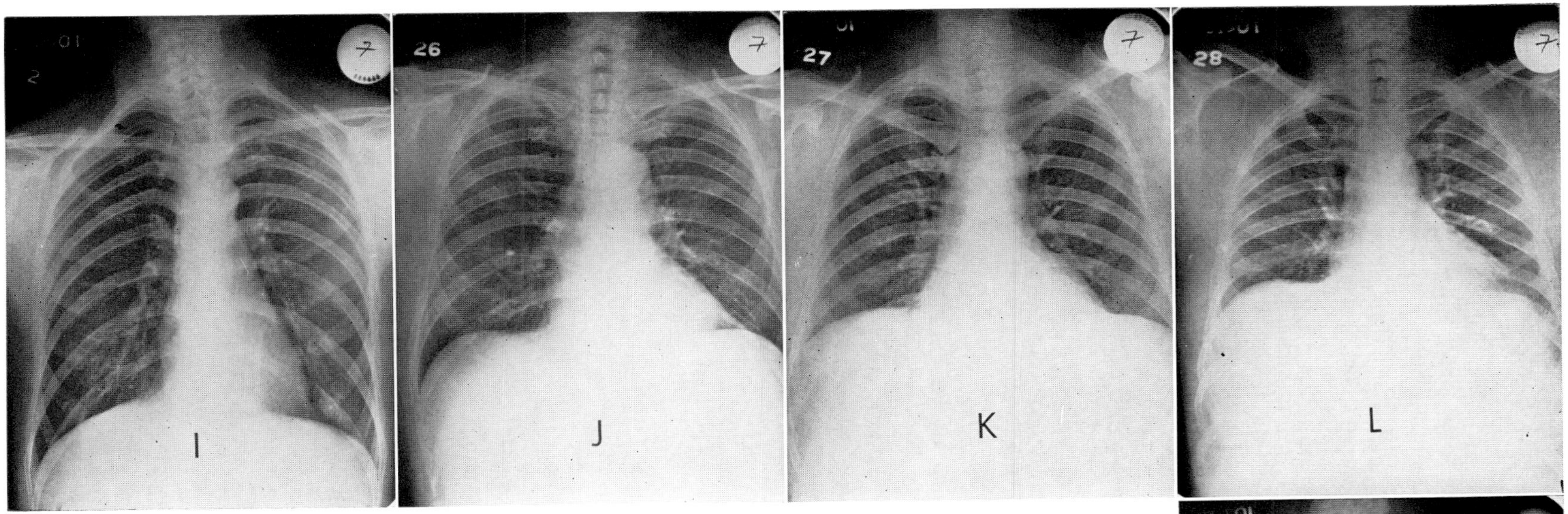

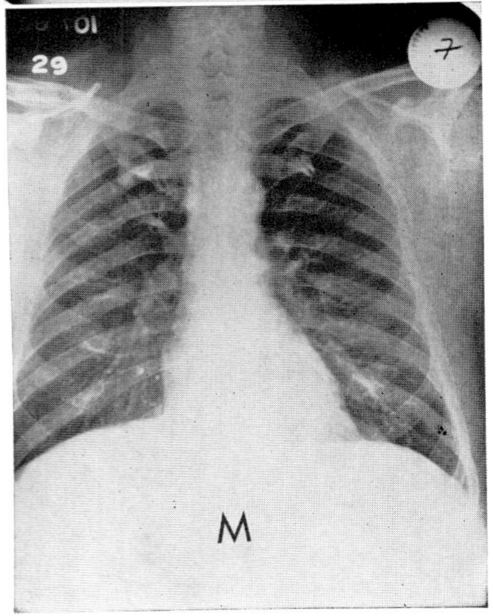

Constant factors				Thickness ranges	A* time	B* time
KvP	80	Cone	To cover area	–17 cm.	1/40 sec.	1/60 sec.
Ma	100	Film	Screen-type	18–19 cm.	1/30 sec.	1/40 sec.
FFD	72″			20–25 cm.	1/20 sec.	1/30 sec.
Screens	Average speed	Developer . . .	Rapid	26–27 cm.	1/15 sec.	1/20 sec.
Filtration . . .	Alum., 1 mm.	Development	5 min. at 68° F	28- cm.	1/10 sec.	1/15 sec.

(Variable Factors: Thickness ranges, A* time, B* time)

* To compensate differences in efficiency of x-ray output in various x-ray generators, it is necessary to establish by trial the time category (A or B) that will produce the desired *radiographic density*. In making the test radiographs, a subject with a 22-23 cm. chest should be radiographed, employing an exposure of 1/20 sec. (Column A). If the density is too great, then 1/30 sec. (Column B) may be used. The density of this second radiograph will usually be satisfactory; on this basis, the time values for the other thickness groups will be found in Column B. The chest radiographs reproduced on this spread were made with the time values listed under Column A.

Figure 119. A typical example of standardized posteroanterior chest technic.

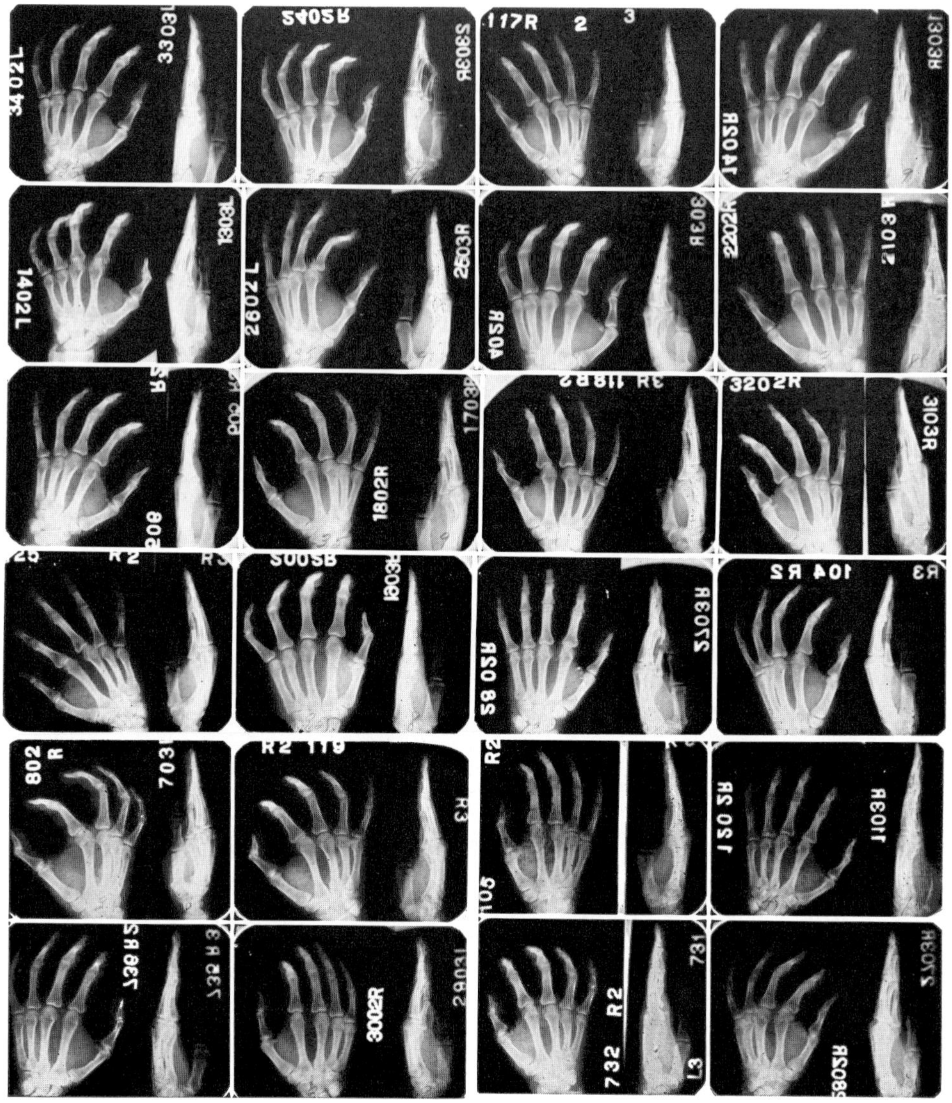

Figure 120. Posteroanterior-oblique and lateral direct-exposure radiographs (unretouched) of various thicknesses of hands that were exposed with identical exposure factors: KvP 50, MaS 50, FFD 36″. The lateral views were made with 80 MaS. Note uniformity of density and contrast.

Density Variations in Average Range

If one were to analyze a series of chest radiographs in the 20- to 25-centimeter range, it would be found that a few 20-centimeter chests possess a higher density than a 23-centimeter chest, and a few 25-centimeter chests have a small loss in density when compared to the 23-centimeter chest. These small differences in density are usually due to a variation in tissue absorption. When these densities are unsatisfactory, a second exposure should be made by employing the MaS value established for the next lower or higher thickness category.

Comment. The above method for changing density can be employed for all projections as long as it is accomplished in a systematic manner. It should be pointed out that *only one exposure factor should be changed at a time* when any exposure technic is to be altered. Changing two factors at a time introduces too many variables that are difficult to control.

OVEREXPOSURE

Overexposure is the most serious exposure fault occurring in the x-ray laboratory. It is often unrecognized that year in and year out the correct radiographic density is seldom obtained because of inattention to the appropriate application of exposure factors. Modern x-ray film, in combination with intensifying screens, is exceedingly fast, so that only relatively short exposures are required to produce radiographs of good quality. These facts are not always fully appreciated, and as a result, overexposure frequently occurs.

To the trained eye, the overexposed radiograph is easily identifiable. One type of overexposure exhibits an over-all grayness with low contrast. This appearance is caused by shortened development of the film, a procedure often followed in an attempt to supposedly correct the error made in th exposure time or to compensate for excessive KvP.

Another type of overexposure produces such a great density of the thinner portions of the part radiographed that they are obliterated. In this case, full development is given, and it usually occurs where time-temperature processing is employed. Regardless of how it is developed, an overexposed film lacks the requisites of ideal radiographic quality—proper radiographic density and contrast—as one or the other is invariably sacrificed. If the kilovoltage is correct, overexposure due to the MaS factor may usually be corrected by making another radiograph with one-half the original MaS (½X). Very frequently, the density of this second radiograph is satisfactory or is so near in quality that if a third radiograph is made, only a minor adjustment of the MaS is needed to secure the most desirable quality.

Example 1. An anteroposterior direct-exposure radiograph of an elbow was made A, Figure 121, with 60 KvP, 36-inch FFD, and 160 MaS. This radiograph proved to be overexposed. A second radiograph (B) was made with one-half the original MaS, i.e., 80. This radiograph was satisfactory.

Example 2. A series of lateral screen-exposure radiographs of the cervical spine, Figure 122, was made employing 85 KvP, and a 72-inch FFD. The initial radiograph (A) was made with an exposure of 10 MaS (X), and the resulting density was excessive. Using the rule of thumb for changing density, a second radiograph (B) was

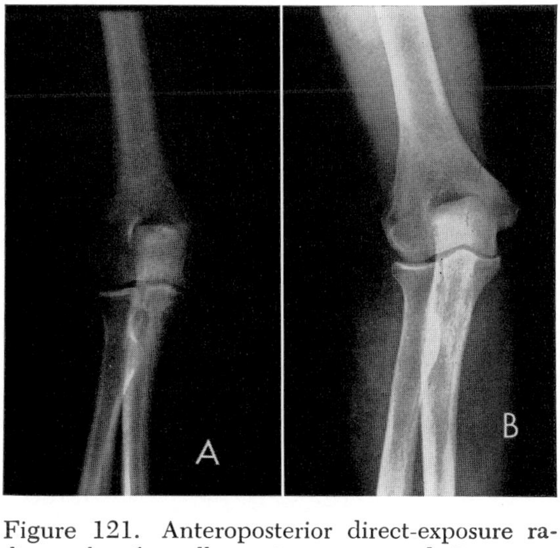

Figure 121. Anteroposterior direct-exposure radiographs of an elbow: A, overexposed; B, correct exposure.

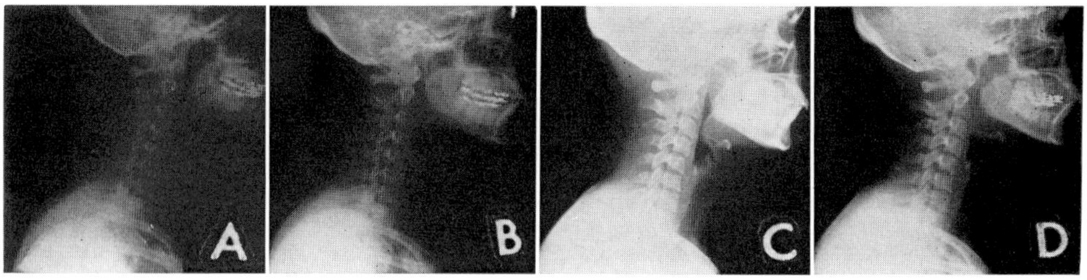

Figure 122. Series of lateral screen-exposure radiographs of the cervical spine to demonstrate influence of MaS factor.

made with 5 MaS (½X), but the density still was excessive. A third radiograph (C) employing 2.5 MaS (¼X) (one-half the exposure for radiograph B) resulted in underexposure. However, the fourth radiograph (D) using 3.75 MaS (⅜X) was satisfactory. This example demonstrates how, with the use of MaS only, a correct result or a basic MaS was finally obtained although the initial radiograph was a total failure.

Example 3. A series of anteroposterior screen-grid radiographs of the lumbar vertebrae, Figure 123, was made with 70 KvP and a 36-inch FFD. The first radiograph (A) was made with a trial exposure of 200 MaS. The density was excessive. Applying the rule of thumb for density, the second radiograph (B) was made with 100 MaS. The density was reduced, but it was still somewhat excessive. The MaS was halved again for the third radiograph (C) but the density became insufficient. A fourth radiograph (D) was made employing 75 MaS, a value midway between 100 and 50 MaS, which yielded a satisfactory image density.

Comment. The three examples cited above illustrate the procedure to be employed in altering density by the rule of thumb method when determining a basic MaS value or making correction for a faulty MaS value. The experienced technician soon recognizes the degree of overexposure and can make short cuts. For instance, in examples 2 and 3, the second radiograph can be eliminated simply by quartering the original MaS and securing a working density that could be easily adjusted, if necessary.

UNDEREXPOSURE

A radiograph is underexposed when important details are lacking because of inadequate radiographic density. Details of thin structures may be visible but those

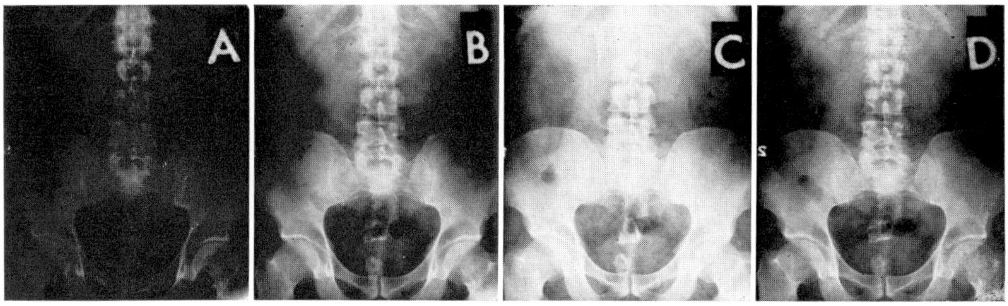

Figure 123. A series of anteroposterior screen-grid radiographs of the lumbar vertebrae to demonstrate influence of MaS factor.

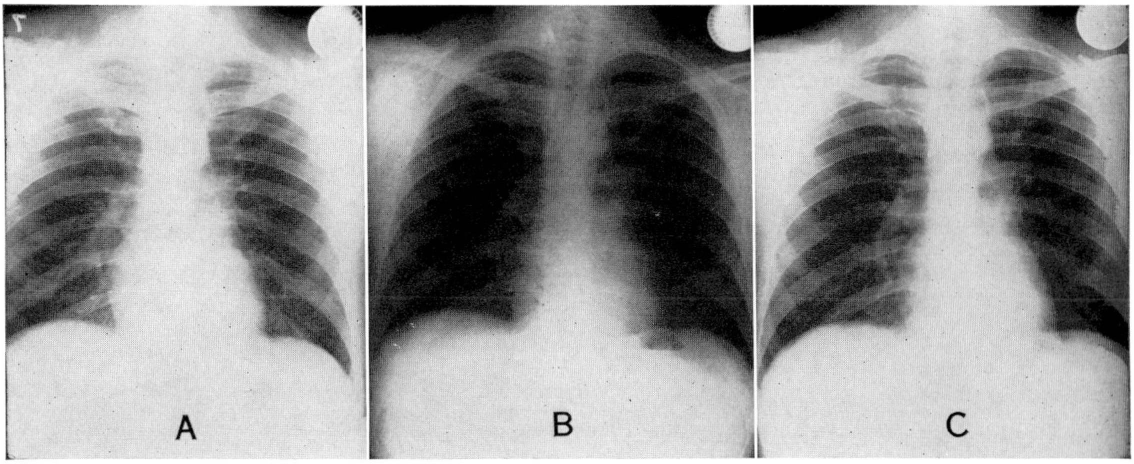

Figure 124. A series of posteroanterior screen-exposure radiographs of the chest to demonstrate the influence of MaS on density.

representing the heavier parts will be absent. When the kilovoltage is of a value to secure proper penetration of the part yet the MaS is insufficient to secure proper density, the radiograph will reveal very faint detail in image areas corresponding to the greater tissue densities. It may be presumed, therefore, that the kilovoltage is satisfactory for the part and that detail may be better visualized if more silver were deposited on the film. To achieve this result, the first step in correction is to *double* the MaS. Usually the density will then be satisfactory. However, a further small adjustment in the MaS may be made, if necessary, to provide a more satisfactory image.

Example 1. A series of posteroanterior screen-exposure radiographs of the chest, Figure 124, was made using 80 KvP; 72-inch FFD; and 3.3 to 6.6 MaS. The first radiograph (A) was made with 3.3 MaS and resulted in an underexposure. The second radiograph (B) was made with 6.6 MaS. The resulting density was excessive. The third and final film (C) was made with an MaS value of 5, approximately midway between the previous MaS values. This exposure may be considered correct.

Example 2. Two lateral screen-grid radiographs of the thoracolumbar vertebrae, Figure 125, were made employing 85 KvP; 36-inch FFD; 100 MaS and 200 MaS; thickness 32 cm. The first radiograph (A) made with 100 MaS was obviously underexposed. By doubling the MaS value to 200 in making the second radiograph (B), a satisfactory over-all density was obtained.

PHOTOTIMING

The use of optimum kilovoltages in ra-

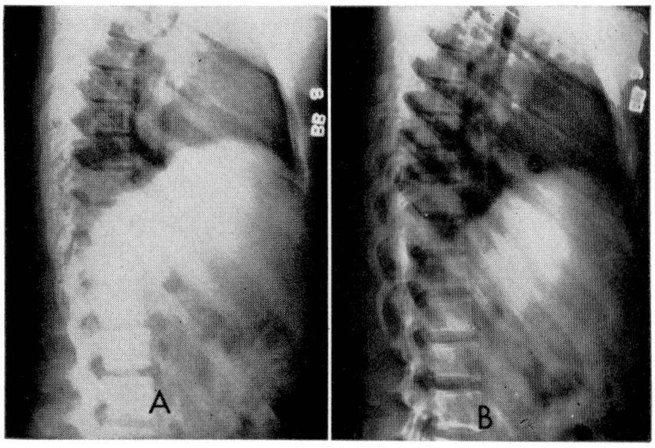

Figure 125. Two lateral screen-grid radiographs of the thoracolumbar vertebrae.

diographic phototiming eliminates many problems in the choice of appropriate factors. Since the focus-film distances are constant for given projections, the burden of placing the correct radiographic density on the film then is on the phototimer which regulates the MaS.

Exposure Tables

The next chapter describes the use of some routine projections that can serve as guides in the development of a comprehensive exposure system employing fixed kilovoltages.

SUMMARY

Knowledge of the function of each exposure factor makes it possible for the technician to predict the quality of any radiograph exposed with a given group of factors. Also, if an error has been made in applying a factor, analysis of the image should readily reveal the exposure factor at fault. Correction can then be made. In establishing a group of factors prior to making any projection, the following routine will aid materially in producing good quality radiographs.

1. Analyze the habitus of the patient and ascertain tissue thickness to be traversed by the central ray.
2. Consult Table IX to determine whether thickness is in the average range.
3. Select the kilovoltage that is considered to be optimum for the projection.
4. Employ the focus-film distance previously selected as a constant for the projection.
5. Affix the appropriate cone in the tube-head and employ a grid, if necessary.
6. Apply the required basic MaS if the part is in the average thickness range; if the thickness is outside the average range, use the value previously selected as appropriate for the thickness.
7. Select the focal spot that is appropriate for the part and the electrical energy to be applied to the tube.
8. After exposure, process the x-ray film according to the requirements of a standardized time and temperature method.

Chapter 16

Exposure Tables and Their Arrangement

It is not possible to construct technic tables that are precisely workable on all types and makes of apparatus which have varying degrees of calibration efficiency. The best that can be accomplished is a compromise in which all factors but one are reduced to constants. The variable factor employed should have only one function—to influence the amount of silver deposited on the film (radiographic density). However, the point of primary importance in selecting exposure factors is to be sure that the kilovoltage being employed provides an x-ray wave length that will accomplish penetration of the thickest and most dense tissue in the part being examined.

No technic table is a cure-all or answer to good radiography. It is only an aid in that direction. Training in positioning and the application of suitable immobilization devices, cones and grids (when employed), all contribute to the quality of the radiograph. Also, clinical experience in estimating the relative x-ray absorption characteristics of the patient as altered by disease, trauma, or age has a decided bearing upon the results. Actually, if the subject matter of the preceding text has been thoroughly assimilated, the x-ray technician should have no difficulty in constructing a working technic table of exposure factors for his use and for others who have occasion to use the same equipment. All technics can be reduced to 4 x 6-inch cards, Figure 126, that can be placed in a Kardex or similar file and hung on the wall adjacent to the control cabinet.

The following tables, designed for use with full-wave rectified equipment, list *suggested* exposure factors for various routine projections. They are printed simply as an aid to the technician when he builds his own charts. The exposure factors may be found practical to adapt to some of the routine radiographic work required by your laboratory. It is most important that the appropriate MaS and KvP values, suffixed by the same symbol, be used together. Also, cones of the correct size must be employed as well as standardized processing with development for 5 minutes at 68° F. The exposure factors listed are based upon the use of Kodak Blue Brand X-ray Film and Kodak Rapid X-ray Developer.

THICKNESS RANGES

The thickness ranges of body parts in the patient are always measured along the course of the central ray. In most instances, three thickness ranges are specified. The first comprises a thickness range for *thin* parts; the second, the *average*

THICKNESS RANGE: CMS	FFD	GUIDE MAS	MA	TIME	MAS	KVP
— 10		.83S	50	1/60	.83S	
11 — 14		1.66S	100	1/60	1.66S	
15 — 17		2.5 S	100	1/40	2.5 S	
18 — 20	72"	3.3 S	100	1/30	3.3 S	80S
21 — 24		5.0 S	100	1/20	5.0 S	
25 — 27		6.3 S	200	1/30	6.3 S	
28 — 30		10.0 S	200	1/20	10.0 S	

LEGEND

F– No screens

S– Screens, aver. speed

G– Grid

CONE NO. 3,5.

DEVELOPMENT: 5 min. 68°F.

CHEST	POST.-ANT.	Film Size 14 X 17	Projection No. 37

Figure 126. Facsimile of 4 x 6-inch card containing the factors for a single projection that can serve as a model for other projections.

thickness range which includes the majority of thicknesses for a given projection; and the third, the thickness range for the *heavy* parts.

Some projections, such as for the chest, require a greater breakdown in thicknesses to attain uniformity in radiographic quality from one thickness to another.

FOCUS-FILM DISTANCE (FFD)

In the tables, the focus-film distances are standardized at 36 and 72 inches. If the FFD is to be changed at any time, the Inverse Square Law should be used to effect the required change in MaS.

GUIDE MaS VALUES

As a starting point in adapting these tables to your requirements, Guide MaS values are listed for various projections. These are trial values but they are quite close to whatever corrected value that the technician will ultimately employ. Adjacent to the Guide MaS column will be found blank columns for Ma, Time and MaS values after the corrected MaS has been determined. These are columns for the technician's own use. Next is the column listing optimum kilovoltages. The kilovoltages listed have been attained by extensive experiment and are premised upon the following criteria:

1. That the wave length generated by the kilovoltage will provide radiation that will penetrate a given part when a practical basic MaS value is used.
2. That the level of secondary radiation fog is such that it will not interfere with the diagnostic quality of the radiographic image.
3. That the image will exhibit a long scale of contrast to assure the rendition of maximum image detail.
4. That the final MaS value selected for the average thickness will provide sufficient translucent over-all image silver to reveal essential details. Since all factors but MaS are constant, it can readily be seen that the level of radiographic density must be regulated by MaS. The kilovoltage should not be used for this purpose.
5. That the focus-film distances listed will assure satisfactory image sharpness.
6. That a minimal object-film distance be employed.

The last column in the tables indicates the appropriate size of film required and the size of the cone needed to enclose the anatomic area specifically required.

In the upper right hand corner of each regional technic page will be found a legend listing the various symbols employed in the tables and their meanings.

USE OF TABLES

Select the projection that is to be standardized. Choose a patient whose thickness is a median in the average thickness range. The thickness should be measured along the course of the central ray. Once the thickness category into which the part falls is determined, note the *Guide* MaS listed for that particular thickness range. Make an exposure of the patient employing the Guide MaS, FFD, KvP, size of film and cone as listed. If the over-all density of the radiograph is greater than desired, repeat the exposure using the Guide MaS value for the next lower thickness category. If the density is less than desired, use the Guide MaS value listed for the next higher thickness. Further small adjustments in MaS can be made to arrive at the exact density level desired. Once the density level for the average thickness is determined, the *percentage* increase or decrease in MaS can be easily determined and the other MaS values corrected accordingly. Simplification of this procedure can be effected by classifying radiography into three types: (1) direct exposure; (2) screen exposure, and (3) screen-grid exposure. By this means only three adjustments in the Guide MaS values need be made for each class of radiography. This essentially consists of determining the percentage increase or decrease in MaS needed for each type of radiography and adjusting the balance of the values by these percentages. This avoids a large amount of needless radiography for all projections.

Example 1. In direct exposure posteroanterior radiography of a 3.5 cm. hand, the Guide MaS for the average thickness range will be found to be 50. If the resulting density is excessive, another exposure should be made employing 40 MaS—the value needed for thinner hands. If the resulting density is satisfactory, the percentage reduction in MaS needed for all direct

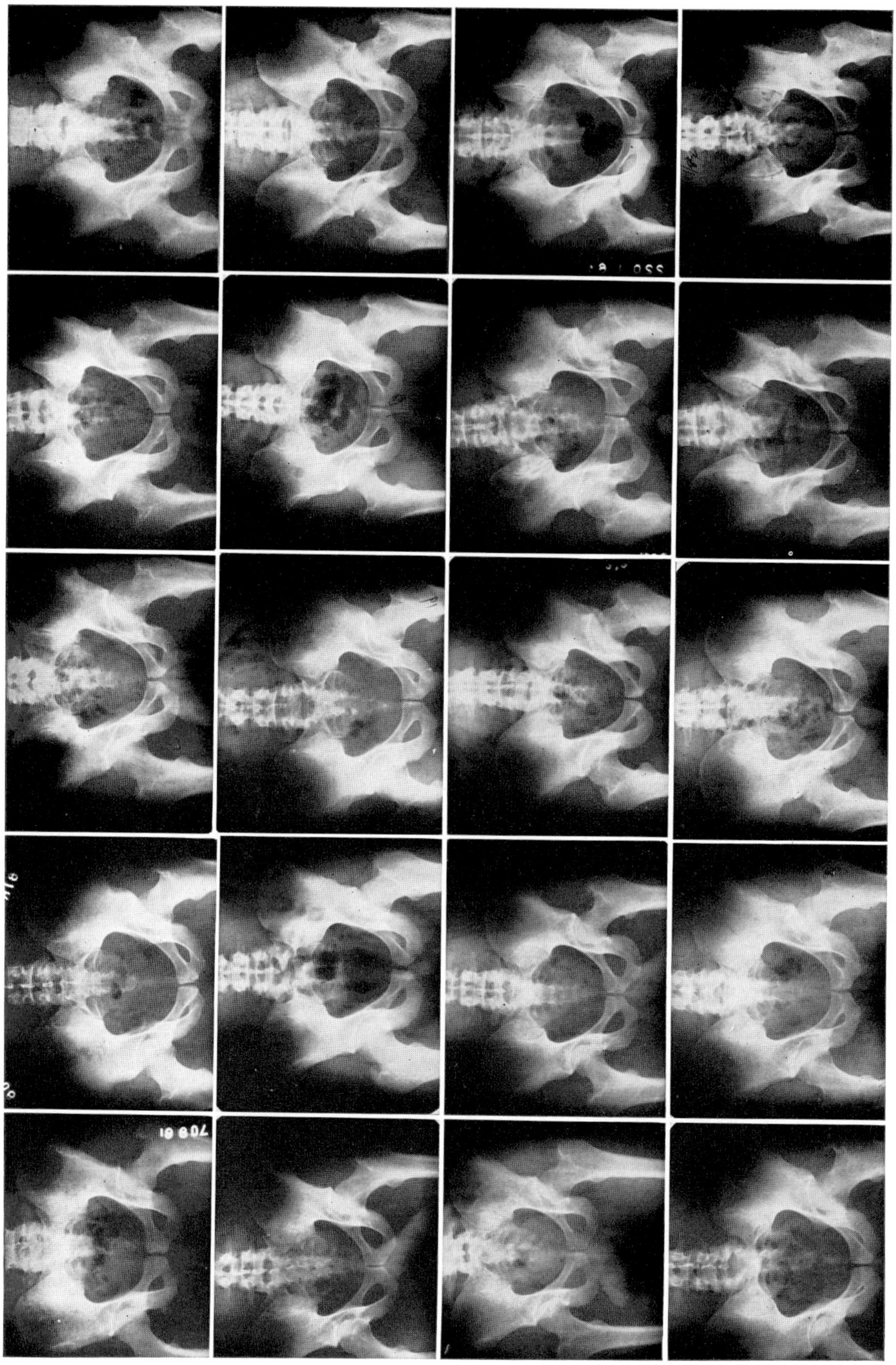

Figure 127. Series of anteroposterior screen-grid radiographs of the pelvis, all of which received the same exposure factors. All patients measured within the average thickness range.

exposures is obtained in the following manner:

Guide MaS	50
Corrected Trial MaS	40

40/50 = .8 = 80% adjustment for other direct-exposure Guide MaS values.

Example 2. Let us select 80 as the Guide MaS for the average thickness in direct-exposure lateral radiography of the elbow.

80% of 80 MaS = 64 MaS. This is the corrected MaS.

In other words, for all direct-exposure radiography, list 80% of each of the various Guide MaS values in the respective vacant MaS spaces. When the resulting MaS value is such that the combination of timer type and Ma stations will not produce the desired MaS value, the nearest value may be employed to suit your apparatus in most instances. This is possible because wide exposure latitude is provided by the various kilovoltages listed. If, in posteroanterior radiography of the hand, the Guide MaS listed is 50*F*, be sure to use the KvP with the symbol "F" following it, i.e., 50F. This indicates that *direct* exposure of the part is to be employed using as factors 50 MaS and 50 KvP. On the other hand, if the symbol is "S," meaning that *screens* are to be used, employ the two factors with the "S" after each—(MaS) 0.5S and (KvP) 60S.

The above procedures can be followed for screen and screen-grid exposures. When completed, the entire chart will have been fairly well adapted to your specific apparatus.

Note. It will be observed that in some projections two different kilovoltages are recommended. For example, 50 KvP is listed for the hand when direct exposure is to be employed. When screens are employed, 60 KvP is recommended. As mentioned previously in this text, the use of screens increases image contrast. In other words, the contrast scale is shortened. By increasing the kilovoltage, one is not concerned with the function of penetration but with the scale of contrast. Increasing the kilovoltage *lengthens* the scale of contrast so that the image exhibits approximately the same contrast scale provided by 50 KvP upon direct exposure. Of course, less sharpness must be anticipated because of the use of screens, but expediency of the occasion is effected by a radical shortening of the exposure time.

In radiography of the chest, 80 KvP with screen exposures is recommended. In radiography of the heavy chest, secondary radiation is excessive. To maintain the same contrast scale and eliminate fog, 100 KvP and a stationary grid is recommended. In other words, the higher kilovoltage is employed solely to extend the contrast scale.

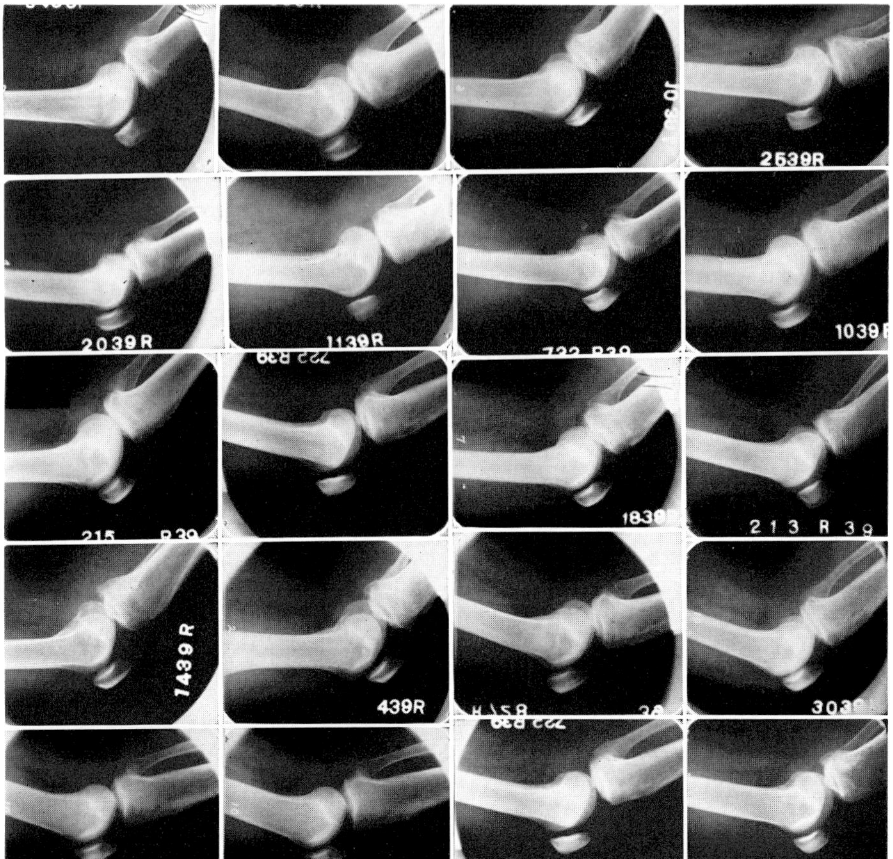

Figure 128. Series of lateral screen radiographs of the knee, all of which received the same exposure factors. All cases measured within the average thickness range.

TABLE XI

TECHNIC FOR UPPER EXTREMITY

No.	Region	Proj.	Thickness Range: Cms.	FFD	Guide MaS	Ma	Time	MaS	KVP	Film Size Cone
1	THUMB-FINGER	AP LAT.	1.5 – 4		30 F 0.4 S					
2	HAND	PA	– 2		40 F 0.25 S					
			3 – 5		50 F 0.5 S					
			6 –		60 F 0.75 S					
3		LAT.	– 6		80 F 1.0 S					
			7 – 10		100 F 1.5 S					
			11 –		120 F 2.0 S				50 F 60 S	8″ x 10″
4	WRIST	PA	– 2		40 F 0.25 S					CONE NO.
			3 – 6	36″	50 F 0.5 S					
			7 –		60 F 0.75 S					
5		LAT.	– 4		80 F 1.0 S					
			5 – 8		100 F 1.5 S					
			9 –		120 F 2.0 S					
6	FOREARM	AP PA LAT.	– 5		40 F 0.75 S				60 F 60 S	10″ x 12″
			6 – 9		50 F 1.0 S					CONE NO.
			10 –		60 F 2.0 S					
7	ELBOW	AP	– 5		60 F 1.0 S					
			6 – 9		80 F 1.5 S					
			10 –		100 F 2.0 S					
8		LAT.	– 6		60 F 1.0 S					
			7 – 10		80 F 1.5 S				60 F 60 S	8″ x 10″
			11 –		100 F 2.0 S					CONE NO.
9	ARM (Distal ⅔ rds)	AP and LAT.	– 6		60 F 0.75 S					
			7 – 10	36″	80 F 1.0 S					
			11 –		100 F 1.25 S					
10	SHOULDER	AP	– 8		1 S 2.5 SG					
			9 – 11		2 S 5 SG					
			12 – 16		3 S 7 SG					
			17 – 18		4 S 10 SG				60 S 80 SG	10″ x 12″
			19 –		5 S 12.5 SG					CONE NO.
11	CLAVICLE	PA	– 12		2 S 5 SG					
			13 – 17		3 S 7 SG					
			18 –		4 S 10 SG					

Legend: F–Film, without screens; S–Screens, aver. speed; G–Grid, 8-1; SG–Scr. + grid.
DEVELOPMENT: 5 min. 68°F.

TABLE XII

TECHNIC FOR LOWER EXTREMITY

No.	*Region*	*Proj.*	*Thickness Range: Cms.*	*FFD*	*Guide MaS*	*Ma*	*Time*	*MaS*	*KVP*	*Film Size Cone*
1	TOES	AP and LAT.	– 2	36″	30 F 0.25 S				50 F 60 S	8″ x 10″ CONE NO.
			3 – 5		40 F 0.5 S					
			6 –		50 F 0.75 S					
2	FOOT	AP and PA	– 5		40 F 0.25 S				60 F 70 S	10″ x 12″ CONE NO.
			6 – 9		50 F 0.5 S					
			10 –		60 F 0.75 S					
3		LAT.	– 5		60 F 0.75 S					
			6 – 9		80 F 1.0 S					
			10 –		100 F 1.5 S					
4	OS CALCIS	AX-IAL	8 – 13		50 F				80 F	8″ x 10″ CONE NO.
5	ANKLE	AP	– 6		80 F 1.5 S				60 F 70 S	10″ x 12″ CONE NO.
			7 – 10		100 F 2.0 S					
			11 –		120 F 2.5 S					
6		LAT.	– 5		60 F 0.75 S					
			6 – 9		80 F 1.0 S					
			10 –		100 F 1.5 S					
7	LEG	AP	– 8		8 S 2.5 SG				60 S 80 SG	14″ x 17″ CONE NO.
			9 – 12		10 S 3 SG					
			13 –		12 S 4 SG					
8		LAT.	– 7		4 S 2 SG					
			8 – 11		6 S 3 SG					
			12 –		8 S 3.5 SG					
9	KNEE	AP and PA	– 9		8 S 4 SG				65 S 80 SG	8″ x 10″ CONE NO.
			10 – 14		10 S 6 SG					
			15 –		12 S 8 SG					
10		LAT.	– 8		3 S 2 SG					
			9 – 13		5 S 3 SG					
			14 –		7 S 4 SG					
11	PATELLA	AX-IAL	–		10 S				80 S	

Legend: F–Film, without screens; **S**–Screens, aver. speed; **G**–Grid, 8-1; **SG**–Scr. + grid.
DEVELOPMENT: 5 min. 68°F.

TABLE XII—*Continued*

TECHNIC FOR LOWER EXTREMITY

No.	*Region*	*Proj.*	*Thickness Range: Cms.*	*FFD*	*Guide MaS*	*Ma*	*Time*	*MaS*	*KVP*	*Film Size Cone*
			– 13		7.5 SG					
12		AP	14 – 17		10 SG					
			18 –		12.5 SG					14″ x 17″
	FEMUR		– 12		5 SG					
13		LAT.	13 – 16	36″	7.5 SG					CONE
			17 –		10 SG					NO.
			– 16		30 SG					10″ x 12″
14		AP	17 – 21		40 SG				80 SG	
	HIP		22 –		50 SG					CONE
			– 19		125 SG					8″ x 10″
15		LAT.	20 – 24		150 SG					CONE
			25 –		175 SG					NO.

Legend: F–Film, without screens; **S**–Screens, aver. speed; **G**–Grid, 8–1; **SG**–Scr. + grid.
DEVELOPMENT: 5 min. 68°F.

* * *

Since going to press, a noteworthy contribution has been made to assist the radiologist to reduce the x-ray dosage to patients in diagnostic radiology. This has been accomplished by the introduction of Kodak Royal Blue X-ray Film which is 50% more sensitive to x-rays than the present Blue Brand film. Therefore, if Royal Blue film is employed with Tables XI through XV, all MaS values should be reduced ⅓. This also applies to the performance of all Experiments cited in the foregoing text. It is well to note that this new film should be handled in the processing room with safelight illumination (6B) emitted by 7½ watt bulbs.

TABLE XIII

TECHNIC FOR CHEST

No.	Region	Proj.	*Thickness Range: Cms*	*FFD*	*Guide MaS*	*Ma*	*Time*	*MaS*	*KVP*	*Film Size Cone*
1	CHEST	PA	Infants	72″	1.66 S				70 S	14″ x 17″ CONE NO.
			– 14		1.66 S				80 S	
			15 – 17		2.5 S					
			18 – 20		3.3 S					
			21 – 24		5 S					
			25 – 27		6.3 S					
			28 – 30		10 S					
2		PA OBL.	19 – 23		5 S				85 S	
			24 – 30		10 S					
			31 – 35		15 S					
3		LAT.	– 26		10 S				90 S	
			27 – 32		13.3 S					
			33 –		15 S					
4		PA	– 14		1.66 SG				100 SG	
			15 – 19		2.5 SG					
			20 – 24		3.3 SG					
			25 – 27		5 SG					
			28 – 30		10 SG					
			31 –		20 SG					
5		OBL.	19 – 23		5 SG					
			24 – 30		15 SG					
			31 – 35		30 SG					
6		LAT.	– 16		5 SG					
			17 – 23		7.5 SG					
			24 – 27		10 SG					
			28 – 29		15 SG					
			30 – 34		20 SG					
			35 – 37		30 SG					
			38 –		40 SG					

Legend: F–Film, without screens; **S**–Screens, aver. speed; **G**–Grid, 8-1; **SG**–Scr. + grid.
DEVELOPMENT: 5 min. 68°F.

TABLE XIV

TECHNIC FOR SKULL AND SINUSES

No.	*Region*	*Proj.*	*Thickness Range: Cms*	*FFD*	*Guide MaS*	*Ma*	*Time*	*MaS*	*KVP*	*Film Size Cone*
1	SKULL	PA	- 17	36″	10 SG				85 SG	10″ x 12″ CONE NO.
			18 - 21		15 SG					
			22 -		25 SG					
2		AP	- 15		15 SG					
			16 - 23		20 SG					
			24 -		30 SG					
3		LAT.	- 12		10 SG					
			13 - 17		15 SG					
			18 -		20 SG					
4		INF.-SUP.	- 19		30 SG					
			20 - 25		40 SG					
			26 -		50 SG					
5	SINUSES	PA FRON.	- 17		10 S 40 SG				70 S 80 SG	8″ x 10″ CONE NO.
			18 - 21		15 S 50 SG					
			22 -		20 S 60 SG					
6		PA MAX.	- 17		10 S 40 SG					
			18 - 22		15 S 50 SG					
			23 -		20 S 60 SG					
7		LAT.	- 12		5 S 10 SG					
			13 - 17		7.5 S 15 SG					
			18 -		10 S 20 SG					

Legend: F–Film, without screens; **S**–Screens, aver. speed; **G**–Grid, 8-1; **SG**–Scr. + grid.
DEVELOPMENT: 5 min. 68°F.

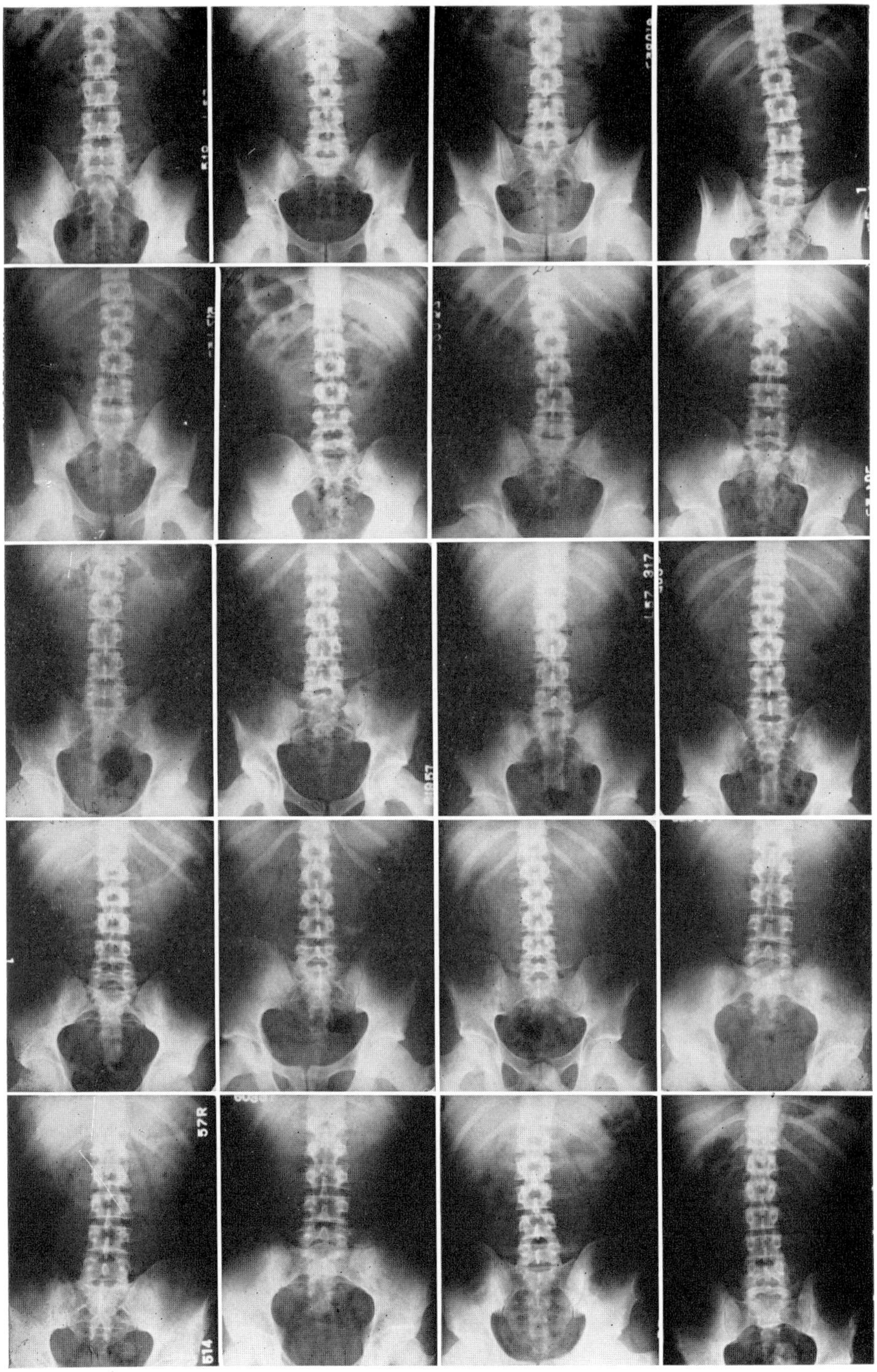

Figure 129. Series of anteroposterior radiographs of the lumbar vertebrae of different patients measuring within the average thickness range. All radiographs received identical exposure factors.

TABLE XV

TECHNIC FOR PELVIS AND VERTEBRAE

No.	*Region*	*Proj.*	*Thickness Range: Cms*	*FFD*	*Guide MaS*	*Ma*	*Time*	*MaS*	*KVP*	*Film Size Cone*
1	PELVIS	AP	– 14		60 SG				65 SG	
			15 – 19		80 SG					14″ x 17″
			20 – 23		100 SG				70 SG	CONE NO.
			24 –		120 SG					
2		AP C1-3	– 11		5 SG					
			12 – 15	36″	7.5 SG					
			16 –		10 SG				80 SG	8″ x 10″
3	CERVICAL	AP and Oblique C4-7	– 10		3.3 SG					CONE NO.
			11 – 14		5 SG					
			15 –		7.5 SG					
4		LAT.	– 9		2.5 S					10″ x 12″
			10 – 13	72″	5 S				85 S	
			14 –		7.5 S					CONE NO.
5		AP	– 19		40 SG					
			20 – 24		50 SG				75 SG	
	THORACIC		25 –		60 SG					14″ x 17″
6	(Patient Breathing)	LAT.	– 30		150 SG	10				CONE NO.
			31 – 34		200 SG	10			80 SG	
			35 –		250 SG	10				
7		AP	– 17		40 SG					14″ x 17″
			18 – 22		50 SG				70 SG	
			23 –	36″	60 SG					CONE NO.
8		Oblique	– 17		50 SG					10″ x 12″
	LUMBAR (Compression)		18 – 22		60 SG				75 SG	
			23 –		70 SG					CONE NO.
9		LAT. L1-4	– 26		80 SG					10″ x 12″
			27 – 32		100 SG					
			33 –		120 SG				85 SG	CONE NO.
10		LAT. L5-S	– 26		180 SG					8″ x 10″
			27 – 32		200 SG					
			33 –		225 SG					CONE NO.

Legend: F–Film, without screens; **S**–Screens, aver. speed; **G**–Grid, 8-1; **SG**–Scr. + grid.
DEVELOPMENT: 5 min. 68°F.

Part II

X-ray Film Processing

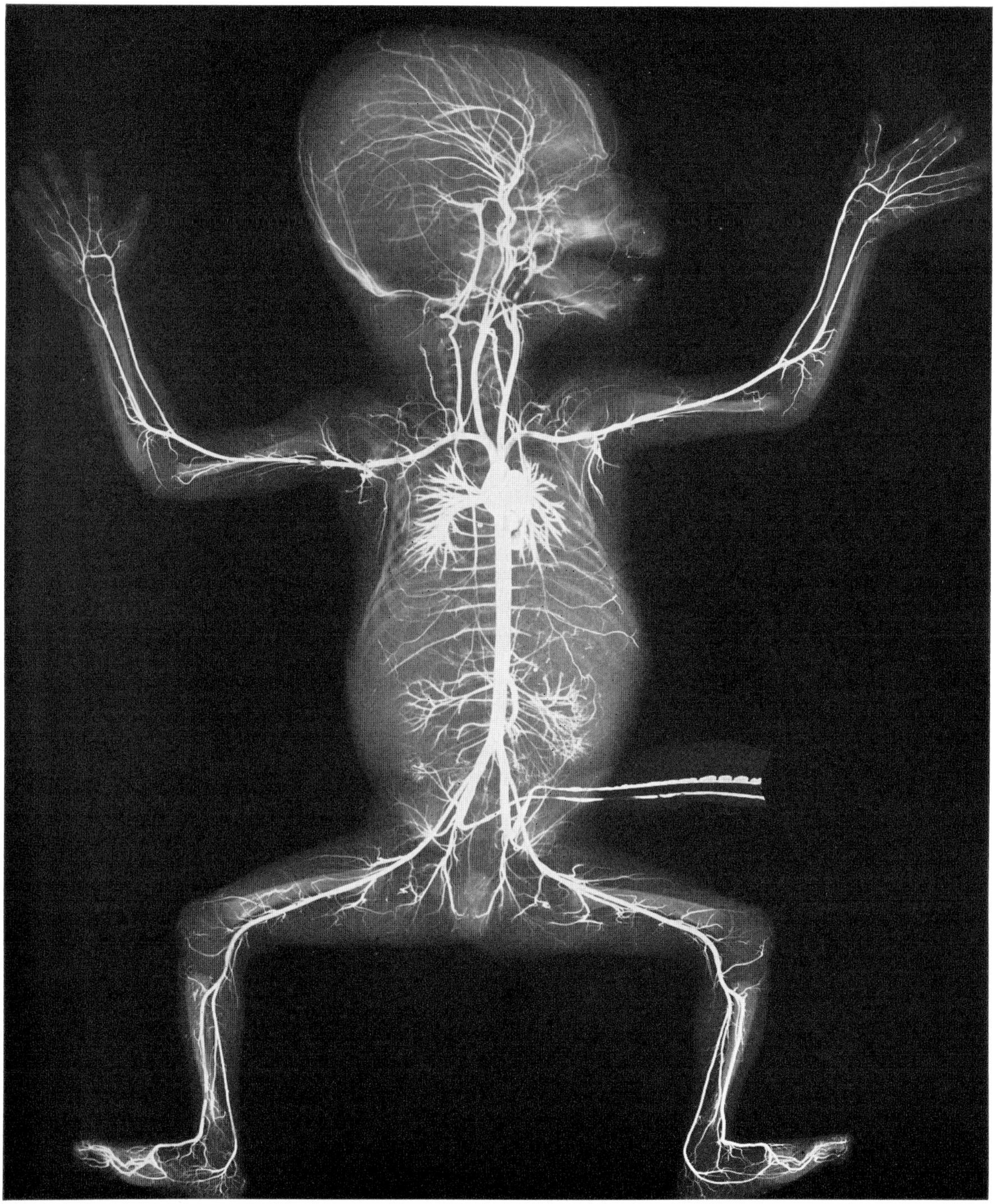

Figure 130. Arteriogram of a 5½-month fetus. Injection was made with a barium sulfate preparation as a contrast medium.

Chapter 17

Processing Procedures

EVEN THOUGH the efficiency of the x-ray apparatus may be high and the best exposure practice employed, the radiograph will be of inferior quality if the processing of the exposed x-ray film is carelessly or slovenly executed. The greatest error in the production of a radiograph often may be a flagrant disregard of the simplest of processing rules. Hence, one of the important operations is the processing procedure that brings about the physical and chemical changes to render visible as a radiographic image, the latent image created by the x-rays. This procedure requires the assistance of photographic chemistry.

PROCESSING FACILITIES

Correct processing is dependent upon the efficiency of layout of the processing room. Normally, the processing room is divided as to function into two areas. The "wet side" or area containing the tanks, Figure 131, Top, and the "dry side" consisting of the loading bench where films are prepared for exposure and processing, Figure 131, Bottom. Details relative to the manner in which a processing room should be constructed may be found in the literature published in the various x-ray journals from time to time. Basic information, however, is contained in the following publications:

Planning Guide for Radiologic Installations. Edited by W. G. Scott, M.D. Published by the Year Book Publishers, Inc., 200 East Illinois Street, Chicago, Illinois, 1953.

Planning the X-ray Processing Facilities and Equipment. Published by the Eastman Kodak Company, Rochester 4, New York. Free, upon request.

STEPS IN PROCESSING PROCEDURE

Processing x-ray film to a radiograph involves at least seven procedures:

1. STORING AND HANDLING X-RAY FILM

The proper storage and handling of x-ray film is an important aspect of radiography. Since film is a delicate material, the manner in which it is stored and handled determines whether the radiograph will be free of artifacts.

2. MIXING SOLUTIONS

The manner in which the various chem-

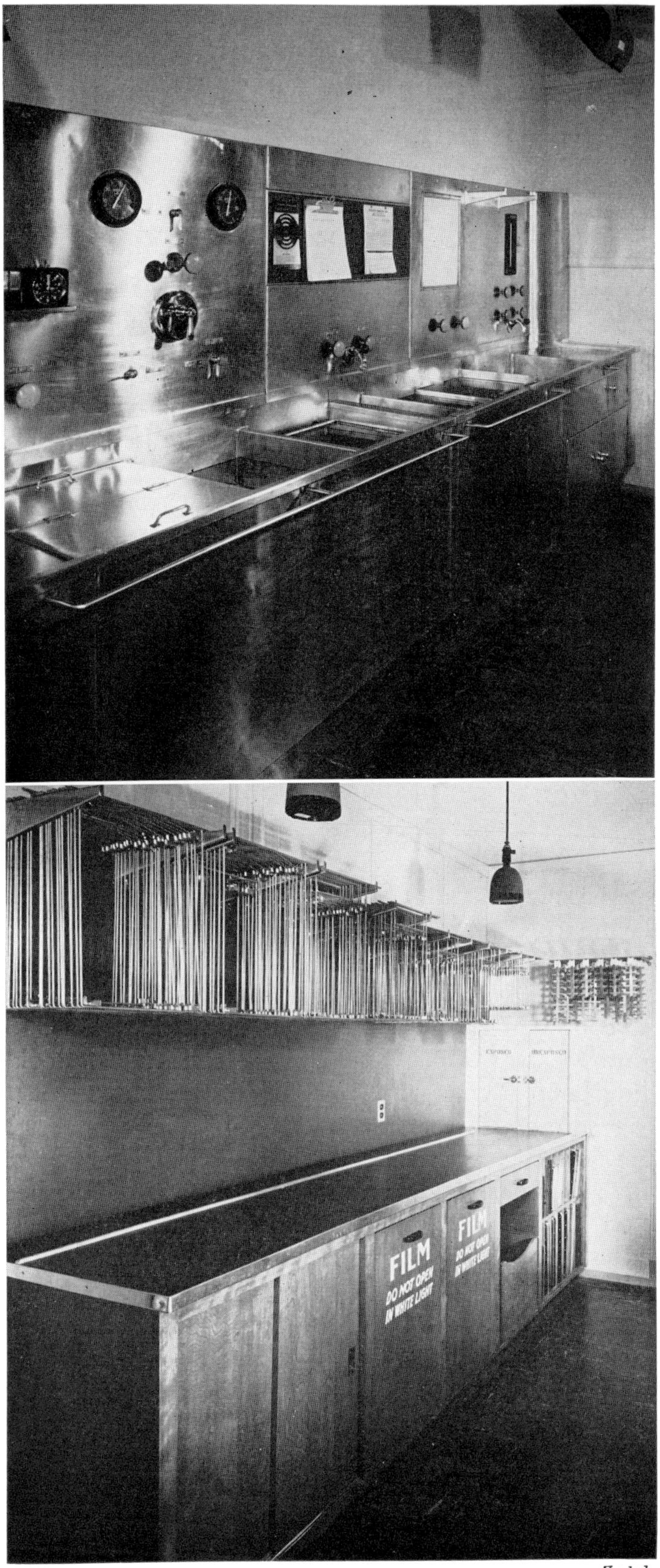

Kodak

Figure 131. Photographs of processing room. (*Top*) Tank or "wet side." (*Bottom*) Loading bench or "dry side."

ical solutions used in processing are mixed is important, since good quality radiographs are only produced when these solutions operate efficiently. Recommended methods for mixing should be carefully followed.

3. DEVELOPMENT PROCESS

Development of the x-ray film changes the silver bromide crystals containing the latent image to black metallic silver that constitutes the visible image. The solution used to effect this change is called a developer.

4. RINSING PROCESS

Rinsing is the operation of removing the excess developer solution chemicals from the film after development and to diminish or halt developer activity. Water is usually employed for this purpose. However, an acid water bath is often used for its greater efficiency. The latter bath immediately stops development and neutralizes the alkalinity of the residual developer solution in the film.

5. FIXING PROCESS

The fixing process involves two activities and is the procedure for removing the unexposed and undeveloped silver bromide from the emulsion and for hardening the soft gelatin emulsion containing the metallic silver image. The chemical solution employed for these purposes is known as the fixing solution.

6. WASHING PROCESS

Washing is the process whereby the soluble fixing bath and silver salts are removed from the film emulsion by means of clean, flowing water.

7. DRYING PROCESS

Drying is the treatment of drying the wet radiographs for permanency and for use by the radiologist.

STANDARDIZATION OF PROCEDURES

The procurement of *uniform* radiographic quality from day to day and year to year should be the ambition of the technician. This can only be achieved, however, through control and standardization of processing procedures. X-ray film is manufactured to produce a consistently uniform degree of density and contrast when correctly exposed and processed according to standard and accepted procedures. Familiarity with the characteristics and performance of a particular film is necessary if any measure of standardized processing is to be obtained. Since the characteristics of density and contrast provided by a particular film and its developer are inherent, they may be considered constant. The sequence of chemical activities in standardized processing is smooth and organized and produces a desired radiographic image.

TANK METHOD OF PROCESSING

There are several ways in which a film may be developed but the standard *time-temperature* tank method is almost universally employed. This method is most efficient, for it is virtually foolproof and provides an excellent means for checking x-ray exposures. The manufacturer formulates an x-ray developer to give the most desirable radiographic quality upon *full* development of the x-ray film within a limited temperature range. Hence, it is understandable that variations from the optimum in temperature or developing time must be carefully compensated to maintain proper quality. Once standardized processing rules are established and followed, over-all changes in density and

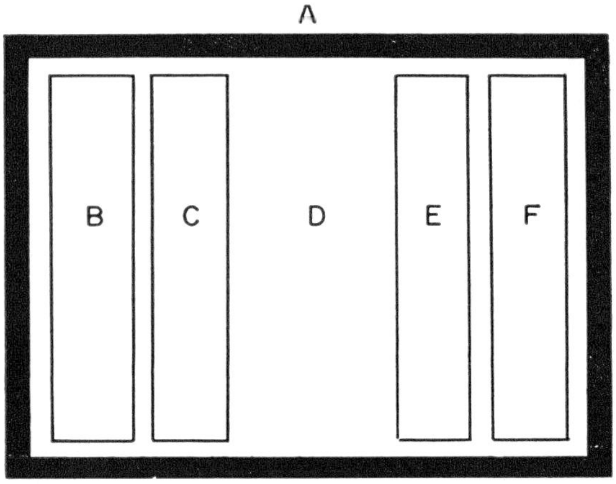

Figure 132. Conventional arrangement of a small tank unit (*top view*).

A. Master tank
B. Developer tank
C. Acid rinse bath, if used
D. Water rinse or washing section
E. First fixing tank
F. Second fixing tank

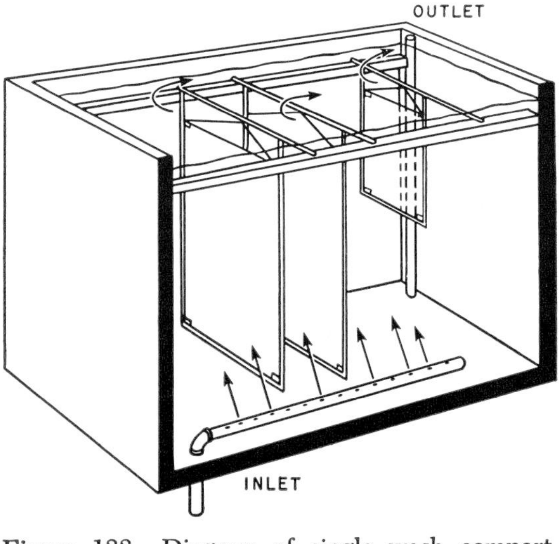

Figure 133. Diagram of single wash compartment. (Arrows indicate water flow from inlet over both film surfaces and to outlet.)

contrast can be attributed to changes in exposure factors. Standardized processing of the film then can become a constant as long as a reasonable measure of discipline is exercised in the processing room.

Photographic research has so standardized processing procedures that operations in connection therewith have virtually been reduced to noting the solution temperature and setting an interval timer according to a time-temperature chart. This procedure, however, is based upon the accumulated knowledge of the many chemical and physical complexities relating to the exposure and development response of the film. Despite the simplicity of a standard processing procedure, it will not work satisfactorily if solutions are improperly mixed, contain poor quality chemicals, or are not used in accordance with the maker's instructions.

The modern method of processing involves the use of a number of solution tanks in which the exposed x-ray film is chemically subjected to treatment that changes the exposed x-ray film to a radiograph.

TANK TYPES

There are two general types of tanks for x-ray processing.

Master Tank

The master tank serves as a water jacket to hold insert tanks and is usually large enough to provide space between the insert tanks for rinsing and washing of films when necessary. When a large washing tank is available, the washing of radiographs is accomplished in this tank.

Insert Tanks

The insert tanks are removable containers for individual processing solutions and are spaced in the master tank.

ARRANGEMENT OF TANK UNITS

The simplest processing tank system usually consists of a master tank containing three solution tanks, Figure 132. If a stop bath is used, the tank total becomes 4. Water in the space between the developer and fixer sections is employed for rinsing purposes or insertion of a tank of stop bath solution, as well as for temperature control. A separate washing tank the same size as the master tank is usually available that is provided with a 2-compartment cascade washing arrangement or a single-compartment tank with overflow compartment. The insert tanks should be arranged in the master tank so that the order of handling loaded hangers is from left to right, the short dimension of the tanks being parallel with the front of the master tank to attain maximum efficiency in operation. Depending upon the volume of work to be accomplished, there are a number of different tank arrangements that can be employed.

Single-Compartment Wash Tanks

When the single-compartment wash tank is used, an overflow pipe is provided, Figure 133. The water flows from the inlet pipe *between* and along the surfaces of the films, then into the overflow pipe. This arrangement permits rapid washing because of the speed and thoroughness with which fresh water is circulated across the film surfaces.

Cascade Wash Tank

Cascade washing of radiographs is the most efficient method because it eliminates fixer solution with a minimum amount of water. Although an additional operation is required for moving the films from one compartment to the next, the cascade system is especially useful in installations handling a continuous volume of films. The tank consists of two washing compartments and an overflow well, Figure 134. The fresh water flows into the bottom of compartment A, passes upward over the partition into compartment B, under the end wall of the tank proper and through the outlet C in the overflow well. Fixer solution is denser than water and normally drifts downward in the washing tank as it is removed from the radiographs. For this reason, preliminary washing should be carried out in compartment B, where the flow of water is downward. The radiographs are then placed in compartment A for the remainder of the washing period. By placing a film first in compartment B, those washing in compartment A are not contaminated, thus overcoming one of the disadvantages of single-compartment washing. The amount of fixer solution carried to the final washing compartment from B is negligible insofar as its effect on the washing time is concerned. The chief purpose of the overflow well in a cascade system is to permit the draining of water from the bottom of the adjacent washing compartment through a standard standpipe or through an overflow pipe in the back of the tank.

TEMPERATURE CONTROL

The temperature of the solutions should be controlled within a close range. The ideal situation would be to maintain both

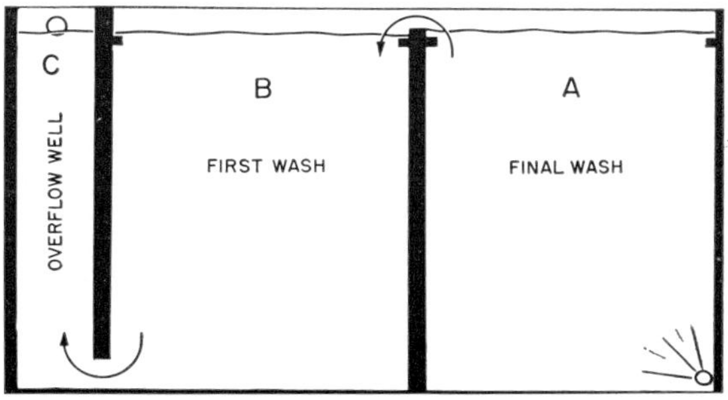

Figure 134. Diagram of cascade system of washing. Flow of water is indicated by arrows.

Figure 135. Radiograph exhibiting typical evidence of fog produced by storing x-ray film in hot basement.

Figure 136. Reproduction of x-ray film that has been subjected to the action of excessive heat and moisture.

the air and the tap water at a temperature of 68° F. Under such circumstances the water jacket and the washing water would remain at a fairly constant temperature, with or without a flow of water. However, the water source is seldom at this temperature for any length of time. In many localities it may closely approach the freezing point in winter, while in summer it frequently rises above 80° F. To maintain an optimum temperature for processing in such instances, necessary amounts of either hot or refrigerated water must be added. Since both may be scarce, some measure of temperature control should be employed that utilizes a minimum of tempered water.

Refrigeration Unit

A detachable or permanent refrigeration unit can be supplied for use with the processing tanks to temper the processing solutions.

Heating Unit

On occasion the temperature of the solutions may drop below safe processing values and it is necessary to raise the temperature to the optimum level. A suitable immersion heating unit can readily raise the temperature of the solution to the required value. The minimum value should be 60° F.

Thermometer

Processing of radiographs requires that an accurate check on the temperature of the solutions be maintained at all times by the use of an accurate thermometer. The optimum temperature as recommended by the American Standards Association has been adopted as 68° F. Do not dip the finger in a solution to judge its temperature for you will be wrong using this method 99 per cent of the time. The temperature of the solutions should *always be checked* when the work is first begun, and at intervals during the day, to be sure the proper temperature is being maintained.

Tank Insulation

Under certain conditions the master tank may require insulation, especially when there are wide differences between the temperature of the air in the processing room and the optimum processing temperature of 68° F. For example, an air temperature of 85° to 90° F. places an increased load upon the refrigerating unit to keep the solutions within the correct processing range if some measure of insulation is not provided. Under these conditions, condensation moisture may accumulate on the outside of the tank and drip to the floor, creating a continual source of annoyance to the technician who must stand close to the tank during the processing of films. Air conditioning solves all of these problems. However, some type of insulation around the master tank is the only alternative. When insulation is applied to metal tanks, it must be done with a tight bond. The sheet insulation must be fastened to the sides and bottom with an adhesive such as asphaltum. Otherwise the moisture works into the insulation and evenutally rots it. Such insulation can be effected in permanent installations.

DETERMINATION OF TANK CAPACITY

Insert tanks are made of stainless steel and are constructed in a standard 5-gallon size. The American Standards Association has determined the inside dimensions of standard 5-gallon tanks to be 20 1/32 inches deep, 14½ inches long, and 4 inches wide. Often the tank capacity is only approximate so its is necessary to compute the actual volume by using the following formula:

$$\text{Capacity (gals.)} = \frac{\text{Width} \times \text{length} \times \text{depth} - 1''}{231}$$

When the inside dimensions of the tank are correct, the solution level is 1 inch below the ledge for the crossbar and the volume of the tank is maintained within plus or minus 5 per cent of its rated 5 gallons capacity. The capacity should be known so that the technician can use the correct amount of processing chemicals when making solutions.

TIME-TEMPERATURE METHOD

In 1929, the work by Martin, Smith, and Hodgson* on a system of standardized tank development did much to advance more uniform radiographic quality. Their system pointed up the advantages of development by time and temperature and a method for adjusting the *time* of development to compensate the progressive exhaustion of the developer with use. They published a chart on which an accurate record of the films developed could be kept. After a certain number of films was developed for a given time and temperature (Period A), the time was increased one minute for a second given number of films (Period B); for a third group of films (Period C), the development time was again increased 1 minute. At the end of this period, the developer was replaced with fresh solution and the cycle repeated. The method, called the *exhaustion* system,

* Martin, F. C., Smith, E. C., and Hodgson, M. B.: A new system of standardized tank development. *X-ray Bull.*, *5*:6-10, 1929.

was readily adopted by the profession and has been in world-wide use since that time.

Since that time, further knowledge regarding the chemistry of development has resulted in a simpler version. This is the *replenisher* system, in which the time of development remains constant and the initial strength of the solution is maintained constant for the life of the solution by the frequent addition of small quantities of a liquid replenisher solution. This solution has all the original chemicals contained in the initial developer except the restrainer —potassium bromide. After a specified volume of replenisher has been employed, the solution is discarded and new solution is made. The replenisher method has been easy to employ and is the answer to true standardization of development.

The tank method of processing is efficient and convenient, and is employed in virtually every x-ray laboratory. Its advantages are many, the most important being that it provides facilities for maintaining constant temperature and for preserving the solutions. In this system, tanks containing the processing solutions are properly located in a master tank containing water at the prescribed temperature. Sufficient space is provided so that a place for film rinsing and washing is available in addition to the solution tanks. Water should be circulated in the master tank at a temperature that should be controlled by a mixing valve (if available) situated in the hot and cold water supply in permanent installation. If the volume of radiographic work justifies it, a separate tank for washing purposes only should be provided.

The chemical reactions involved in the processing procedure take place within a limited time and temperature range for optimum results. Although the exposure latitude of the film will compensate in a measure for some errors in exposure, good quality radiographs cannot be consistently secured if processing is not standardized.

Uniformity in radiographic densities and equal densities that are desired in comparative films are only obtained when the standard, *time-temperature* method of development is employed. When the time and temperature of development are optimum, films lacking density are the result of underexposure, not underdevelopment; and those having excessive density are the result of overexposure and not overdevelopment. Results of this nature make possible suitable changes in the exposure factors so that good quality radiographs can be secured.

* * *

A new method of x-ray film processing was announced in 1957 that is solving a major problem of the larger x-ray laboratory. This method is called the X-Omat System for automatic rapid processing of x-ray film. Employing an entirely new series of chemical solutions at higher than usual temperatures, the exposed x-ray film is automatically processed in six minutes. X-ray films, 5 x 7 to 14 x 17 inches can be easily fed into the processor one after the other. Developing hangers are not used. The System facilitates the rapid production of dry radiographs for diagnosis shortly after the x-ray examination, case by case. This processing method is of particular value in cases of trauma, pyelography, cholecystography, angiography and like situations where immediate radiographic information is required by the medicosurgical team. All radiographs are available for interpretation the same day so that reports can be sent to the referring physician shortly thereafter.

Chapter 18

Packing, Storage and Handling X-ray Film

X-RAY FILM is a delicate material and it should not be handled carelessly or roughly. It is sensitive to treatment of any kind—and heat, light, x-rays, radium, chemical fumes, pressure, rolling, bending, etc., are capable of adversely affecting the emulsion. Fortunately, it can be handled safely and swiftly in accordance with all the various radiographic needs as long as the technician knowns what he must do to avoid the production of foreign marks (artifacts) on the film. The increased speed of film in late years has made it a bit more sensitive to handling operations, and greater care must be exercised.

Safety x-ray film is in common use today. It represents no greater hazard in the stock, radiographic, processing or filing rooms than would an equal quantity of paper records. Radiographs made with this film can be stored on open shelves, in manila envelopes. Discarded film boxes may be stood on end and employed for filing radiographs.

PACKING

X-ray film is packed in hermetically sealed metal foil and paper wrappings to protect it from light and moisture. Packaged in quantities of 25 and 75 sheets, the relatively dry film is enclosed in a folder of chemically pure interleaving paper. Each unit quantity of 25 or 75 sheets is placed between cardboard and wrapped in black protective paper. The package is then placed in a metal foil bag that is hermetically sealed under conditions that insure approximately 50 per cent humidity *inside* the package. The package is then inserted in a cardboard carton.

Packed under these conditions, x-ray film will be free from any defects that may be due to conditions of humidity, as long as it remains in the foil wrapping. When overseas shipments are made, each carton should be sealed in heavy waterproof paper for additional protection.

Some of the reasons for wrapping each film in interleaving paper may be of interest. The pulp from which the paper is made is very carefully selected and manufactured under rigid conditions of cleanliness. The interleaving paper is soft, nonabrasive and chemically inert. It has a matte surface which serves to prevent very close contact with the film. Thousands of tiny points in the paper surface prevent this. These characteristics tend to reduce the possibility for generation of static electricity when the films are packaged and subjected to some measure of pressure or friction.

During all operations a temperature of 50° F. and 50 per cent humidity is constant. A water vapor balance between the film and the paper is maintained within the heat-sealed bag. The residual moisture cannot get out and none can get in it. Until the package is opened, the film is stored under ideal conditions provided the temperature is optimal. The constant moisture level in the heat-sealed bag is best for good keeping and prevention of fog.

STORAGE

Unexposed and unprocessed x ray film should always be kept in a cool, dry place. It should never be stored in basements or near steam pipes or other sources of heat. In extremely warm climates only small quantities of film should be ordered at one time, so that a rapid turn-over takes place.

HEAT

High temperatures exert injurious effects on the emulsion causing loss of contrast and the production of fog. Unexposed x-ray film should not be expected to be usable more than a few weeks after subject to temperatures of 90° to 100° F.; or more than a few days at 110° to 120° F. A relatively brief period of excessive heat in transit or storage may ruin the film regardless of how well it is protected during the major portion of its life. Because x-ray film is packed in hermetically sealed containers does not mean that it no longer requires care or protection. Such packing does protect film from moisture, both from humid air or actual water immersion, and from other contaminants—as long as the package is *unbroken*. However, it does *not* provide protection from high temperatures.

An approximate guide to usability of film under various temperature storage conditions and approximately 60 per cent humidity is as follows. If film is to be used in 2 months, it can withstand temperatures up to 75° F. without deterioration. If stored at 60° F., it can be kept 6 months in storage; at 50° F., for 1 year. Ideal storage conditions will prevail at temperatures of 50° to 70° F. and 40 to 60 per cent relative humidity.

X-RADIATION

Film must be suitably protected from the unwanted action of x-rays or radium by lead-lined walls or chests (see Figure 137). Film bins located in the processing room should be protected by sheet lead.

FUMES

X-ray film must never be stored in drug rooms or other places containing fumes of any kind. Illuminating gas, formalin, ammonia, volatile oils, sewer gas, etc., will fog film in opened packages if it is stored in an atmosphere containing these substances.

PRESSURE

Film should never be subjected to extreme pressure such as wrinkling, bending, or rolling because changes take place in the emulsion which, upon development, appear as artifacts on the finished film. To avoid pressure markings, packages of unexposed x-ray film should always be stored on edge; they should never be stacked one upon another.

EXPIRATION DATE

All film should be used before its expiration date because film aging causes loss in speed and contrast.

REFRIGERATION

Storage of unopened packages of x-ray

film in refrigerators is satisfactory provided packages are removed 24 to 36 hours before they are used. This procedure is necessary to avoid the production of condensing moisture on the film when each sheet is removed from the package under high atmospheric temperatures. Open boxes of x-ray film should not be stored in refrigerators wherein conditions of high humidity usually prevail. Once a box of film is opened it should be used as soon as possible. If opened boxes of film must be contained in refrigerators, no other materials should be stored therein and some type of dehydrator should be placed in the refrigerator to reduce the humidity.

HANDLING

In handling x-ray film, the technician should avoid touching the film surfaces. Film should be held as near the edges as possible with clean dry hands. X-ray film is very sensitive to almost all forms of energy. When it is properly handled, exposed and processed, a satisfactory image free of artifacts * will result.

It is well to remember that any form of white light creeping into a processing room through cracks around the edges of partitions, windows, doors, or open film bins many fog x-ray film. Be sure that all white light is turned off in the processing room when handling film. When white light is on, film bins should be tightly closed and the tops secure on all film boxes, Figure 138. White light should never be turned on while films are developing because films will be fogged in the tank, Figure 139.

SAFELIGHT ILLUMINATION

X-ray films are sensitive to white light and must be handled either in darkness or under safelight illumination of the proper quality. The processing room should be adequately provided with both white-light and safelight illumination. White-light is necessary to perform many activities such as the mixing of chemicals, cleaning of tanks, caring for intensifying screens, placing films in the dryer, and unloading film hangers. Fixtures for white-light should be properly located to afford general illumination when films are not being developed.

Safelight illumination should be furnished in the working areas by hanging "direct" or "indirect" type lamps. Film exposed with x-ray intensifying screens is approximately 8 times more sensitive to safelight illumination than unexposed film. Because films are subjected to safelight

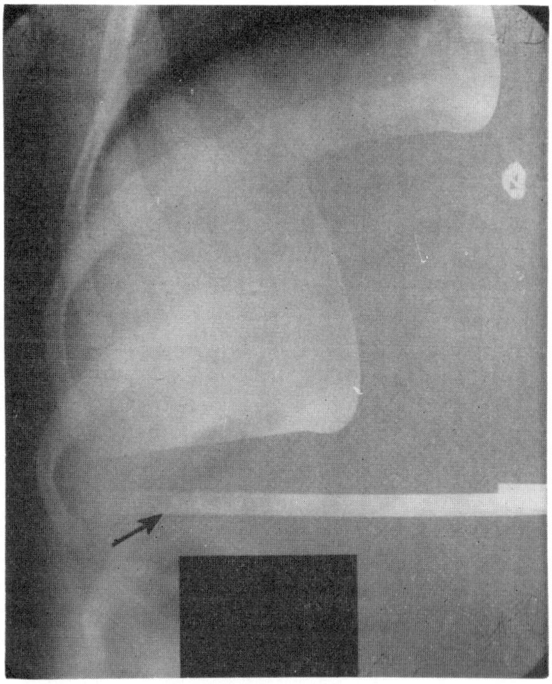

Figure 137. Radiograph made with film from a box that had been inadvertently exposed to x-rays in a laboratory. Note radiographic image of lead foil band that is normally incorporated in cardboard box.

* In a radiographic sense, an artifact is a mark foreign to the x-ray image, and which is not necessarily imposed on the film by the action of x-rays.

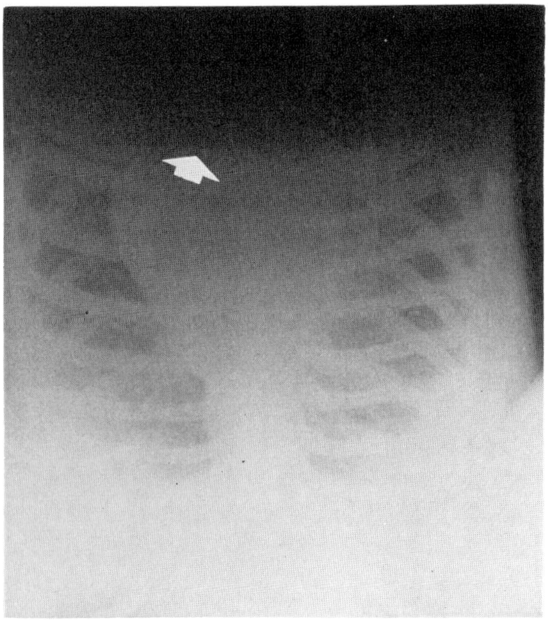

Figure 138. Posteroanterior radiograph of chest showing fogged area produced when white light was turned on in the processing room while film box was uncovered.

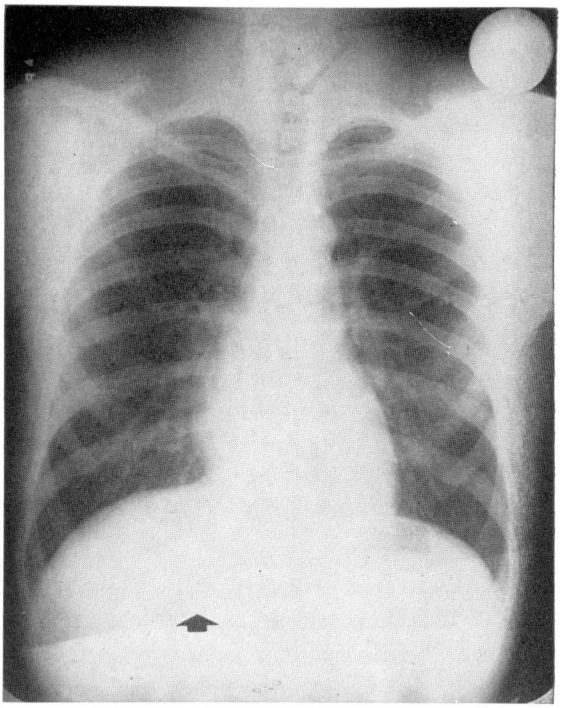

Figure 139. Radiograph exhibiting safelight fog because exposed film was laid on loading bench too long and partially covered by a piece of paper.

illumination at the loading bench for a longer period than in any other zone, direct-type safelight lamps over this area are liable to raise the amount of postexposure fog to an undesirable degree. For this reason, the loading bench should be illuminated by an indirect safelight lamp. No film should be exposed to the safelight lamp for a period longer than it takes to unload a film, place it in its hanger, and immerse it in the developing solution.

Safelight illumination is designed to give enough visibility in the processing room for the technician to accomplish all necessary duties in connection with the handling and processing of x-ray film without harmful effect to any unprocessed film that may be exposed. No safelight is safe if the standards of safety are abused. Film left out under a safelight lamp too long will fog, Figure 139. If film cannot be processed at once, it should be stored in a light-tight container. When loading films in hangers, preparatory to group development, it is important that they be protected from direct radiation from the lamps. *Exposed* films being more sensitive to safelight illumination should be set to one side away from the direct beam of a safelight lamp or, better still, placed under or behind a protective screen. If the films cannot be covered, the safelight lamp nearest the stacked films should be turned off.

Improper safelight illumination is a common cause of film fog. Excessive examination of films under a safelight during development as well as holding them too close to the safelight causes aerial fog and/or light fog on film. Therefore, certain considerations must be kept in mind in connection with safelight lamps and safelights.

1. The illumination will be safe only if bulbs of the wattage indicated on each lamp are used.

2. All safelight filters are safe only as long as specific conditions prevail. The standard of safety for all safelights is such that unexposed x-ray film may be safely handled in the light at a distance of 3 feet, for 1 minute. These factors apply to the use of safelights, Series 6B, with *unexposed* x-ray film.

Safelight Lamps

Safelight lamps are an indispensable item in every processing room. Safelights, Figure 140, are lamphouses equipped with filters that provide photographically *safe* illumination in a processing room while handling and developing unprocessed film. The light emitted by a safelight is of such spectral quality and intensity that it does not fog film handled under it for a reasonable handling period and yet the illumination provided by it is as high as possible consistent with safe handling of the film. As far as practicable, the general illumination should be made indirect by suspending from the ceiling one or more safelight lamps of appropriate design and size. If the walls and ceiling are painted with a light colored paint, the entire room will be well lighted with safe illumination. For light in specific sections of the processing room, there are safelight lamps of various designs. The choice and arrangement of safelight lamps should depend upon the amount of illumination desired and the angle at which it must fall.

Blackout conditions in the permanent processing room are neither necessary from a technical standpoint nor desirable from a psychologic one. A dark colored wall finish will absorb much of the safelight illumination. If the quality of the light from a safelight lamp is "safe," the illumination reflected from any surface is also "safe" regardless of its color. Nor does the reflected light gain in intensity over the direct or incident light beam. The wall finish, should, therefore, reflect the maximum amount of safelight illumination and the color should be attractive and pleasant. In order to appear bright, the wall color must reflect rather than absorb light from the safelight lamp.

The best processing room illumination is that transmitted by a series 6B safelight, using a tungsten light source. The light emitted is in the yellow and yellow-red portion of the spectrum. Therefore, maxi-

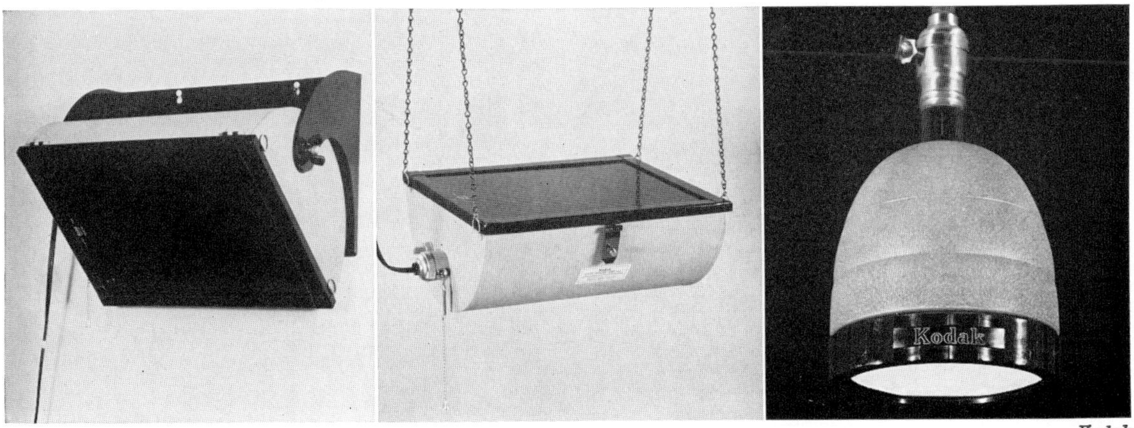

Kodak

Figure 140. Various types of safelight lamps employed in processing rooms equipped with Series 6B safelights.

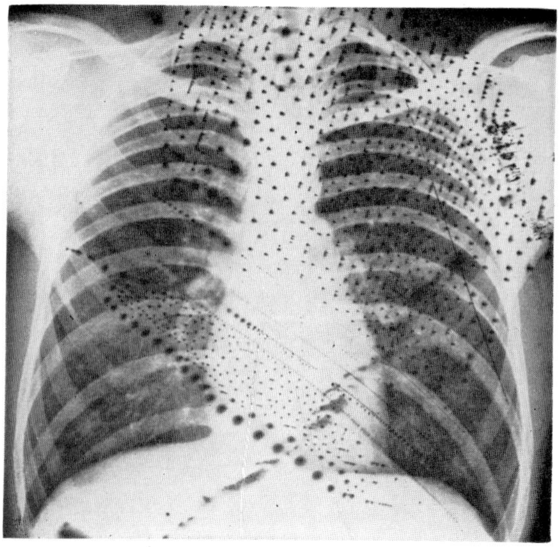

Fig. 141. Radiograph exhibiting various artifacts resulting from static electric discharges to the film.

mum reflection under safelight illumination is achieved if the wall finish is either a color within this same spectral range, or a light enough shade of any other color. It is desirable also to have a color that is pleasing under white light as well as safelight illumination. In permanent installations, the ceiling and the upper 18 inches of the side walls should be painted white to provide maximum reflection of white light. For the remainder of the side walls, warm tones such as ivory, cream, and buff, or extremely pale shades of any desired color, are generally more pleasing than white, which is apt to be too glaring and shows soil quickly.

Checking Safelight Illumination

A simple method of checking the safety of illumination is to cover part of an unexposed film and expose sections of the remainder for different lengths of time in the place where films will be uncovered in handling. This test film is then given standard development. If no fog shows on the parts that receive a reasonably long exposure, as compared with the covered part, the lighting may be assumed to be safe. If fog does appear, the distance of the safelights from the film should be increased. All safelight lamps should be tested periodically for white light leaks, fading of filter, and excess wattage of bulbs.

STATIC DISCHARGES

Every precaution in the manufacture and packing of x-ray film is employed to avoid the accumulation of static electricity on the film surfaces. Whenever two dissimilar surfaces are pressed together and separated, static electric charges develop. The electric charge becomes appreciable when one or both surfaces are nonconductors and when the atmospheric humidity is low. The quantity of the charge depends partly upon the electrical storage capacity possessed by the total surface of the area involved and the spacing of the charged parts and the insulating strength of the intervening medium.

A static electric discharge emits visible light capable of exposing the film, and the resulting artifacts assume various shapes, Figure 141. They are usually treelike or bushlike in appearance (the point of discharge always has the greatest density) with fingerlike processes emanating outward from the point of discharge. Often static marks assume the character of black smudges. Discharges are most likely to occur in cold, dry periods and it is then that particular care must be taken to handle film carefully and avoid friction on its surface. The loading bench in the processing room should be grounded so that in the handling of the cassette any static charges that are built up can be dissipated before the cassette is opened.

Prevention of static sparks can be effected by grounding the location where static charges may develop and by increasing the humidity. To raise the humidity of the air in the x-ray and processing rooms, the use of a commercial humidifier will assist in maintaining a satisfactory humidity level. Remember that the danger point for static production occurs when the humidity is 60 per cent. As the humidity gets less and less, static electric accumulations grow.

In the emulsion-coating operation during manufacture, static electricity is removed by ingenious and complicated methods so that static charges have no opportunity to accumulate on the film and

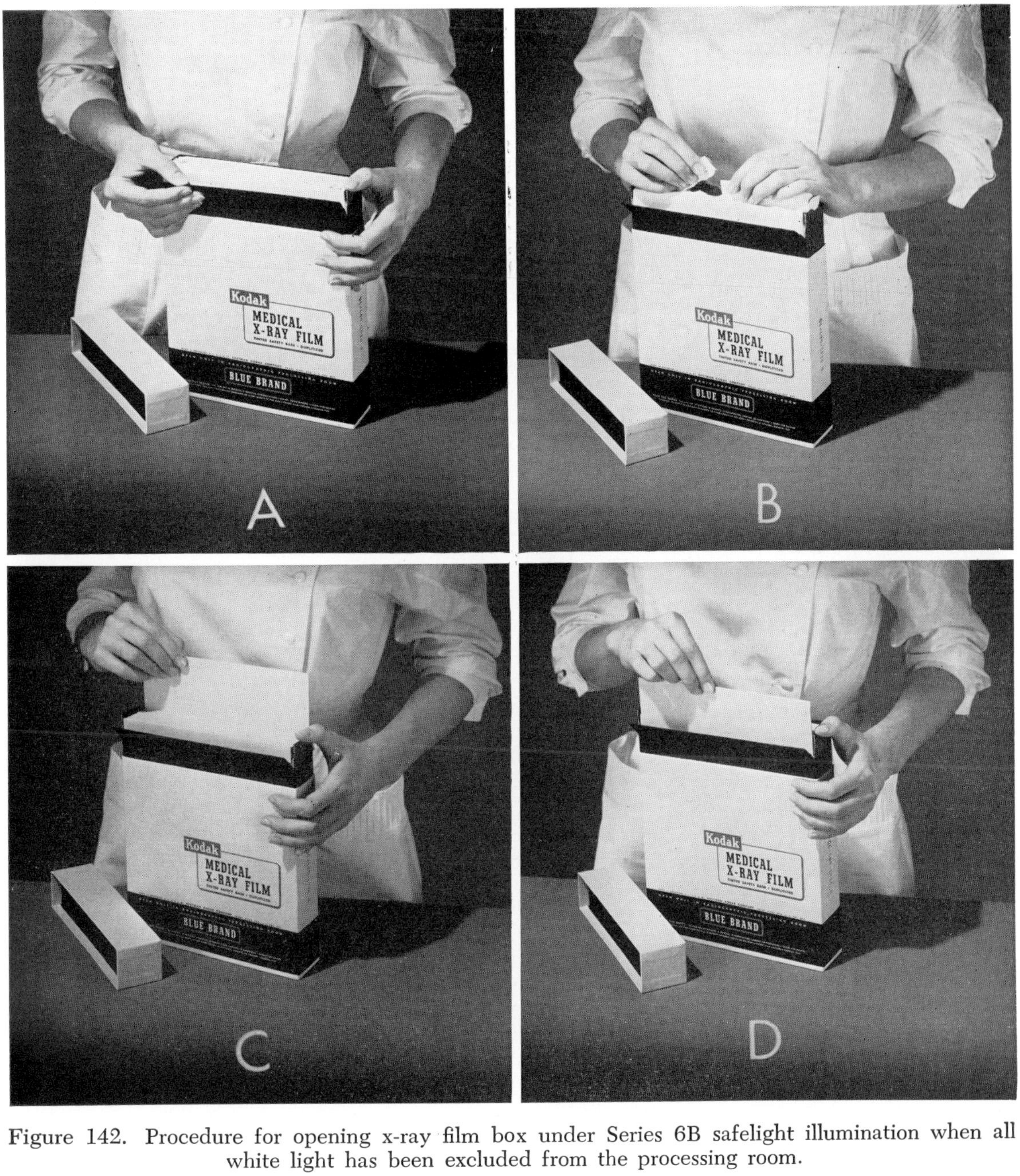

Figure 142. Procedure for opening x-ray film box under Series 6B safelight illumination when all white light has been excluded from the processing room.

lead to artifacts on the finished radiograph. The fact that the film is coated and dried in an atmosphere free of dust and at an optimum and constant temperature and humidity, serves to keep the formation and production of static electricity to a minimum.

REMOVAL OF FILM FROM CARTON

When obtaining x-ray film from a new carton, the film should always be removed with its folded paper wrapper. Rapid movement should be avoided as a protection against the production of static electricity or pressure artifacts. The proper procedure in opening the film carton is illustrated in Figure 142.

The box of film is placed on the loading bench, the paper retaining strip at the edge of the cover is cut and the cover lifted from the box top, Figure 142A. All white light in the processing room is turned off and the 6B safelight illumination provides ample light for opening the film box. When the cover of the box is removed, the serrated edge of the heat sealed bag is exposed. One side of the box near its top is scored so that about one inch of the box can be folded down. This will help to remove the films later (A). The flap on the bag should be stripped by tearing it at its center and stripping the top away to each side (B). The package of film in its yellow interleaving paper then becomes visible. The two cardboard stiffeners are removed (C) and the film may then be easily removed (D).

LOADING AND UNLOADING FILM

There are two types of containers in which medical x-ray films can be held during exposure—cardboard exposure holders and cassettes. The choice depends upon the exposure technic to be employed. In the direct exposure technic, the film enclosed in its interleaving paper is placed in the exposure holder which comprises a light-tight envelope mounted between two pieces of radioparent paperboard that are hinged together, Figure 143; in the double-intensifying-screen technic, the film is placed between two x-ray intensifying screens that are mounted in a cassette, Figure 145. In loading and unloading x-ray film, all white light must be extinguished in the processing or loading room.

LOADING THE EXPOSURE HOLDER

An x-ray exposure holder consists of two pieces of x-ray transparent paperboard that comprise the covers; they are held together with heavy binding cloth. To one cover, a metal clip is attached on a pivot; laminated to the inside of the cover is thin lead foil that protects the film during the x-ray ex-

---

→

Figure 143. Procedure for loading unexposed x-ray film in exposure holder.

A. Unlatch clip of exposure holder; raise back of holder and open paper envelope.
B. Remove film in its protective paper folder from carton with right hand and hold it vertically.
C. Grasp film and paper at lower center margin with left hand and, without bending or crimping bring it to horizontal position over exposure holder with the aid of the right hand.
D. Carefully lay film in its paper folder in envelope.
E. Fold large end flap of envelope into place.
F. Fold over top and side flaps of envelope.
G. Lower back of holder.
H. Latch holder together with metal clip.

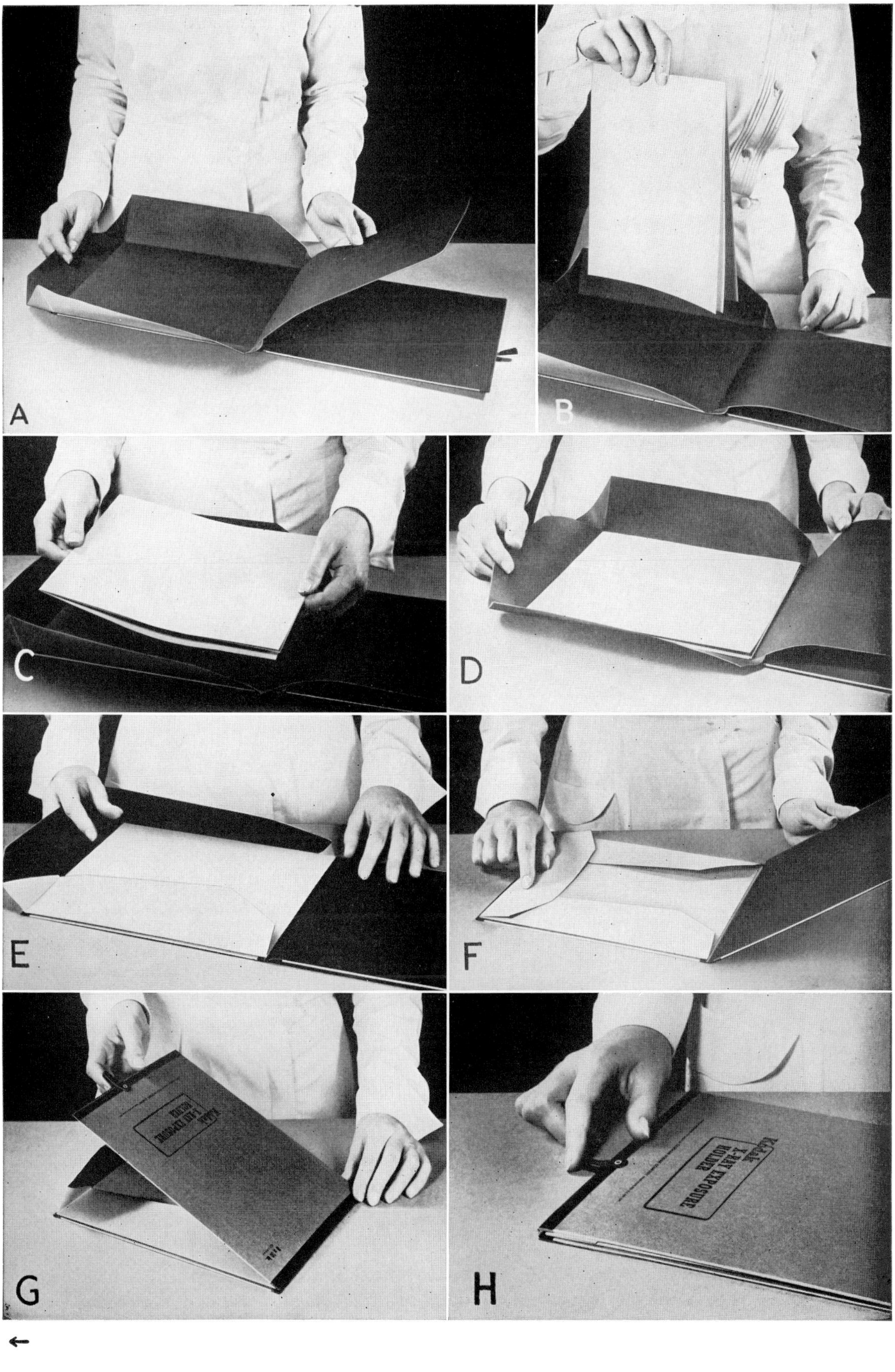
A
B
C
D
E
F
G
H
X-RAY EXPOSURE
HOLDER

←

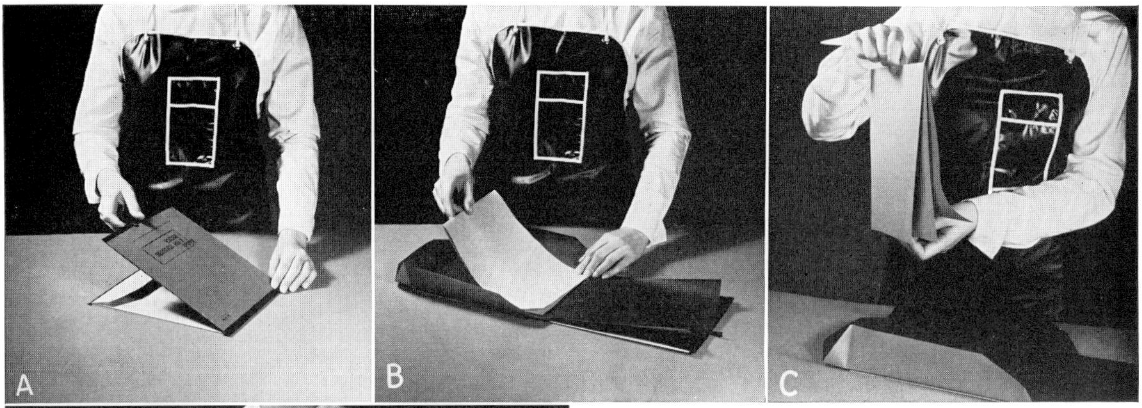

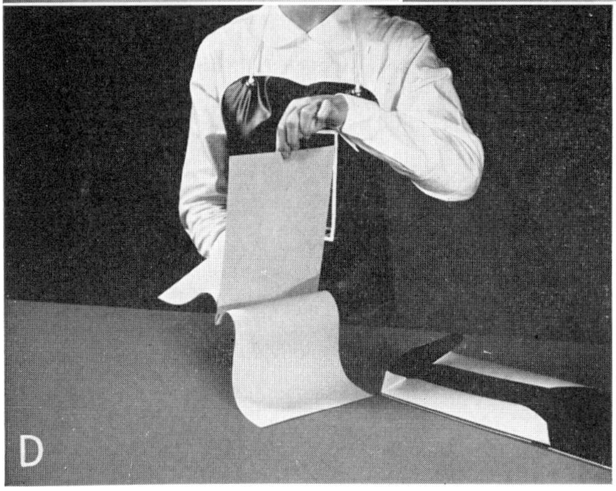

Figure 144. Procedure for removing x-ray film from exposure holder after exposure.

A. Open metal clip and lift back of holder.
B. Unfold envelope; grasp folded edge of interleaving paper with right hand and lift paper and film together.
C. Hold paper and film vertically; with left hand separate film from paper at bottom and grasp edge of film.
D. Turn edge in left hand clockwise so that paper drops away from film. Film is now ready to be loaded in processing hanger.

posure from back-scatter of secondary radiation. Affixed to the inside of the other cover is an envelope that folds around the film and excludes all light.

The correct procedure for loading an exposure holder with film is shown in Figure 143. In loading, the film *enclosed in its paper folder* is placed in the open exposure holder; next, the large flap of the envelope is turned down, then the side flaps are brought over, followed by the end flap. The final step is to bring together the covers and fasten them with the clip. It is most important that this procedure for protection of the film be followed if light-fog is to be avoided. The holder is now ready for use. Since the back of the exposure holder contains a thin sheet of lead to prevent secondary radiation backscatter, it must not be interposed between the part and the film. This would cause an underexposure by reason of the absorption of the radiation by the lead. The cover of the film exposure holder upon which is printed "tube side" should be uppermost and face the x-ray tube during exposure of the film.

UNLOADING THE EXPOSURE HOLDER

After exposure of the film, the film is removed from the exposure holder. In this procedure, be sure that the film is not buckled in handling. The correct procedure for this operation is shown in Figure 144.

LOADING THE CASSETTE

When the film in its paper folder is removed from its carton, it should be held vertically at the middle of the top border with the finger tips of the right hand, Figure 145. The open paper leaves at the bottom can then be carefully separated

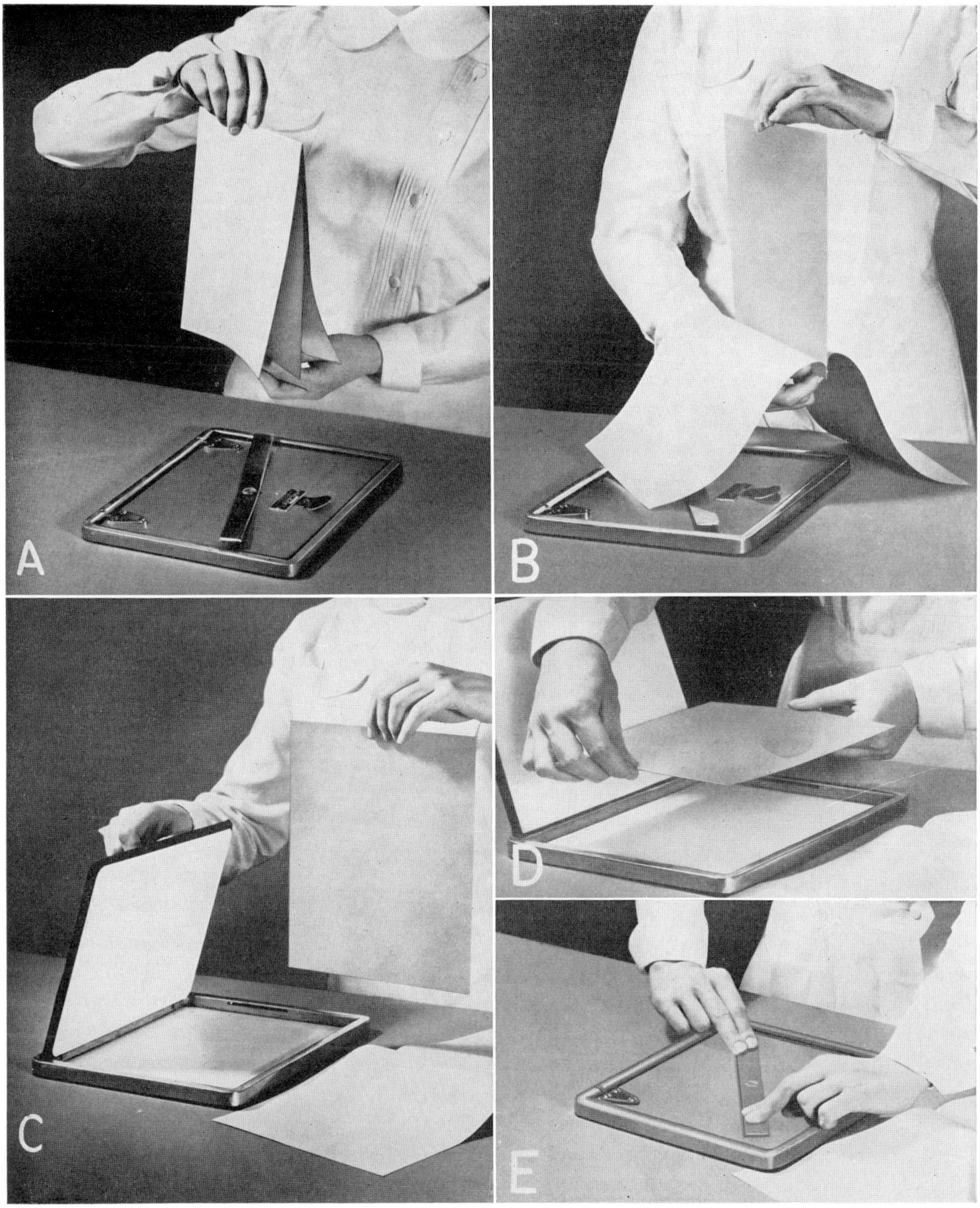

Figure 145. Procedure for loading film in cassette containing x-ray intensifying screens.

A. Unlock cassette; remove film in its paper folder from carton and hold it vertically with finger tips of right hand. Separate film from paper with left hand and grasp lower edge of film with thumb and forefinger.

B. With left hand still holding its lower edge, turn film 180° clockwise so that paper falls away.

C. Discard paper and raise cassette lid with right hand.

D. Grasp film at center of lower edge with finger tips of right hand, and without bending, lay it flat in cassette.

E. Close and lock cassette lid by spring lever.

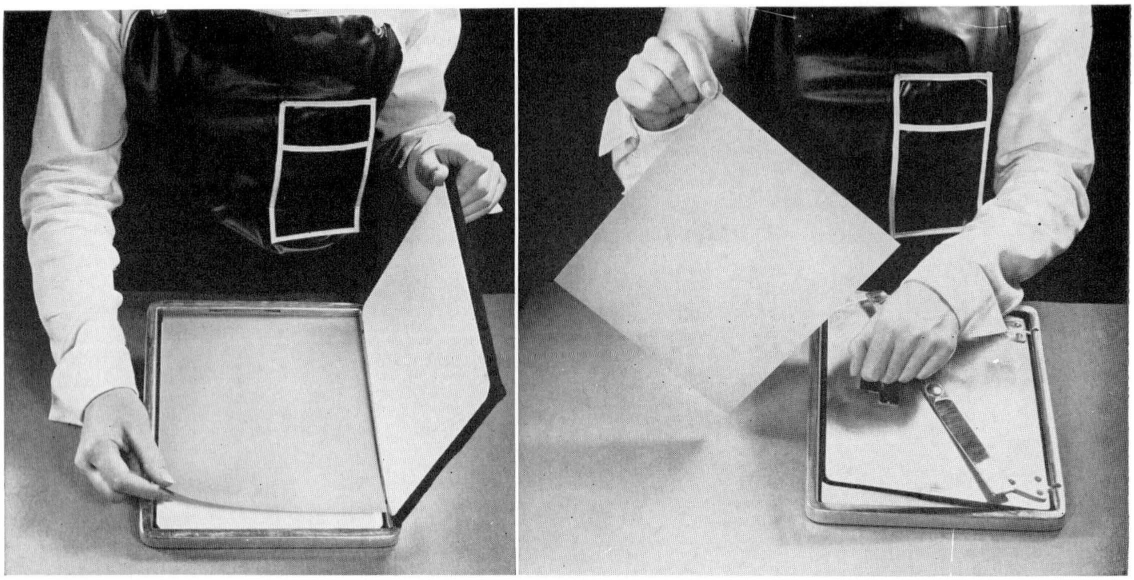

Figure 146. Procedure for removal of exposed x-ray film from cassette.

(*Left*). Open and raise cassette lid; grasp right upper corner of film with right forefinger and thumb. (*Right*). Lift film from cassette and hold vertically while closing lid with left hand. Before placing in processing hanger, grasp opposite corner of film with left hand.

from the film with the left hand. In this operation the lower border of the film is grasped by the fingers of the left hand and the ensemble rotated 180° vertically. The paper will then fall away easily from the film. The lower edge of the freely suspended film is then grasped by the finger tips of the right hand and rotated so that the plane of the film is taut and horizontal. It is then placed in the cassette on the front intensifying screen. The lid carrying the back screen is gently closed and locked by means of the back springs. When placing the film in the cassette, care should be exercised to avoid scraping or sliding the film over the edges of the cassette or surface of the screen. The procedure for correctly loading a cassette is illustrated in Figure 145.

UNLOADING THE CASSETTE

The correct procedure for removal of the film after exposure in the cassette, is shown in Figure 146. Be sure that in this operation the hands are dry and chemically free and that they do not come in contact with the x-ray intensifying screens.

LOADING THE PROCESSING HANGER

The processing hanger is an invaluable processing accessory, for it provides a means for securely holding the film during the processing procedure. After the film is removed from the cassette or exposure holder, it is loaded into a stainless steel developing hanger that consists of a rigid frame to which are attached four clips, two of which are mounted on a bow spring welded to a top crossbar. When the exposed film is removed from the cassette or exposure holder, it is held vertically with the left hand at upper left corner while a hanger of proper size is taken from the storage rack. The upper left corner of the film is inserted in the bottom left clip, and the right film corner in the right bottom clip. The hanger is then inverted, making certain the film does not buckle and the procedure repeated. The bow spring serves to keep the film taut and straight during processing. The procedure for loading the hanger is shown in Figure 147.

The film is now ready to be developed, but before immersing it in the developer, the surface of the film should be checked to see that it is taut and does not bulge. If bulging is present, one of the upper bow spring clips should be loosened and the film reinserted in the clip after the slack is carefully taken up. Since cleanliness is of importance and the presence of extraneous marks or artifacts on the radiograph are objectionable, residual gelatin or dirt in the clips should be removed periodically.

Immersion of Hangers in Solutions

When placing hangers loaded with film in solutions either singly or in groups, do so as a unit. They should be immersed quickly and carefully so that the film surfaces are uniformly bathed with solution and are not endangered by adjacent hangers. Immediately after complete immersion of the films, they should be raised several times about two inches out of the solution and then lowered. This action serves to remove air bells and to bathe completely the surfaces of the film with solution. Hangers should then be separated by about three-fourths of an inch. Hangers should never be removed entirely from the solution until they are ready to be subjected to succeeding processing operations. By keeping the level of the solutions one inch below the top of the tanks, the crossbars of the hangers are not covered by the developer or fixer solution. When in the wash water, fresh water should flow over the hanger crossbars.

Bow springs of hangers that have been used for an extended period gradually lose their original tension and, instead of producing tautness in the films, permit them

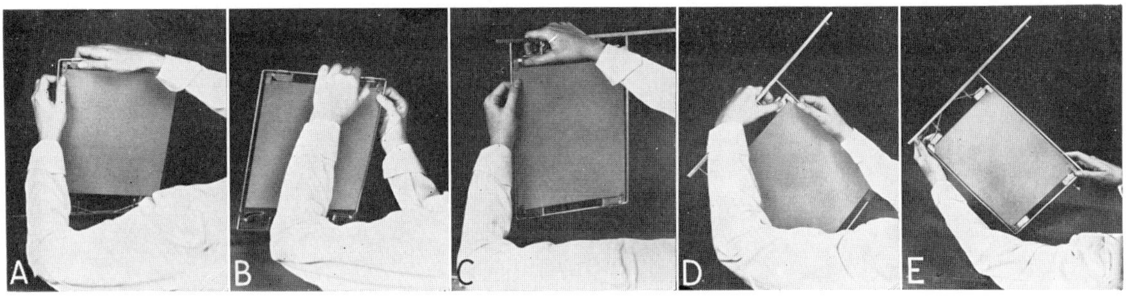

Figure 147. Procedure for loading exposed x-ray film in a processing hanger; when unloading hanger, the above procedure is reversed.

A. Hold frame of hanger bottom-side up and edge of film near film clip at corner with left hand; open jaws of clip with right forefinger and thumb, and engage corner of film; release spring tension.

B. Slide finger along bottom of hanger to other film clip, while right thumb and forefinger guides other corner of film into clip; left hand squeezes clip and engages film. Be sure that film is taut across bottom edge.

C. Invert hanger so that hanger bar is uppermost. Grasp edge of film with left hand and guide it into clip mounted on bow-spring that is pushed into position by right hand; clip is opened and engages corner of film.

D. The fourth clip engages the remaining corner of the film to complete the operation. Be sure that the film is held tautly in the frame.

E. Completed action for correctly loading x-ray film in the hanger. Note that the surface of the film is held flat and taut by the hanger. Film is now ready for processing.

to bulge. When several hangers exhibiting this deficiency are placed in the processing tank, areas of the films they hold may touch or even adhere to one another, preventing complete development and resulting in artifacts in the radiographs. To correct the condition, the springs may be bent until the distance between the opposite top and bottom clips, when not supporting a film, is slightly greater than the length of the film intended to be hung in the space. This can be readily accomplished by the following procedure. Place the hanger on the loading bench. Insert in the jaws of the lower clips a sheet of cardboard from a box of x-ray film of the same size as the hanger. Bend the bow springs upward until the lower tips of the clips attached to them are about one-eighth inch above the top edge of the cardboard. When this adjustment has been made, films that are placed in the hanger will again be held taut.

Chapter 19

Mixing Processing Solutions

Processing chemicals today are compounded as dry chemicals according to very precise formulae. The correct amount of each chemical is mixed together so that by merely adding water the correct solution is obtained. No longer is it necessary for the technician to prepare a solution by weighing out the necessary quantities of individual chemicals according to an antiquated formula. To make a solution from prepared and packaged processing chemicals, the technician need only read the instructions on the package and mix the bulk chemicals accordingly. It is most important, however, that these instructions be read and followed exactly so that a properly functioning solution is obtained. The manufacturers of packed chemicals have expended a great deal of effort in making these instructions simple and easy for the technician to follow. *Be sure to read the label on the chemical containers.* Formulae for these prepared powders are not available for use by the technician. However, they usually do provide better solutions than any that can be prepared from raw chemicals employing any published formula.

IMPORTANCE OF CLEANLINESS

The procedure employed for processing radiographs involves chemical reactions between the various processing solutions and the x-ray emulsion. As in any chemical reaction, its success depends upon the purity of the solutions employed. Consequently, the cleanliness and care exercised in the preparation of the solutions and their subsequent use is of paramount importance. The processing room, as well as the accessories and equipment, must be kept scrupulously clean and used only for the purposes intended. Spilled solutions should be wiped up at once; otherwise, upon evaporation, the chemicals may dust into the air and later settle on film or screen surfaces that may result in artifacts on the radiographs. When mixing chemicals, be sure to turn off any electric fans, for chemicals may be blown about the proc-

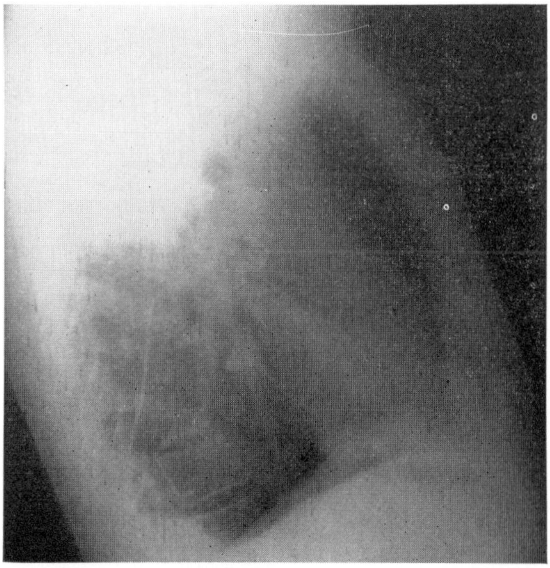

Figure 148. Radiograph exhibiting black spots caused by developer dust that was blown around processing room and into cassette by an electric fan.

essing room and contaminate the loading bench, screens, etc., Figure 148. Hands that are wet with chemicals should never be used for handling films, screens, or other allied accessories.

WATER

Since water is the solvent for all processing solutions, care should be exercised in choosing its source. Most city water supplies are suitable but they should be checked for high concentrations of various salts before use. In general, any potable water is usually satisfactory.

PURE WATER

Distilled water, since it does not contain dissolved chemicals, is pure and ideal for mixing purposes. It is not always easy to obtain this type water but if available, rain water or distilled water melted from clean ice or snow are good substitutes.

WATER IMPURITIES

The chief kinds of impurities found in water usually comprise—

Suspended Material

Suspended material may consist of decayed animal or vegetable matter, mud, rust, and sulfur. Filtration will remove the majority of these substances.

Dissolved Chemicals

Chemicals found freely in nature that have been dissolved by water. Such chemicals cause hardness of the water and are composed of calcium and magnesium salts in the form of bicarbonates, chlorides, and sulfates. These salts are not injurious to the image but may produce a scum on the surfaces of the film that reduces its transparency. It must and can be removed before drying by squeegeeing the faces of the radiographs with cotton or a photographic spone. The hardness of the water may be eliminated by circulating the water through a water softener.

Coloring Matter

Coloring matter of vegetable or animal origin, usually yellow or brown, may stain the film. Such water should be avoided.

Dissolved Gases

Various gases often become dissolved in water. These gases may be carbon dioxide or hydrogen sulfide. The latter is particularly objectionable because it reacts with the silver image and ultimately discolors it. These waters should be avoided.

MIXING SOLUTIONS

The first step in the processing procedure is the proper preparation of the processing solution with water. When mixing the chemicals to be made into solutions, the manufacturer's directions found on the label of the container should always be carefully followed if best results are to be obtained. There are, however, some general recommendations which it is necessary to observe when making up solutions.

MIXING TEMPERATURE

The temperature of the water in which the chemicals are to be dissolved should never exceed that shown on the label of the package.

MIXING UTENSILS

The containers for mixing chemicals should consist of corrosion-resistant materials such as good enamel or glazed earthenware, glass, hard rubber, or Types 316 and 317 stainless steel. Vessels con- the solution will fog film during the development period. Two stainless steel pails to hold two gallons each of solution and a taining tin, copper, zinc, aluminum, or galvanized iron should never by used because small quantities of these metals in stainless steel or plastic funnel are important items of the mixing equipment. Separate stainless steel mixing paddles for the developer and for the fixer should be employed, after which they should be washed with clear warm water and hung up to dry.

VOLUME OF SOLUTIONS

To insure the proper concentration of solutions, the *volume* in gallons of the tank used should always be mathematically computed, this being easily accomplished by dividing the product of the inside dimensions of the tank (width, breadth, and depth minus 1 inch) by 231. Processing tanks should be thoroughly cleaned before fresh solutions are placed in them.

MIXING PROCEDURE

When mixing chemicals, the water should always be poured into the tank or pail and the chemicals added *slowly* while the mixture is stirred vigorously, permitting the chemicals to go into solution quickly without "caking" and "lumping" of the ingredients. The creation of clouds of chemical dust by rapid pouring of the dry chemical into the water should be avoided. When the chemicals are entirely dissolved, sufficient cold water should be added to bring the solution to the correct volume and temperature; thorough stirring being necessary to mix the cool water with the chemically laden solution already present. Solutions should not be used until all the chemicals are thoroughly dissolved and at the optimum temperature of 68° F.

SOLUTION STORAGE

If the solution is not for immediate use, it should be placed in a clean bottle of the proper size, well stoppered and labeled plainly. Developer should be stored in brown bottles, away from radiators, for heat may cause deterioration of the solution.

MIXING WITH SEA WATER

There may be occasions when fresh water for processing is exceedingly scarce. While not recommended as a routine procedure, sea water can be utilized in the same quantities as fresh water, to compound x-ray developers and fixing baths. The resulting solutions are turbid but will clear on standing. If time permits, it is best to allow the solutions to stand overnight, and to decant the clear fluid for use. If turbid solutions are utilized, however, it is essential that the surfaces of the films be carefully wiped off with a soft wet photographic chamois or cellulose sponge after washing and before drying to remove any deposit.

Chapter 20

Development Process

THE PURPOSE of development is to convert chemically the invisible latent image to the visible silver image by means of a developer solution. In the conversion of the exposed silver bromide crystals to metallic silver, the film is immersed in an alkaline developer solution that softens and swells the gelatin so that ionization of the exposed silver bromide crystals occurs and the reducing agents transform the silver ions into clumps of black metallic silver. The unexposed silver bromide is unaffected by this treatment during the development period required by the exposed crystals.

TYPES OF X-RAY DEVELOPER SOLUTIONS

There are two general types of x-ray developer solutions each possessing essentially the same chemicals but differing in their activity. For purposes of discussion in this text, one developing solution is commonly referred to as "regular x-ray developer." Its activity or development potential is average in character because of the use of sodium carbonate as the alkali. The second solution is referred to as "rapid x-ray developer" because of its greater activity than the regular x-ray developer. Rapid x-ray developer has a high development potential because of the use of the chemical *kodalk* (sodium metaborate) as the alkali. Sodium hydroxide is also used for this purpose. These chemicals have greater alkalinity than sodium carbonate and are able to penetrate the emulsion swiftly, thereby providing a more rapid action of the reducing agents on the exposed silver salts.

DEVELOPER CONSTITUENTS

Conversion of the silver bromide to metallic silver must be accomplished by the many chemicals contained in the developing solution and it is necessary that the developer formula be standardized with all chemicals in balance so that the results will always be the same. Each film manufacturer, however, recommends formulae that produce the best results with that manufacturer's film and the compounded chemicals are packaged in convenient units so that they are easy to mix into solution form. The formula for a typical regular x-ray developer is printed below.

X-Ray Developer (*Kodak D-19b*)

Water, about 125° F.	2½	gallons.
Elon	1½	ounces.
Sodium sulfite, desiccated	3	pounds.
Hydroquinone	6	ounces.
Sodium carbonate, desiccated	2	pounds.
Potassium bromide	3	ounces.
Water to make	5	gallons.

Note. Dissolve chemicals in order given.

An x-ray developer usually contains five types of ingredients, Table XVI:

1. **Solvent.** Chemical reactions that occur in development require that all chemicals be dissolved in water. Besides acting as a solvent for the chemicals and as a means for their ionization, water aids in softening the gelatin emulsion.

2. **Reducers.** The purpose of a reducing agent is to convert the exposed silver bromide crystals to black metallic silver. A reducing agent cannot be a developer unless it reacts more rapidly with *exposed* silver bromide crystals than those that are unexposed. However, the exposure must be of a degree that will cause a satisfactory image to be formed in a given development period at a given temperature. In a properly exposed radiograph, this action is usually completed upon full development and *before* the unexposed crystals have an opportunity to develop to any perceptable degree. Reducing agents commonly employed are *elon* and *hydroquinone*. The activity of these chemicals requires their presence in an alkaline* solution. Each of these chemicals functions differently in attacking the emulsion. The elon starts development by attacking the exposed silver bromide crystals swiftly, with resultant production of low contrast in the image. Elon is little affected by temperature changes, whereas hydroquinone ceases its activity below 50° F.

The activity of the hydroquinone is slower but it serves to build up the required image contrast. Together, the reducers produce an image with satisfactory contrast in a minimum of time provided the temperature of the solution remains in the optimum range. Reducers are not stable in the presence of oxygen, for they can readily absorb it from the air or the water. The reducing action of hydroquinone on silver bromide in development is shown in the following chemical equation:

$$2\,AgBr + C_6H_4(OH)_2 \rightarrow 2\,Ag + 2\,Br^- + C_6H_4O_2 + 2H^+$$

Silver Bromide	Hydro-quinone	Free Silver	Bromine Ions	Quinone	Hydrogen Ions

3. **Activator.** The *activator* or alkali *softens* the gelatin of the emulsion and provides the necessary alkaline medium to the solution, so that the developing agents can diffuse into the gelatin emulsion and attack the exposed silver bromide crystals. In general, the more alkaline the developer the more powerful and rapid is its action. The chemicals most frequently used are sodium carbonate and kodalk.

Sodium Carbonate. Sodium carbonate is the alkali usually found in regular x-ray developer. It has been used for many years but there are some disadvantages to be recognized in its use. When a film is processed in a warm x-ray developer containing sodium carbonate and then transferred to a cool acid fixing bath, tiny bubbles of carbon dioxide gas may form in the soft gelatin. As the bubbles escape, they form tiny craters or pits in the emulsion thereby breaking up the normal character of the silver image. The finished film or radiograph then is said to have been blistered. To overcome this occurrence when sodium carbonate developers are employed, the temperatures of developer, rinse, and fixer solutions should be approximately the same.

Kodalk. Kodalk is a highly alkaline chemical activator (sodium metaborate)

* In chemistry, there are two types of solutions—alkaline and acid. Developers are usually alkaline in solution; and fixers, acid in solution.

TABLE XVI

CONSTITUENTS OF AN X-RAY DEVELOPING SOLUTION AND THEIR FUNCTIONS

<table>
<tr><th>Chemical</th><th>General Function</th><th colspan="2">Specific Function</th></tr>
<tr><td>Elon</td><td rowspan="2">Developing or reducing agents.</td><td>Builds up detail quickly in first half of development period.</td><td rowspan="2">Developing agents reduce exposed silver bromide crystals in emulsion to black metallic silver constituting the image.</td></tr>
<tr><td>Hydroquinone</td><td>Builds up contrast slowly during development period.</td></tr>
<tr><td>Sodium sulfite</td><td>Preservative</td><td colspan="2">Prevents rapid oxidation of developer.</td></tr>
<tr><td>Sodium carbonate</td><td>Alkali or activator</td><td colspan="2">Governs reducing activities of developing agents; provides necessary alkaline medium and swells gelatin emulsion so that reducing agents can attack exposed silver bromide crystals.</td></tr>
<tr><td>Potassium bromide</td><td>Restrainer</td><td colspan="2">Controls activity of reducing agents and tends to prevent fog.</td></tr>
</table>

found in rapid x-ray developer. It has the same function as sodium carbonate. It is more capable of being used when high temperatures are encountered since it does not cause gas formation in the emulsion when the film is immersed in a cooler fixer. It is the most efficient activator available today.

4. Preservative. The function of the preservative is to retard the activity of the reducing agents to within controlled limits so that the "life" of the developing solution is maintained over a reasonable period of time. As mentioned previously, the reducing agents react quickly with oxygen and if this reaction is not controlled, the developing solution would not last very long. The chemical, *sodium sulfite,* is used as a preservative since it serves to retard oxidation of the reducing agents and prevents the formation of stain on the film. It has an affinity for oxygen and reacts with the oxygen of the air or solution forming sodium sulfate thereby extending the life of the reducing agents.

5. Restrainer. The restrainer is employed to limit the action of the reducing agents to the breaking up of the *exposed* silver bromide crystals only, without attacking the unexposed crystals in the emulsion during the normal course of development. This function is quite important if a satisfactory image is to be produced, for if the restrainer is omitted the unexposed crystals would also develop, and a veil of "fog" (silver deposit) would be deposited over the image. *Potassium bromide* is, therefore, added to the developing solution as a restrainer.

The following data is based upon the use of screen-sensitive x-ray film. When direct exposure (no-screen) x-ray film is employed, characteristics are sufficiently different to require development according to the manufacturer's directions.

INFLUENCE OF DEVELOPMENT TIME

The time of development given to an exposed x-ray film materially affects the amount of silver deposited on the radiograph. As the time of development in-

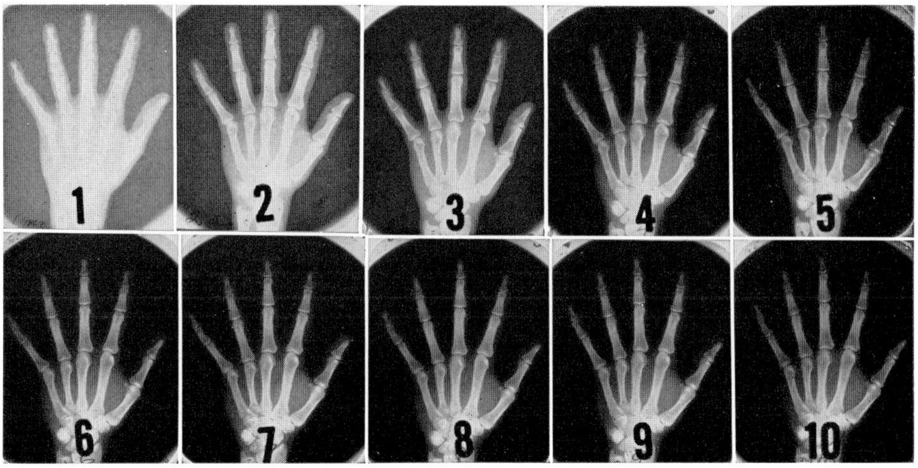

Figure 149. Series of radiographs developed in *regular* x-ray developer for 1 to 10 minutes at 68° F. The numbers on the radiographs represent minutes of development time.

creases up to a certain point, the amount of silver deposit increases; as the time decreases, the quantity decreases. In general, the time required to develop a film in a given developer depends upon the emulsion and its thickness. To assure accurate timing of all processing procedures, it is necessary to use a well functioning interval *timer*. The influence of the *time* of development on the latent image at a given temperature is illustrated in Figures 149 and 150. A series of ten (10) correctly exposed hand radiographs was made employing identical x-ray exposure factors. Films were developed at one-minute intervals at a constant temperature of 68° F. in *regular* x-ray developer, Figure 149.

1. Radiograph 1, developed for 1 minute, shows only slight traces of silver deposit. Image detail is lacking and the contrast is low. Note the streaked back-

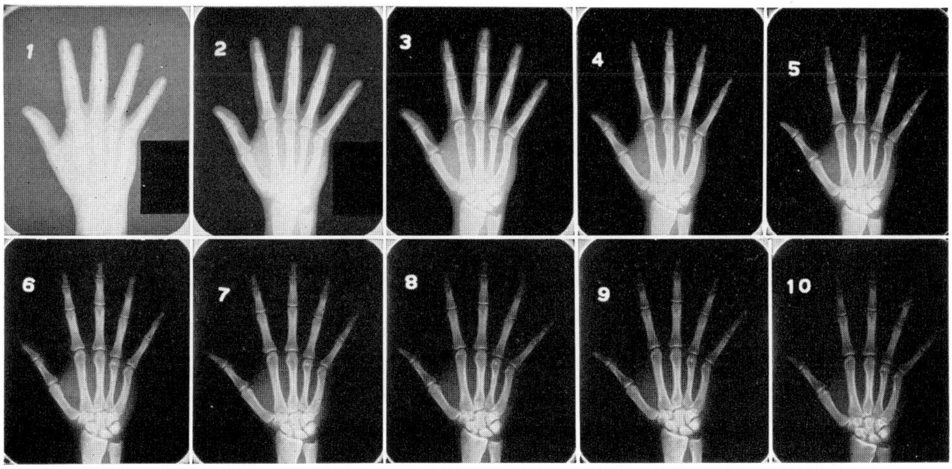

Figure 150. Series of radiographs developed in *rapid* x-ray developer for 1 to 10 minutes at 68° F. Note the higher over-all contrast exhibited in this series when compared with Figure 149. The numbers on the radiographs indicate minutes of developing time.

ground density which is characteristic of the underdeveloped radiograph.

2. No. 2, developed for 2 minutes, shows some of the important features of the image and a greater over-all deposit of silver may be noted. Image detail and contrast are somewhat improved.

3. No. 3, developed for 3 minutes, shows more silver deposited but the image is still somewhat weak.

4. No. 4, developed for 4 minutes, shows a fairly well defined image.

5. No. 5, developed for 5 minutes, shows all essential details, for the maximum practical amount of silver has been deposited on the film. The x-ray exposure was such as to provide a satisfactory image when developed for 5 minutes. The amount of silver deposit with longer development times, however, is not sufficient to justify extension of the development time beyond the basic 5-minute period.

6. Nos. 6-10, developed for 6 to 10 minutes, show little gain in density.

A similar series, Figure 150, was also exposed and developed in *rapid* x-ray developer for 1 to 10 minutes at 68° F. Note the higher contrast in this series.

The time of development has a direct relation to the activity of the developer during its life. For example, the reliability of the recommended normal development intervals for an x-ray film is valid only as long as the solution has a reasonable measure of its original developing power. Since the activity of the chemicals is gradually diminished through their action on the films, it is necessary to increase the time interval so that succeeding radiographs show as satisfactory development as the initial ones in fresher solution. Or, when using the replenisher system, the development time should remain the same at a given temperature for the life of the solution as long as the activity is restored by *frequent* additions of a replenisher solution.

BASIC TIMES OF DEVELOPMENT

Development time intervals should never be guessed. There are two *basic* times of development for both types of developing solution. One produces an image with average speed and contrast while the other provides maximum speed and contrast. Irrespective of the type of developer used, the longer development period in each instance will always provide a better radiographic quality than the shorter interval because full development is always secured and the maximum exposure benefit is assured.

1. Regular X-ray Developer

The first basic time of development provides a short time that requires an addition of 25 per cent more x-ray exposure for compensation; the second is a longer time but the x-ray exposure should be 25 per cent less than the former. When employing regular x-ray developer, the time of development to provide average speed and contrast is 4½ minutes at 68° F., to secure maximum speed and contrast, the development period is 6 minutes at 68° F.

2. Rapid X-ray Developer

When employing rapid x-ray developer, to obtain average speed and contrast, the development time is 3 minutes at 68° F.; to obtain maximum speed and contrast, the time is 5 minutes at 68° F.

INFLUENCE OF DEVELOPER SOLUTION TEMPERATURE

Chemical reactions are stimulated or retarded with temperature. Since processing is essentially a series of chemical reactions, the temperature of the solutions assumes major importance. Variations in temperature require adjustment in the development time factor so that uniform densities may be maintained. Temperatures should never be estimated and a good thermometer, Figure 152, is essential to determine the correct solution temperature. The temperature should always be checked when development is first begun, and at intervals during the course of the day's work. The optimum temperature as recommended by the American Standards Association has been adopted at 68° F.

The influence of developer *temperature* on the density of the radiograph is demonstrated in a series of radiographs of the hand, Figure 151, Top, when times of exposure and development are held constant.

1. Radiograph A was developed for 5 minutes at 60° F. Note the weak image and the lack of silver deposit (density), as well as the low contrast within the image.
2. Radiograph B was correctly developed for 5 minutes at 68° F. Note the satisfactory gradation of densities and contrast of the image.
3. Radiograph C was developed for 5 minutes at 75° F. Note the higher density.
4. Radiograph D was developed for 5 minutes at 80° F. Note the excessive density of the image. The presence of excessive density and fog tends to produce unsatisfactory radiographic quality.

In Figure 151, bottom, radiographs D-F demonstrate that temperature differences require adjustment of the development time to secure comparable densities. These radiographs exhibit approximately the same over-all density.

1. Radiograph A was developed at 60° F. for 8½ minutes. Note that density is almost comparable to that of radiograph B.
2. Radiograph B was developed for 5 minutes at 68° F. and exhibits normal density and contrast.

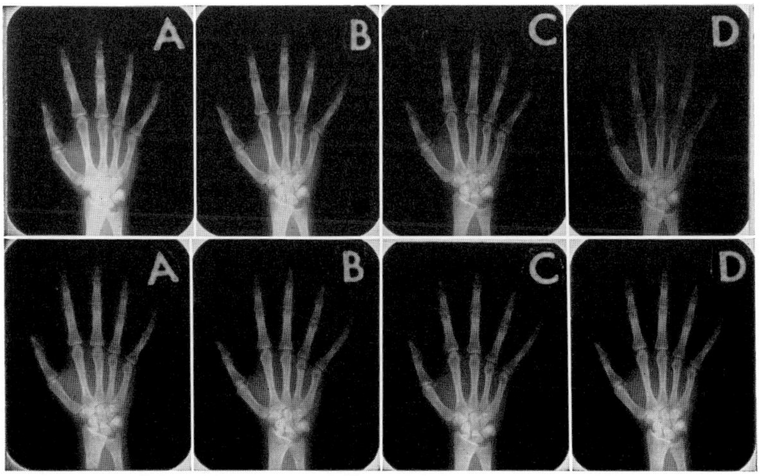

Figure 151. (*Top*) Series of radiographs developed for 5 minutes demonstrating influence of developer solution temperature on image-density when all other factors are constant. A—60° F.; B—68° F.; C—75° F.; D—80° F. As the temperature increased, radiographic density increased. (*Bottom*) Series to demonstrate how the time of development can serve to balance densities when the temperature varies. A—60° F., 8½ minutes; B—68° F., 5 minutes; C—75° F., 3½ minutes; D—80° F., 2 minutes.

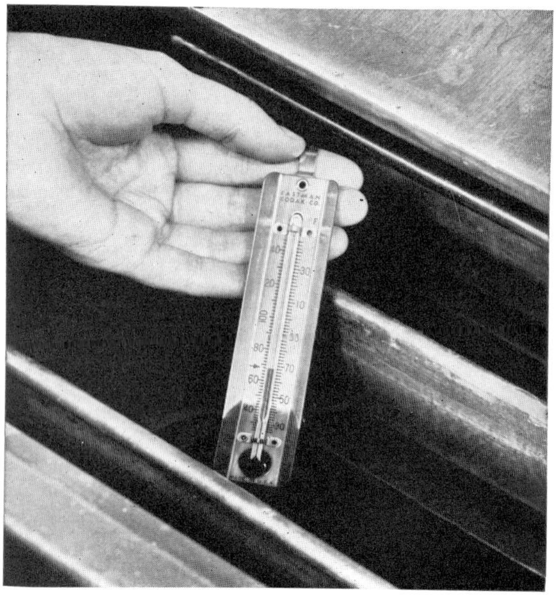

Figure 152. The use of a good thermometer assures the employment of the correct developing time for a given temperature.

3. Radiograph C was developed for 3½ minutes at 75° F. and is comparable to B.
4. Radiograph D was developed for 2 minutes at 80° F. Note that the image is fairly comparable to B, yet a slightly higher density is present because of the greater activity of the developer at this temperature and, as the solution ages, chemical fog would accrue to increase the density.

TIME COMPENSATION FOR TEMPERATURE CHANGES

Although processing solutions should be maintained at the optimum of 68° F., for the best quality, there are occasions when it is necessary to process films at other temperatures. Some compensation can be made for temperature variations *within limits* by increasing or decreasing the time of development in accordance with Tables XVII and XIX. It may be seen therefrom that for the higher temperatures, shorter developing times are necessary to maintain uniform radiographic density. The ideal method is to employ the time-temperature system that accurately compensates for temperature differences with the correct time of development. It is true that x-ray film may be developed satisfactorily without special treatment at any temperature between 60° and 75° as long as the temperature differences are compensated by appropriate development times. The lower temperatures in this optimum range require longer development times and the higher temperatures, although permitting shorter development times, are closer to the zone where processing defects may begin to appear on the radiograph. In general, a rise of 10° doubles the speed of the chemical action.

Low Temperatures

Temperatures below 60° F. actually inhibit the activity of one of the reducing agents. In winter weather, underdevelopment often occurs when the temperature of the solutions has been unwittingly permitted to fall. Even if new solutions are employed at temperatures below 60° F., radiographs will be underdeveloped. If the technician is not certain of the temperature, the appearance of the film is likely to lead him to believe that insufficient exposure has been given. Hence, the exposure time is usually increased in a futile attempt to increase radiographic density, and a cycle of overexposure and underdevelopment occurs resulting in poor radiographic quality. If the solutions gradually warm up to a more normal temperature and the fact is not observed, the sequel is that no compensating reduction in exposure time is made. Overdevelopment of an overexposed film ensues and results in the deposit of excessive densities on the radiograph. The remedy is obvious; know the correct temperature at all times so that optimum developing times and correct exposures can be employed.

High Temperatures

A developer at 80° F. will require less time to produce a satisfactory image, but the density of the image is liable to be excessive; and, as the solution ages, chemical fog appears. Also, the emulsion may melt from the film base, Figure 153, unless the solutions are specially treated. When it is found that development must take place with temperatures above 75° F., the special processing procedure as described in Chapter 25 must be employed.

FACTORS INFLUENCING DEVELOPER ACTIVITY

The importance of a well functioning developer in the production of good quality radiographs is well known. Developer begins to age as soon as it is mixed. It is fresh only while the active chemicals are still in approximately the same concentration as when the solution was originally mixed. Each film that is developed not only removes solution by absorption and surface cohesion, but also weakens the developer left in the tank. Initially, the degree of exhaustion progresses so slowly that many radiographs can be developed at the standard time without apparent loss in radiographic density. However, the chemicals are gradually used up and a decrease in radiographic density occurs. As a consequence, the time of development must be increased to compensate for this loss in density. After more radiographs are developed it becomes necessary to again increase time of development for another quantity of films. Since the developer has deteriorated materially at the end of this last period, it becomes good practice to discard the solution and mix a new one.

The developer solution should never be used beyond the exhaustion limit or after 3 months because a weakened solution will produce weak images and may also cause chemical stain or fog. During development, several chemical reactions take place which tend to exhaust the solution. For example, if the developer remains uncovered, the developing agents and preservative are slowly oxidized by the air. In use the developing agents are destroyed by their action in reducing the exposed silver bromide crystals of the emulsion to black metallic silver. The by-products of these chemical reactions accumulate and the soluble bromide and oxidation products, in particular, slow up the speed of development. The amount of bromide produced is proportional to the amount of silver reduced from the silver emulsion. Other factors that shorten the usefulness of the developer are high temperatures, dilution with water, and contamination.

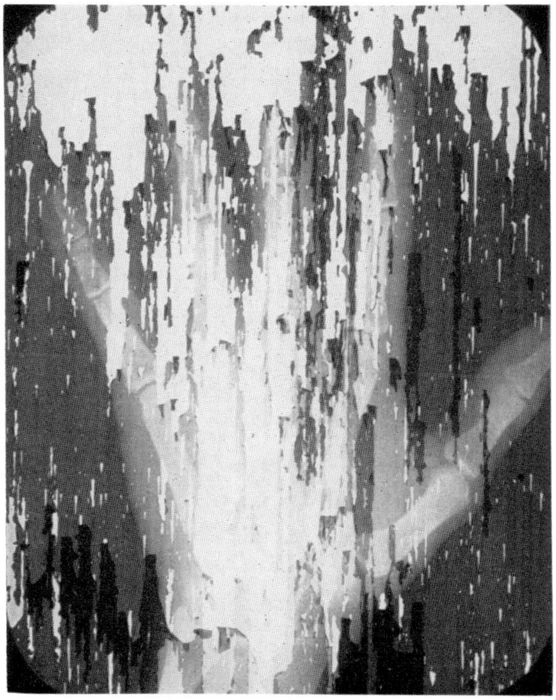

Figure 153. Radiograph exhibiting melted emulsion caused by incorrect high-temperature processing.

RATE OF DEVELOPMENT

The rate of development is affected by the activity of the developer. This activity is determined by the type and quantity of the ingredients employed in making the solution, the dilution and alkalinity of the solution, the degree of its exhaustion, and the temperature.

DILUTION

The dilution of the solution is often influenced by a disregard of the instructions published by the manufacturer in regard to the correct method for mixing the developer chemicals into a solution. Poor radiographic quality also results from using solutions that do not have the required strength; also because the processing tanks have a greater capacity than is supposed. Many so-called "5-gallon" tanks actually have a capacity of 6 or more gallons. Hence, although one adheres strictly to the time-temperature method of development, actually the radiographs obtain 20 to 25 percent less than normal development because of developer dilution. Whenever this condition exists, the exposure given all films must be invariably greater than normal to compensate for the lack of proper development.

Every technician should measure the tanks he is to use to determine exactly their volumes and employ a sufficient quantity of processing chemicals to provide a correctly balanced volume of solution. Dilution of the developer also takes place because of the poor practice of using water to maintain the required level of the solution. If the developer level is low, the correct level should be maintained by adding *fresh developer* solution kept on hand for that purpose.

SOLUTION LEVEL

For efficient time-temperature processing, the level of the developer in the tank should be kept at a fairly constant point. The absorption of the developer solution by the dry film after immersion, and the carry-over of the developer to the rinse bath gradually reduces the level of the solution. When radiographs are removed from the developer, the amount carried away by the film depletes the volume of solution and the surface level drops below the top level of the films contained in the processing hangers. (At least 3 ounces of solution, for example, is contained in the emulsion of a developed 14 x 17-inch film). Before the level reaches this point, however, new solution must be added to maintain the original level. If solution is not added, the upper portion of the film is not developed. The addition of developer also revives the solution to some extent. The volume of solution lost should be restored by the frequent addition of fresh developer or replenisher depending upon the processing system employed. Water should never be used to maintain the solution level, for dilution would occur and proper development would not take place.

AGITATION OF DEVELOPER SOLUTION

To assure uniform activity over the entire surfaces of the x-ray film during processing, it is necessary after a period of inactivity to thoroughly stir the developer and also the fixer solutions with *separate* paddles so that all solutions are uniform in concentration and temperature. This is particularly important with the developer. When the developer solution is not stirred in the tank, there is a tendency for the lower areas of the film to receive less development than the upper areas because the temperature of the solution is usually less at the bottom of the tank. The lower temperature and concentration of reaction products cause unequal development of the film.

During the course of development, some agitation of the developer should be made by moving the hanger up and down several times during the development period. This is necessary because as development takes place, reaction products diffuse out of the emulsion and flow downward over the film surface and affect the development of areas of the film over which they pass. Some agitation of the film serves to disperse the reaction products throughout the solution as fast as they emerge from the emulsion and to prevent local or unequal development of the film.

EXHAUSTION

The exhaustion of a developing solution is affected by the rate of oxidation (aerial or by use), the number of films processed and their average density, the introduction of contaminating substances and accumulation of the by-products of the development reactions and secondary changes in the developer of mechanical or chemical origin such as the formation of sludge, accumulation of insoluble matter, etc.

The manner in which exhaustion of the developer solution diminishes its activity is illustrated in the chemical reaction previously cited. This reaction shows that during development of the silver bromide emulsion the development agent is oxidized; acid substances are released in the form of hydrogen ions that tend to reduce the alkalinity of the solution; and bromine ions that accumulate in the solution to lessen its activity. All of these changes lowers the activity of the developer. To maintain developer solution with good working properties to the end of its useful life, either of two systems is employed—the *exhaustion* system or the *replenisher* system (preferable).

TABLE XVII

DEVELOPMENT TIMES FOR EXHAUSTION SYSTEM AT VARIOUS TEMPERATURES AND EXHAUSTION PERIODS WHEN SCREEN-TYPE FILM IS USED

Temperature	*Regular X-ray Developer*			*Rapid X-ray Developer* — *Basic Development Time of 3 min. at 68° F.*			*Rapid X-ray Developer* — *Basic Development Time of 5 min. at 68° F.*		
	Exhaustion Period			*Exhaustion Period*			*Exhaustion Period*		
	A	*B*	*C*	*A*	*B*	*C*	*A*	*B*	*C*
F.	*min.*	*min.*	*min.*	*min.*	*min.*	*min.*	*min.*	*min.*	*min.*
60°	6¾	7½	8½	5½	6½	7½	8½	9¾	11
62°	6	6½	7½	4¾	5½	6½	6¾	8	9½
64°	5½	6	6¾	4	4½	5½	6¼	7	8½
66°	5	5½	6	3½	4	4½	5½	6¼	7½
68°	4½	5	5½	3	3½	4	5	5¾	6¾
70°	4	4½	5	2½	3	3½	4½	5¼	6
72°	3¾	4	4½	2¼	2¾	3	4¼	4¾	5½
74°	3¼	3½	4	2	2½	2¾	3¾	4½	5
75°	3	3¼	3¾	1¾	2¼	2½	3½	4	4¾

Note: Maintain solution level with *fresh* developer.

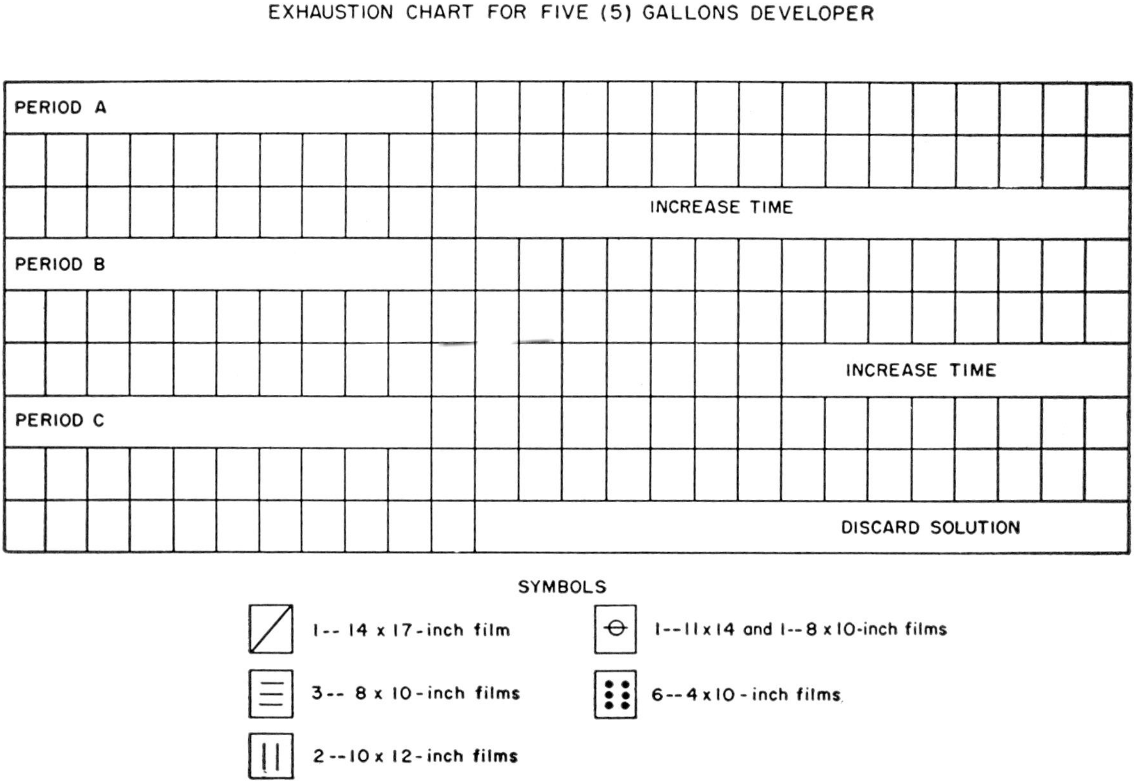

Figure 154. X-ray film developer exhaustion record sheet.

EXHAUSTION SYSTEM OF DEVELOPMENT

The exhaustion system requires that: as certain quantities of films are developed, the time of development must be increased in compensation to maintain uniform radiographic density; after development, *films must be thoroughly drained back into the developer solution;* and the developer should be discarded when the maximum number of films is developed in accordance with the predetermined film area as related to volume of solution. As radiographs are developed, the gradual loss and exhaustion of the developer occasioned by the carry-over of films from developer to rinse and accumulation of by-products, necessitates the adoption of a system for compensating the lower chemical activity of the developer and maintaining its level in the tank. When this is accomplished by adding fresh developer, it is still necessary to increase the time of development according to the number of films developed to produce a revival of activity, as indicated in Table XVII.

After a certain number of films has been developed and the exhaustion point reached, even prolonged development will not produce a well developed radiograph. The solution must then be changed using as a basis the exhaustion rate of the x-ray developer as determined by Table XVII. From Table XVII an *exhaustion record chart,* Figure 154, can easily be constructed, based on the capacity of the developer tank, Table XVIII. It is then possible for the user to accurately forecast the

TABLE XVIII

TABLE LISTING NUMBER OF 14 x 17-INCH FILMS OR THEIR EQUIVALENT IN FILM AREA THAT CAN BE DEVELOPED IN THE RESPECTIVE EXHAUSTION PERIODS.

Exhaustion period	*Number of 14x17-inch films or their equivalent film area to be developed in tanks of varying capacity in each exhaustion period.*			
	5 gal.	*10 gal.*	*15 gal.*	*20 gal.*
A	53	106	159	212
B	60	120	180	240
C	53	106	159	212
Total....	166	332	498	664

point where an increase in the time of development (based on the temperature) should occur and when the solution should be discarded.

OPERATION

The use of an exhaustion record chart aids in securing good quality radiographs at all times. Since the chart is based upon the *area* of film actually developed, a record can easily be kept by noting the sizes of the films processed and tabulating them with the aid of symbols. Since each square on the chart represents a film area equivalent to one 14 x 17-inch film, the symbol employed for this size film can be a *diagonal mark.* The 8 x 10-inch films can be represented by horizontal marks—three of which represent in area one 14 x 17-inch film; 10 x 12-inch films are represented by *vertical* lines—two of which represent in area a 14 x 17-inch film. The 4 x 10-inch films may be represented by dots, six of which would represent the area of one 14 x 17-inch film. Dental films need not be counted.

Based on the use of 5 gallons of regular developer, it may be seen, Table XVII, that in period "A," development is for 4½ minutes at 68° F. Reference to Table XVIII will show the number of 14 x 17-inch or their equivalent film area that should be developed in the various periods when employing 5, 10, 15 or 20 gallons of solution. After 53 14 x 17-inch films or equivalent have been developed period "B" begins and the time is incerased to 5¼ minutes. When 60 14 x 17-inch radiographs have been developed in period "B," period "C" begins and the time is increased to 6¼ minutes. When 53 additional 14 x 17-inch films have been developed in "C" period, the solution is discarded and new solution is made. Table XVIII indicates the change in time required after specific areas of 14 x 17-inch films have been developed employing one or the other of two types of developer in 5-, 10-, and 20-gallon quantities at a given temperature.

REPLENISHER SYSTEM OF DEVELOPMENT

The function of a replenisher developing solution is to restore the concentration of the developer chemicals to that of the original solution. Replenisher also compensates for reduced alkalinity and overcomes the accumulation of bromide released during the development process.

The success of the replenishment method is dependent upon the procedure followed when the radiograph is removed from the developer. The object is to remove the film from the developer as rapidly as possible. This requires that the film be drained to the waste or rinse section of the master tank and *not* into the developer tank. The largest quantity of drainage of this partially exhausted surface solution occurs immediately following the removal of the film from the developer.

Correct replenishment requires the frequent addition of small quantities of replenisher solution to the developer to maintain the original solution level. The rate depends upon the amount of work

TABLE XIX

DEVELOPMENT TIMES FOR REPLENISHER SYSTEM AT VARIOUS TEMPERATURES WHEN USING SCREEN-TYPE X-RAY FILM

Temperatures	*Regular X-ray Developer*		*Rapid X-ray Developer*	
	Basic Development Times at 68° F.		*Basic Development Times at 68° F.*	
	4½ min.	*6 min.*	*3 min.*	*5 min.*
F.	*min.*	*min.*	*min.*	*min.*
60°	8½	8¾	5½	9
62°	7	8	4¾	7½
64°	6	7¼	4	6½
66°	5½	6½	3½	5½
68°	4½	6	3	5
70°	3¾	5½	2½	4¼
72°	3¼	5	2¼	3¾
74°	2¾	4½	2	3¼
75°	2½	4¼	1¾	3

Note. Maintain solution level by *frequent* additions of replenisher solution. *Do not add while films are developing.*

TABLE XX

DEVELOPMENT TIMES FOR REPLENISHER SYSTEM AT VARIOUS TEMPERATURES USING DIRECT-EXPOSURE (NO-SCREEN) X-RAY FILM

Temperature	*Rapid X-ray Developer*	
	Basic Development Times at 68° F.	
	5 min.	*8 min.*
F.	*min.*	*min.*
60°	8½	16
62°	7¼	13¼
64°	6¼	11
66°	5½	9¼
68°	5	8
70°	4½	7
72°	4	6¼
74°	3½	5¾
75°	3¼	5½

Note. Maintain solution level by *frequent* additions of replenisher solution. *Do not add while films are developing.*

done by the developer. The higher the density of the radiograph (grid radiographs of spine) the more silver bromide there is to be reduced to metallic silver and the greater the work performed by the developer. If high density films predominate, more replenisher is required than for lower density films (screen radiographs of chest).

Since a solution of greater activity is employed, in the replenisher system, the developing time can be kept *constant* throughout the life of the developer. Since all x-ray developer chemicals are available in package form, chemicals for replenishers for each type and kind of developer are also available in package form. The appropriate replenisher for its companion developer should always be used. A developer of one manufacture and a replenisher of another should not be employed since the compounding formula may not be appropriate. The development times used at various temperatures when employing the replenisher system and two types of developing solutions are shown in Table XIX.

OPERATION

With the replenisher system, films should be removed from the developer quickly, and *the excess solution should not be allowed to drain back into the developing tank.* It should be drained to the *waste* outlet. Normally, this procedure will carry out about the proper amount of solution for efficient use of the replenisher system. Approximately one gallon of replenisher should be added for every forty 14 x 17-inch films, or their equivalent area. If sufficient solution has not been drained to the waste by the films, it may be necessary to dip a measured quantity of developer from the tank and add a comparable amount of replenisher to maintain normal developing activity. However, by the *fre-*

quent addition of small quantities of replenisher solution, the proper level of the developer and the activity of the solution can easily be maintained. This procedure relieves the technician of computing the actual quantities needed for replacement, but a record of the volume of replenisher used must be maintained.

A rough estimate of the number of films that can be developed in a properly replenished developer has been determined to be 125 14 x 17-inch films per gallon of solution or 625 per 5 gallons of solution. Obviously, it is not practical to continue replenishment indefinitely, and the solution should be discarded when the volume of replenisher used equals three or four times the original quantity of developer as indicated by the manufacturer's instructions for replenishment on the label of the container. It is also recommended that the solution be discarded at the end of a 3-month period because oxidation of the reducing agents results in a decline of developer efficiency. This procedure is necessary even though the total amount of replenisher had not been used during this period.

Note: Never add replenisher solution to the developer while films are developing. Streaks of high density will be produced, Figure 155.

DEVELOPMENT BY INSPECTION

Development by inspection opens avenues of error through which the quality of the finished radiograph may become impaired. It is a characteristic of x-ray film emulsions that the silver bromide crystals are packed more closely together than in the usual photographic emulsion. Depending upon the type of radiographic exposure given, the visual appearance of the developing image may be comparatively different.

In radiographs exposed with x-ray intensifying screens, the exposure effect occurs chiefly in the crystals at or near the surface of the emulsion. This occurrence is due to the fact that exposure is made chiefly by the fluorescent light emitted by the x-ray intensifying screens. As a consequence, the image appears to flash up quickly in the developer and the developed crystals at the surface prevent one from estimating the degree of over-all development in the body of the emulsion. It is, therefore, largely a matter of guesswork as to the time development is judged to be complete. Very frequently, the radiograph is removed from the developer before complete development of the entire image takes place because the image appeared to the eye to possess a very high density. This results in underdevelopment.

In the case of direct exposure of the x-ray film, the x-rays penetrate the entire emulsion layer fairly equally. As a con-

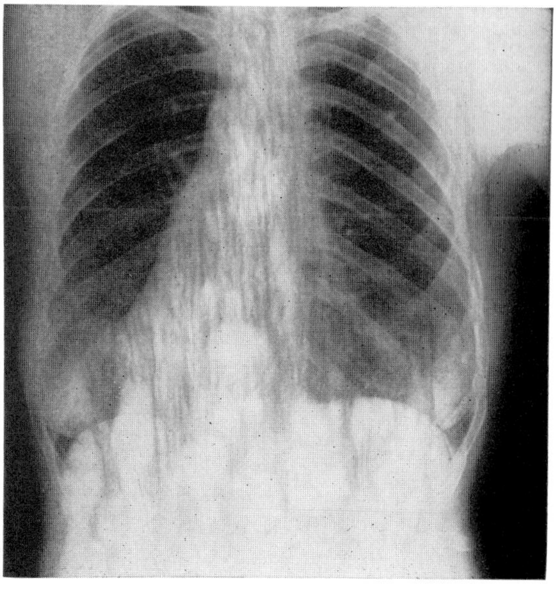

Figure 155. Radiograph exhibiting irregular areas of high density caused by the addition of replenisher during development.

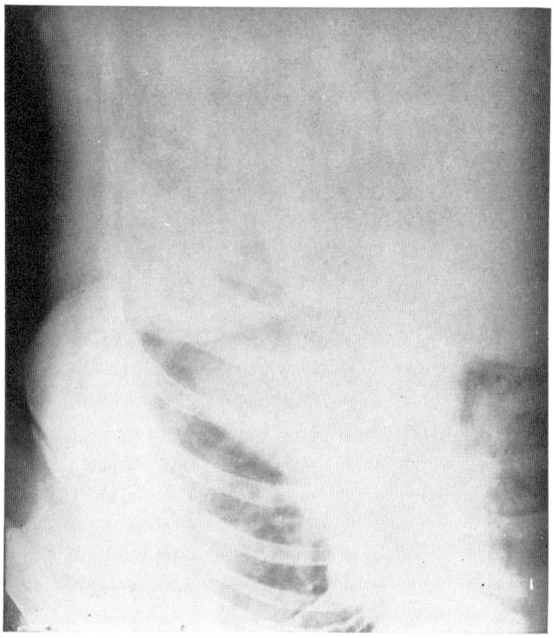

Figure 156. Radiograph fogged by safelight lamp and aerial oxidation during inspection development.

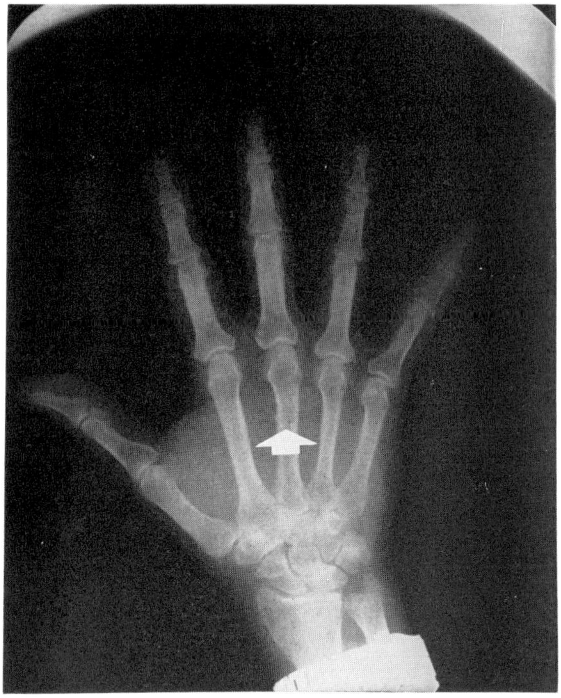

Figure 157. Radiograph showing higher density areas due to developer splash on exposed film prior to development.

sequence, the emulsion develops slowly. The developing image is ill-defined at first, but it gradually builds up to the point where the *well-accommodated* eye sees what may be construed to be a well-defined image. Frequently, however, an error in judgment is made and full development is not given.

Sight development requires a large amount of experience before a measure of proficiency occurs, and even then, there are a number of physiological factors that tend to degrade the efficiency of the method. The degree of fatigue of the technician is a major factor that lessens eye acuity in sight development as well as poor inherent ocular adaptation. Passage from a brightly lighted exposure room to the dark processing room requires a period of adaptation that in some instances may require 15 to 30 minutes. Also, the frequent inspection of the developing radiograph in front of the safelight together with the action of aerial oxidation frequently fogs the film. To avoid the foregoing disadvantages, a standardized time-temperature processing procedure should be employed and *films should not be developed by inspection.*

METHOD OF CHOICE

Full development is always to be recommended for production of the best radiographic image. When it is a matter of choice, the replenisher system is better than the exhaustion system because a constant time of development at a given temperature need be employed for the life of the developing solution, more efficient use of the chemicals is secured, and the deleterious effect on the radiograph of an accumulation of oxidation products is reduced to a minimum.

SECONDARY DEVELOPER CHARACTERISTICS

Secondary characteristics of developer solutions frequently cause difficulties that may be considered as those that affect the chemical balance and composition of the solution and the effects of these conditions on the radiograph.

EFFECTS ON SOLUTION

The effects on developer solution may be noted as those that influence the activity, the formation of sludge and slime.

Activity

Lessened activity may be the result of incorrect mixing, an error in dilution, or low temperature. An unusual drop in activity may be attributed to addition of water instead of fresh developer to raise the solution level, contamination from fixing solution or acid rinse bath, or inadequate replenishment. The remedy is adherence to a correct processing routine.

High activity is seldom encountered, but it may occur by reason of high temperature or the addition of more replenisher solution than is necessary. The remedy is to follow time-temperature processing and a correct replenishment routine.

Crystallization of Chemicals

Crystallization of chemicals is caused by insufficient dilution when mixing or storing the solution at low temperatures. Proper dilution should be maintained when mixing the solution. If crystallization takes place because of low temperatures, the crystals may be redissolved by warming the solution to 125° F.

Sludge

With use of the developer solution, sludge gradually accumulates at the bottom of the tank. This sludge may consist of insoluble calcium and magnesium salts, originally obtained from the water source; metallic silver reduced and removed from the emulsion by the developer; gelatin; and dirt particles. The sludge does not interfere with development unless it is present in large volume. It may be easily siphoned from the bottom of the tank.

Slime

Some kinds of bacteria grow on the accumulated gelatin in the developing solution despite its high alkalinity. Evidence of this growth is in the form of slime on the walls of the tank. Sometimes the slime floats freely in the solution and it then adheres to the surfaces of films being developed. The remedy for this condition is

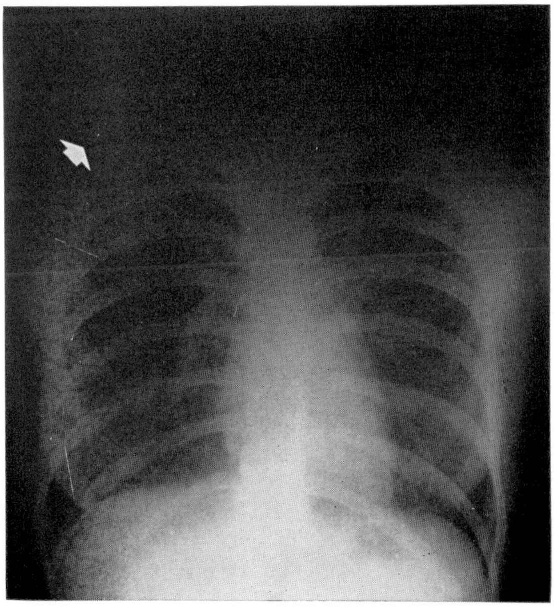

Figure 158. Posteroanterior radiograph of chest showing fogged area at top of film that had been fogged by white light during development.

to thoroughly clean the tank before making each new solution. After cleaning it should be sterilized with a solution of sodium hypochlorite and rinsed thoroughly.

EFFECTS ON RADIOGRAPHS

Some of the effects on radiographs are uneven development, fog and stain, scum, blisters, and reticulation.

Uneven Development

Evidence of uneven development may appear in the form of streaks. Probable causes may be the use of a very short development time, insufficient agitation during development, incorrect high temperature processing procedures, use of exhausted acid rinse and fixing solutions, or failure to agitate films when first immersed in fixing bath. The remedy lies in the use of correct processing methods.

Chemical Fog and Stain

Chemical fog and stain are usually the result of using exhausted developer solution and contamination from the fixing bath and dirty developing hangers.

Blisters and Reticulation

The formation of blisters and reticulated emulsion is usually the fault of improper high-temperature processing. Reticulation is largely the result of transferring a film between solutions possessing wide temperature differences. Physical distortion of the emulsion usually takes place under such treatment.

SUMMARY

The amount of silver deposited by development depends upon the amount of exposure of the silver emulsion to x-rays; the length of time of development; and the temperature of the developing solution. In other words, as the time and/or temperature of the developer increases, the amount of silver deposited increases and vice versa. Since radiographic density, as well as other film characteristics, is materially influenced by the time of development and the temperature of the solution, adequate density control may be obtained by standardization upon full development of the film. Once this is exercised, radiographic density as influenced by development may be considered a constant. When it is a matter of choice, the replenisher system is better than the exhaustion system because a constant time of development at a given temperature may be employed for the life of the developing solution; more efficient use of the chemicals is secured; and the deleterious effect on the radiograph of an accumulation of oxidation products is reduced to a minimum. *Full* development of the exposed x-ray film is always to be recommended for production of the best radiographic image and to take advantage of a lesser exposure value.

Chapter 21

Rinsing Process

WHEN THE x-ray film is removed from the developer, the gelatin emulsion is swollen and, like a sponge, it is saturated with all the soluble chemicals contained in the developer solution. These chemicals include unoxidized developing agents, sodium sulfite, sodium bromide, sodium iodide, and various oxidation products of the development reaction. Besides these chemicals, the gelatin contains the black metallic silver image and unexposed, undeveloped silver bromide crystals.

The bulk of the soluble developer chemicals should be removed from the x-ray film before it is placed in the fixing bath, and replaced by either fresh or acidified water. Such treatment is necessary to stop the reaction of development, and to neutralize the alkalinity of the residual developer, as well as to remove the oxidation products of development. There are two methods to employ for removing these chemicals—rinsing the film in fresh water and rinsing in acidified water.

WATER RINSE BATH

After development, the x-ray film should be rinsed for 30 seconds in circulating fresh water to remove not only the soluble chemicals of the developer retained on the surface of the film but also those in the pores of the emulsion. It is estimated that the emulsion on a 14 x 17-inch x-ray film holds at least 3 ounces of developer. To stop development, it is necessary that the residual developer be quickly diluted with water. The use of a rinse is necessary, for if films are insufficiently rinsed and repeatedly placed directly in the fixing bath, the chemical balance of the fixer is eventually disturbed and its useful life materially shortened.

Poor rinsing practice causes the acidity of the fixer to be rapidly reduced, the hardening action to be destroyed, and stains may appear on the radiograph. Still water should not ordinarily be employed for rinsing. An accumulation of developing solution in the rinse bath eventually oxidizes and, when carried over to the fixing solution, streaks and stains are produced on the radiographs because the fixing solution has been contaminated.

OPERATION

When employing the exhaustion system of development, films should be removed after development and held above the *developer* tank to permit drainage of excess solution. When the replenisher system is used, the films are drained immediately to the *waste* outlet. In each case, they are then immersed in circulating water for 30 seconds. On removal from the rinse bath, they are drained and then placed in the fixing solution.

ACID RINSE BATH

The use of an acid rinse bath serves to prolong the life of the fixer; and also insures that the hardening action is maintained. An acid rinse bath eliminates the need for running water as required by a water rinse bath. The most efficient rinse (stop) bath is one consisting of a dilute solution of acetic acid in water made according to the following procedure: Add 2½ quarts of 28 per cent acetic acid to 1 gallon of water. Stir thoroughly. Then add sufficient water to make 5 gallons of solution. This bath can be made in a 5-gallon tank and placed between the developer and fixer solution tanks. The function of the bath is to immediately stop development of the emulsion, and to neutralize the alkali in the developer contained in the emulsion.

OPERATION

Radiographs should be rinsed in the acid rinse bath for 30 seconds, but there is no harm in leaving them in the bath for as long as 1½ minutes. It is important not to overwork the acid rinse bath. When the acidity of the solution becomes reduced, its continued use will accentuate rather than prevent staining or streaking. The acid rinse bath will operate satisfactorily within the normal range of processing temperatures when *rapid* x-ray developer is employed. When using *regular* x-ray developer, however, it should not be employed when the temperature of the solution rises above 70° F., or when there is a wide difference in temperature between the various solutions. During the useful life of the acid rinse bath, it will rinse about 200 14 x 17-inch films or their equivalent in film area per 5 gallons of solution. The exhaustion of the bath may be easily determined chemically by the use of a testing outfit for stop and fixing baths.

PREFERRED METHOD

A combination of water and acid-rinse bath procedure is the most efficient method. In the tank compartment provided for running rinse water place a small tank containing an acid rinse bath. After development, the films should be thoroughly rinsed for 5 to 10 seconds in running water. This treatment removes or dilutes the bulk of the developer on the surface of the film. The film is then placed in the acid rinse bath for 15 to 30 seconds to quickly neutralize the alkalinity of the residual developer and stop development. It is then removed and placed in the fixer solution.

Chapter 22

Fixing Process

THE DEVELOPMENT process reduces only a portion of the silver bromide emulsion to metallic silver. The remaining unused silver bromide must be removed, for it would impair the diagnostic and photographic character of the silver image. Subsequent chemical treatment known as the fixing process serves to *clear* the film of this unwanted silver bromide without damage to the image and, to *harden* the gelatin emulsion.

The solution employed for fixation is known as a fixing solution and is composed of a number of chemicals in balance with one another. A typical formula is shown below:

Kodak Fixing Solution F-10

Water, about 125° F	2½	gallons.
Sodium thiosulfate	13¾	pounds.
Sodium sulfite, desiccated	5	ounces.
Kodalk	1¼	pounds.
Acetic acid, 28 per cent*	45	fluid ounces.
Potassium alum	15	ounces.
Water, to make	5	gallons.

* Dissolve each chemical in order given. Make sure that each chemical is dissolved completely before adding the next. To make approximately 28 percent acetic acid from glacial acetic acid, dilute three parts of glacial acetic acid with eight parts of water.

FIXER CONSTITUENTS

The constituents of a fixing solution and their functions in the fixation process are as follows, Table XXI.

1. **Solvent.** The solvent employed in mixing the chemicals of a fixing solution is *water.*

2. **Acidifier.** *Acid* serves a double purpose for it permits the use of potassium alum as a hardening agent and neutralizes

TABLE XXI

CONSTITUENTS OF AN X-RAY FIXING BATH AND THEIR FUNCTIONS

Chemical	*General Function*	*Specific Function*
Sodium thiosulfate (hypo)	Fixing Agent	Dissolves unexposed silver bromide crystals. Does not affect reduced metallic silver of image.
Sodium sulfite	Preservative	Maintains equilibrium of chemicals in solution.
Potassium alum	Hardening Agent	Shrinks and hardens emulsion.
Acetic Acid	Acidifier	Provides acid medium and neutralizes developer carried over in film.

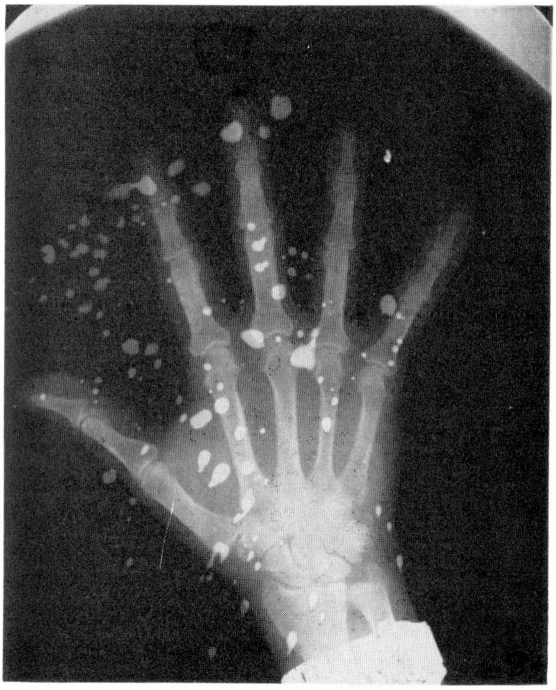

Figure 159. Radiograph exhibiting areas of translucence caused by fixer splash on film before development. The fixer dissolved out the silver emulsion thereby making impossible development of these areas.

any alkaline developer that may be carried over from the developing solution.

This latter action quickly stops development and prevents the formation of stain. The acid usually employed is *acetic acid.*

3. Clearing Agent. The function of the *clearing agent* is to change the residual unexposed and undeveloped silver bromide crystals in the emulsion to soluble silver salts that are readily removed by washing the film in water. This is accomplished without damage to the silver image. If the film is not properly cleared, the remaining silver bromide crystals will darken on exposure to light and obscure the radiographic image. The usual chemical employed for this purpose is *sodium thiosulfate* or ammonium thiosulfate—commonly known as "hypo." The former provides a satisfactory concentration to meet normal radiographic needs; the latter has the ability to react more completely with the silver bromide, and its comparable concentration is approximately two-thirds that needed when sodium thiosulfate is employed as a clearing agent. The clearing action involves a chemical reaction between the sodium or ammonium thiosulfate and silver bromide in the emulsion wherein silver thiosulfate is formed and remains in solution.

4. Hardening Agent. The *hardening agent* is used to decrease the possibility of physical injury to the gelatin emulsion. A swollen emulsion is easily scratched or distorted by physical means during the washing and drying processes. The hardener restrains swelling of the gelatin and hardens it so that it can withstand the normal effects of processing. The most effective chemical employed for this purpose is *potassium alum.*

5. Preservative. The *preservative* prevents decomposition of the clearing agent by the acid with a resultant precipitation of sulfur at normal temperatures. It assists in clearing the film and prevents the residual developer carried over in the film from oxidizing and discoloring the fixing bath. The chemical used is *sodium sulfite.*

PROCESS OF FIXATION

When the film is placed in the fixing solution it is milky in appearance because of the residual unexposed and undeveloped silver bromide crystals but, as it is moderately agitated until both film surfaces are completely bathed by the solution, this milkiness gradually disappears. The action of the acidifier immediately neutralizes the residual alkaline developer and any continuing development action ceases. Since the gelatin is still swollen and porous, the clearing agent dissolves out the unexposed and undeveloped silver bromide crystals, leaving untouched the developed silver image. This is the *clearing action.* As clearing abates, the *hardening action* begins, resulting in shrinking and hardening of the gelatin emulsion containing the silver image. This hardening action is most important, since it prevents swelling of the emulsion to any marked degree in the later washing operation. It is advisable not to turn on the white light in the processing room until the film is entirely clear; otherwise it will become streaked (fogged).

INFLUENCE OF TEMPERATURE

As with most chemical reactions, the higher the temperature the greater the speed of fixation; the lower the temperature, the slower the speed of fixation. In fixer solutions, however, there is an optimum range of temperatures that should be used; i.e., 60° to 75° F. With higher temperatures, a fixing solution tends to sulfurize thereby shortening its life. It must, therefore, be specially treated when high temperatures prevail.

INFLUENCE OF TIME

The duration of fixation is dependent upon several factors, such as the strength and nature of the fixer employed; the temperature of the solution; the amount of film agitation; the volume of fixing solution as related to the number or surface area of the films being fixed; and the emulsion thickness. The total *fixing time* is made up of the duration of time needed to *clear* the film and that required to harden the film. For best results, the film should remain in the fixing bath at least for *twice* the time necessary to clear the film. Although radiographs may be safely left in the fixer for a slightly longer period, it is not wise to do so, for it will later take longer to wash them free of residual silver and fixing bath salts. An important point to remember in this connection, however, is that the hardness of the emulsion in a given fixing solution decreases with its exhaustion, and the initial fixing time must be extended as the solution is used to maintain normal hardening.

EXHAUSTION OF FIXING SOLUTION

Normally, the usefulness of a single tank fixer ends when the bath loses its acidity or when more than twice the normal time is required to remove the unexposed silver salts from the film. The bath should then be discarded, especially when it becomes turbid. An exhausted fixing bath permits abnormal swelling of the emulsion due to deficient hardening action. Consequently, drying is prolonged and reticulation or sloughing of the emulsion may take place. Also, neutralization of acid in the bath invariably causes certain types of stains on the radiograph. A good rule to follow is to change the fixing bath when fresh developer is made. When exceptionally high temperatures prevail, the fixing bath should be changed *twice* during the life of the developer. This assures maximum hardening of the emulsion and freedom from hot weather troubles.

TABLE XXII

LIFE OF UNREPLENISHED FIXING SOLUTION IN A SINGLE 5-GALLON TANK. TEMPERATURE RANGE: 60° TO 75° F.

Number 14 x 17-inch Films Fixed	*Clearing Time (min.)*	*Fixing Time (min.)*
0–50	1¼–3	5–6
51–100	3–5	6–9½
101–150	5–8	9½–16

Note. Make new fixing solution.

TABLE XXIII

REPLENISHMENT OF X-RAY FIXING SOLUTION IN A 5-GALLON TANK

Number 14 x 17-inch films fixed	*Clearing time (min.)*	*Fixing time (min.)*	*Replenishment*
0- 50	1½–2¾	5	Remove 2 qts. old solution; replace with 2 qts. replenisher.*
51-100	1¾–3	5	Remove 2 qts. old solution; replace with 2 qts. replenisher.*
101-150	2–3	5	Remove 2 qts. old solution; replace with 2 qts. replenisher.*
151-200	2–3½	6	Remove 2 qts. old solution; replace with 2 qts. replenisher.*
201-225	2½–3	7	Remove 2 qts. old solution; replace with 2 qts. replenisher.*
226-250	3–4	8	Discard fixer solution; make new solution.

* Replenisher is made by dissolving sufficient dry chemical normally used to make 1 gallon fixing bath in 5 pints of water; or chemical for 5 gallons in 12½ quarts of water.

Caution: This is a concentrated solution of fixing bath to be used only as a *replenisher.*

SINGLE-TANK FIXING SOLUTION

Most processing tank systems only provide for a single tank of fixing solution. Unfortunately, the use of a single bath is not the most efficient nor economical method for fixing purposes. The gradual accumulation of silver salts in the bath makes longer washing times necessary because of the difficulty encountered in replacing these salts with pure water.

REPLACEMENT

When the volume of the fixing solution is the same as that of the developing solution, the fixing solution should be changed twice during the life of the developer to insure satisfactory clearing and hardening of the emulsion. The exhaustion chart, Table XXII, may be employed as a guide for determining the clearing and fixing time and to determine the exhaustion point. The most efficient procedure when employing a single-tank fixer is to use double the volume employed for the developer solution. If a 5-gallon solution of developer is used, then 10 gallons of fixing solution should be employed. When the developer solution is exhausted and then changed, the fixer solution should also be changed.

REPLENISHMENT OF SINGLE-TANK FIXING SOLUTION

A fixing solution with use gradually loses its acidity because of the carry-over of the alkaline developer by the film. It also becomes diluted by rinse water carried into the solution from the rinse bath. As a consequence, its hardening properties and fixing rate are gradually affected (Table XX). The exhaustion of the thiosulfate reduces its ability to dissolve silver salts. The loss in function of the fixing solution, however, can in some measure be restored by replenishment.

ADVANTAGES OF REPLENISHMENT

There are definite advantages to be gained by replenishing the fixing solution.

1. Fixation times may be kept to a minimum.

2. In the first half of the life of the solution, the clearing and fixing time may be kept relatively constant; in the latter half of its life, the fixing time is slowly increased to its exhaustion limit.

METHOD OF REPLENISHMENT

In replenishing a 5-gallon tank of fixing

solution, 2 quarts of the solution are removed and discarded; a volume of 2 quarts of fixer *replenisher* solution is then added to the original bath, etc. (see Table XXI).

TWO-TANK FIXING SOLUTION

One of the quickest and most economical ways to remove silver salts from radiographs is the use of a *two-tank* fixing bath. This bath consists of two tanks of equal volume of fixing solution. The No. 1 tank is reserved for clearing the film and the No. 2 tank for hardening of the emulsion. Radiographs are taken from the rinse bath and placed in the first tank where most of the silver salts are removed during the clearing time. As soon as the film is cleared, it is removed to the second bath where the emulsion is hardened. Because of this procedure, the second bath always has a very low concentration of silver salts and the diffusion of any residual salts from the radiograph is exceedingly rapid. Since a very few silver salts are carried over to the washing tank, the washing time can be materially reduced.

REPLACEMENT

When the equivalent in film area of 180 14 x 17-inch films has passed through the No. 1 tank, the solution should be discarded. No. 2 tank is then removed into the original position of No. 1. New solution is then made in No. 1 tank that now becomes No. 2 tank. The original No. 2 tank hardens the equivalent of 180 14 x 17-inch films and when used as the No. 1 tank for clearing purposes, its life will be expended after an additional equivalent area of 180 14 x 17-inch films has passed through it—a total of 360 14 x 17-inch films. Once the routine has been established, this system of rotation between tanks will assure the production of well-fixed films indefinitely.

SECONDARY FIXING CHARACTERISTICS

Any discussion of fixing solutions is incomplete without some mention of secondary characteristics that may pose problems during the fixing process.

SLUDGING

An excess of developer carried over into the fixer solution tends to precipitate some of the hardening agent. The result may be a white sludge in the solution, or a white scum on the films. This sludging may be prevented if films are thoroughly rinsed in flowing water between development and fixation. The films should then be adequately drained so that only a minimum of developer-contaminated rinse water is transferred to the fixer. The use of Kodalk in an x-ray fixing solution helps to prevent possible sludging of the solution and reduces its odor.

STREAKINESS

Uneven density or streakiness in uniformly exposed areas also may result if films are not rinsed before fixation and agitated during fixation. This is due to the fact that one or two minutes may elapse before the alkali in the developer carried over by the films is neutralized by the acid in the fixer solution. During this time, development of the film may continue unevenly in the fixer solution, resulting in streaks. The importance of adequate rinsing cannot be too strongly emphasized. The use of an acid stop bath will tend to eliminate this fault.

OPALESCENCE

Sometimes a film viewed immediately after fixation in a fresh solution appears opalescent. The condition, however, is transient, disappearing when the film is washed and dried. It is caused by the reaction of the gelatin of the emulsion to the high concentration of sodium thiosulfate in the fixer. This condition frequently occurs when the solution has been freshly mixed.

Chapter 23

Washing Process

WASHING OF RADIOGRAPHS must be regarded as a chemical operation, the object of which is to remove residual processing chemicals and silver salts from the radiograph. Proper washing insures the permanence of radiographs as records. If these chemicals are not removed, the image will discolor or fade and the entire film may deteriorate. Normally, x-ray films should be washed in running water so circulated that the entire emulsion area, as well as every portion of the wash tank, will receive frequent changes. There are occasions when a radiograph may be insufficiently washed. But, as long as the film is not subject to high heat and humidity conditions, it may be thoroughly washed later provided rewashing takes place within a period of 3 to 6 months after the film is processed, and staining has not occurred. With this fact in mind, a shorter washing time may be used if the circumstances demand it.

Generally speaking, if a radiograph is to remain in a temperate zone, less washing can be given a film than if it is to remain in a tropical or sub-tropical region. However, there is no likelihood that one can determine where the radiograph will ultimately be stored when it is made; therefore, every effort should be made to properly wash the film during its initial processing. In tank processing, the bar of the hanger and the top clips should always be completely covered by the water.

WATER SOURCES

Any water declared to be potable by competent authority is satisfactory for film processing purposes. Occasionally, an abundance of microscopic plant and animal matter is contained in tap water or other water sources. The bulk of this matter should be removed by filtration. Several thicknesses of gauze placed over the outlet of the water supply will provide some measure of filtration if none other is available. The gauze filter will need to be renewed or cleaned daily.

A generous supply of water is in some measure a necessity for film processing. However, there will be some occasions when the source of supply becomes inadequate, contaminated, or extremely meagre in quantity.

NEED FOR ADEQUATE WATER SUPPLY

An adequate water supply assures the removal from the radiograph of the soluble silver and fixing bath chemicals. When silver salts remain in the emulsion, the image will discolor and a brown stain of silver sulfide will eventually occur. This condition becomes exaggerated when the radiographs are stored under conditions of high temperature and humidity. The prevalence of atmospheric hydrogen sulfide in coal burning or sulfur spring areas very often contributes to staining. The removal of fixing bath salts is also as important as the removal of the silver salts, for residual fixer salts will, in time, cause the image to discolor and fade. Washing the radiograph must therefore accomplish the removal of both silver and fixing solution chemicals. Also, as the fixing solution approaches the exhaustion point, the concentration of silver salts becomes so high that the washing process should be most thorough at this time.

WASHING TIME

The time required for adequate washing depends principally upon the type of x-ray film to be washed; the rate at which the water flows through the tank; the temperature of the water and the type of fixing bath employed. The following rates apply when a sodium thiosolfate fixer is employed. When an ammonium thiosulfate fixer is used the washing time is approximately one half.

WASHING IN SINGLE TANK

The usual arrangement for a single tank washer is shown in Figure 133. The flow of water through the tank is quite important for most of the soluble chemicals must be eliminated if the radiograph is to have some measure of permanence. When the hourly flow of water through a single tank is 4 gallons, 30 to 40 minutes is required for washing x-ray film if the temperature of the water is about 70° F. When the flow is 8 gallons per hour, the washing time is 15 to 20 minutes. Shorter intervals should not be used no matter how frequently the water in the tank is changed. If the flow of water through the tank is very slow, the films should remain in the water even longer than the above specified periods. The washing time should be measured from the immersion of the *last* film in the wash water, since washed and partly washed films absorb fixing bath chemicals from water contaminated by fixing solution previously carried over, as well as release them in fresh water. The direct-exposure film requires twice the above washing times because of its thicker emulsion.

During the washing process in a single tank, films should initially be placed near the *outlet* end of the tank. As more fixed films are put in the wash tank, those already partially washed should be moved nearer the *inlet* end so that the final part of washing is done in fresh uncontaminated water.

CASCADE WASHING

A most efficient method of washing is to employ the two-stage cascade system, Figure 134. In this system, the water flows in a direction opposite to the flow of films. In other words, the flow of water is from right to left, while the flow of films in normal processing is from left to right. The film laden with fixing bath salts is placed in the *first* compartment of the tank. Washing in this compartment removes about 90 per cent of soluble salts and the rate of washing is very rapid. When the flow of water is at the rate of about 8 gallons per hour, the radiograph remains approximately 5 minutes in the first compartment and is then placed in the second compartment where it is bathed with uncontaminated fresh water for an additional 5 minutes—a total of 10 minutes washing time. At no time should a film fresh from the fixing solution be placed in the second compartment.

TEMPERATURE OF WASH WATER

The temperature of the wash water is important. Wash water within the temperature range of 68° to 70° F. is about 40 per cent more efficient than at 40° F. Water with a temperature of 75° F. and higher, has a tendency to soften the gelatin emulsion to the point where it may be damaged or, as in some instances, it may actually slough away from the film support. Washing should, therefore, take place in a minimum of time and in the 65° to 70° F. range if possible. Washing under high temperature conditions is not to be recommended unless the films have had special prior treatment that would insure adequate hardness of the emulsion. In general, the temperature of the wash water should approximate the temperature of the other processing solutions.

USE OF SEA WATER

When an inadequate source of fresh water exists, radiographs may be safely washed in sea water. Afterward, however, they should receive an additional *final* washing in *fresh* water for 5 minutes. This step is extremely important to prevent the rapid fading of the image caused by residual salts from the sea water; and to prevent the absorption of moisture by hygroscopic salts absorbed by the emulsion. The chemicals of the processing solutions are removed from the film more rapidly with sea water than with fresh water; consequently, the washing time with sea water may be one-half of the usual time. Washing in sea water may be carried out at lower temperatures than when fresh water is used. Temperatures of 50° F. or lower are feasible. When processing solutions have been mixed with sea water, it is advisable to wipe the surfaces of the radiographs with a soft wet cloth after washing to remove any chemical deposit that may be present.

Chapter 24

Drying Process

DRYING OF THE radiograph is the simplest, yet an important final, step in the processing procedure. It contributes to the excellence of the radiograph when properly accomplished. The most common procedure is the use of a rapid flow of air passing over the edges of the film surfaces with or without the aid of heat.

The success of any drying operation lies in the rapid removal of water from within and without the emulsion and, in most instances, it takes more time than all the other operations together. This delay frequently constitutes a "bottleneck" to the rapid flow of radiographs through the processing room. Also, the prevention of excessive swelling of the emulsion during the processing procedure effectively tends to accelerate the rate of drying. During the drying process, the radiographs are wet and vulnerable to damage. Dirt from dusty air may become imbedded in the emulsion or the film may become scratched and abraded if not carefully handled. Radiographs should never be removed from their hangers unless they are dry.

DRYING AIDS

Since the process of drying should be accelerated, certain aids can be safely employed when available.

PREVENTION OF EMULSION SWELLING

The speed with which x-ray film dries is dependent upon the quantity of water to be evaporated from the emulsion. This speed is proportional to the combined thicknesses of the emulsions. It is, therefore, necessary to prevent excessive emulsion swelling. The use of a good fixing bath at all times aims to keep swelling to a minimum by shrinking and hardening the emulsion. It is essential to remember that the emulsion should be hardened effectively *before* excessive swelling takes place. Hardening of a swollen emulsion raises its melting point but does not necessarily greatly reduce its thickness. Consequently, development and fixation should take place in solutions possessing a temperature within the optimum range.

The above precautions should be considered when processing is to take place in hot, humid climates where drying always tends to be prolonged. Another point to observe is that washing of the film should be adequate but not prolonged. When processing temperatures over 75° F. are employed, special treatment serves to keep the emulsion hard, provided short washing times are employed.

WETTING AGENT

The use of a photographic wetting agent aids in shortening the drying time. A wetting agent is a detergent whose function is to reduce the surface tension of water so that the water can drain more rapidly from the surfaces of the radiograph after washing. It also serves to eliminate drying marks. There are a small number of wetting agents that are safe to use for photographic purposes. They are available and labeled under various trade names such as *Photo-Flo.* A separate 5-gallon tank of dilute wetting agent in water to be used as a final rinse after washing is prepared by adding 2½ ounces of the detergent to 5 gallons of water. After washing, the radiograph is immersed in this solution for 30 seconds and then drained. The radiograph may then be placed in the dryer. When 400 14 x 17-inch films or their equivalent in film area have passed through the solution, it should be replaced with a new one.

ALCOHOL

The use of alcohol for drying is recommended only when some emergency requires the use of a dried radiograph in a minimum of time after processing. Any good grade of denatured alcohol may be employed for drying films, provided that when diluted with water it does not turn milky. The alcohol concentration should be not greater than 70 per cent by volume if opalescence of the emulsion or deformation of the base is to be avoided. After washing, the radiograph is thoroughly drained. Then, the film is immersed in a tray of alcohol for 2 minutes at temperatures under 70° F. The tray should be rocked while in the alcohol to assure uniform bathing of both film surfaces and prevent the film from sticking to the bottom of the tray. This operation causes the water to diffuse from the pores of the emulsion and be replaced by the alcohol. Thus, the bulk of the water is removed and the film is then immersed in a second and final tray of alcohol to remove any residual water. The film is then drained. The alcohol will rapidly evaporate to leave a dry emulsion.

DRYERS

Most processing installations are provided with cabinet dryers equipped with a fan and heating elements. The dryer should always be vented to the outside of the processing room to prevent excessive heat and humidity of the air. Drawers are provided in which the films are hung in their hangers. Ordinarily, radiographs should be dried with air moderately warmed. Heat should be used cautiously when drying films in hot, humid weather because the water-laden gelatin emulsion may soften and ruin the radiographic image. Under these conditions, it is safest to use only the dryer fan. Overheating of the dryer should be avoided because very rapid drying is apt to cause distortion in the radiograph.

As a precaution, the heating elements are connected to the fan circuit to prevent turning on the heat without activating the fan. The dryer is usually ducted to the outside atmosphere. This serves also to prevent the accumulation of excessive atmospheric moisture in the room. Where only a small number of films are processed daily, a convenient rack for holding hangers during drying can be made by drilling ⅜-inch holes about 4 inches apart in a 1 x 3-inch board of a length that will fit any space where it can be mounted. When the rack is placed high on a wall, the films can be suspended by inserting the crossbars of the film hangers in the holes. This obviates danger of striking the radiographs while wet, or spattering water on the drying surfaces and spotting them.

The small processing room in which only a few films are processed daily usually does not justify the installation of a hot-air film dryer. In such instance a commercially available drying rack on which the x-ray film hangers are hung by one end of the hanger crossbar is adequate. This rack is best placed on the wall over the washing tank, sink, or drainboard. When drying is to be accelerated, a flow of air from an ordinary electric fan can be directed toward the edges of the films in their hangers.

The drying unit may be installed along the wall at one end of the processing room or underneath the loading bench. The drying of films is usually considered a "wet-film" operation and the placement of the dryer on the "dry" side of the room may at first seem a violation of the rule to keep "wet" and "dry" operations separate. In actual practice, however, if the films and hangers are drained first, and if a moderate amount of care is exercised, there is little likelihood that water will be splashed on the loading bench.

A uniform air flow is secured when the air is drawn *into* rather than blown through the dryer. The dryer should deliver a minimum air flow of 450 to 500 cubic feet per minute to the radiographs. In general, the *lowest* heat possible should be used to maintain the air temperature at approximately 120° F. inside the dryer. In order to prevent accidental overheating of the films, the circuits should be designed so that the heating elements cannot be activated unless the fan is operating.

Suitable insulating material is placed around the dryer so that heat cannot escape to raise the room temperature or affect unprocessed films on top of the loading bench. The dryer should be vented *outside* the processing room. The drip pan underneath each film drawer should be kept clean and free of dust and debris.

DRYING TIME

The time required to dry a radiograph is dependent upon the efficiency of the hardener in the fixing solution; the amount of water retained in the gelatin emulsion after washing; the velocity and temperature of the drying air; the humidity of the atmosphere; and the use of a wetting agent. Water absorption is reduced to a permissible minimum by the use of a reasonably fresh fixing solution that will assure proper hardening of the emulsion. The humidity of the air should ideally be below 50 per cent and the temperature under 90° F. When films are dried in cabinet dryers, the heat should be adjusted so that drying takes place in from 10 to 20 minutes. High temperature drying is to be avoided even though the radiographs may be dried more quickly, for brittleness of the film may occur. The use of infrared lamps for drying is not recommended for they cause *unequal* drying of the film surfaces.

SUMMARY OF TANK PROCESSING

The steps employed in tank processing of x-ray film are summarized in the following paragraphs.

1. Stir the developer and fixer solutions with *separate* paddles to obtain a uniform temperature. Check the temperature of the solutions and adjust, if possible, to 68° F. before development. Be sure to maintain solution level by adding sufficient

developer or replenisher. Do not add to solution while films are developing.

2. Exclude all white light in processing room and turn on 6B safelights.

3. Remove exposed film from its holder and clip into a developing hanger and set interval timer so it will ring at end of desired period of development. Consult Tables XVII or XIX.

4. Immerse film smoothly in the developer solution and start the timer. Agitate film hanger by raising and lowering it several times to break up residual air bells and permit solution to bathe both surfaces of the film. Agitate films several times during course of development. Remove hanger from developer when bell rings indicating the termination of the development period.

5. Immerse the film in circulating rinse water or acid rinse bath and agitate.

6. After rinsing, place the film in the fixer solution and agitate until fixer has thoroughly bathed both film surfaces. *Do not expose to white light until the film has cleared.*

7. Upon completion of fixation, remove film to the washing compartment. Let it remain until it is completely washed in circulating water.

8. After washing, drain the film in its hanger and place in Photo-Flo solution for 1 minute. Then, hang up to dry or place in a dryer that supplies circulating, clean dry air.

9. Remove the dry radiograph from the hanger by *opening* the clips which release their grip on the corners. Do not pull film from clips since clips may be broken or portions of film remain to clog them later when another film is to be processed.

10. The corners of the radiograph should be rounded and the radiograph placed in a filing envelope.

Chapter 25

High Temperature Processing

IF IT IS NOT possible to cool the solutions and wash water to 68° F., a number of general precautions may be exercised to lessen the difficulties of processing x-ray film at higher temperatures. For temperatures in the neighborhood of 75° F., the development times should be those as indicated in the development time-temperature Tables XVII and XIX. The *rapid* type of developer is preferable for best results. Films should be fixed for fully 15 minutes to insure maximum hardening and the fixing solution should be renewed frequently. A good practice is to use a volume of fixing solution that is twice the volume of the developer and to change the fixer whenever the developer is changed. The washing time should be limited to 15 minutes. Proper development, thorough fixation, and minimum washing all help to prevent excessive softening and swelling of the gelatin of the emulsion.

TEMPERATURES ABOVE 75° F.

For processing at temperatures above 75° F., further precautions may be taken. The use of regular developer is preferable. It is not generally advisable to employ solutions at temperatures above 95° F. because of the possibility of emulsion damage. The recommended processing times for development, hardening, and fixing of x-ray film is indicated in Table XXIV. Between development and fixation, the films should be rinsed in an emulsion hardening bath (Kodak Hardening Bath SB-4).

TEMPERATURES ABOVE 90° F.

When the temperature of the processing solutions is 90° F. or above, sodium sulfate should be added to the developer solutions as indicated in Table XXV. When the temperature is 95° F., sodium sulfate should also be added to the hardening bath. *Once the sodium sulfate has been added, the bath should not be allowed to cool; if its temperature falls 5 to 10°, the sodium sulfate may crystallize.* The hardening bath should be mixed fresh every 24 hours because, when partially used, the bath loses its hardening properties rapidly.

HARDENING AND FIXING

X-ray films should remain in the hardening bath for 3 minutes; during the first minute they should be agitated frequently to prevent the formation of a precipitate

TABLE XXIV

HIGH TEMPERATURE PROCESSING TIMES

Temperature	*Development—regular x-ray developer*	*Hardening—Kodak SB-4*	*Fixation*
80° F.	2½ min.	3 min.	10 min.
90° F.	2½ min.	3 min.	10 min.
95° F.	2¼ min.	3 min.	10 min.

Kodak Hardening Bath SB-4[1]

Water . . . . 1 gallon.
Potassium chrome alum . . . . 4 ounces.
Sodium sulfate desiccated[2] . . . . 8 ounces.

[1] The same proportions of ingredients should be used for making larger or smaller quantities of solutions, i.e., for 5 gals. multiply above quantities by 5.

[2] If crystalline sodium sulfate is used in place of the desiccated, increase the quantity in the above formula by 2¼.

on the film surface. Next, the films should be transferred to the fixing solution. In order to minimize the exposure to the air, the films must be transferred quickly from one solution to the other.

WASHING

In washing the films the flow of water should be sufficient to permit washing for a period not exceeding 10 minutes, since prolonged washing may cause the gelatin in the emulsion to swell excessively. In a single wash tank, the hourly flow of water should be at least 15 times the volume of the tank. In the two-compartment cascade washing system, the hourly flow of water should be at least 8 times the volume of one compartment.

TABLE XXV

TABLE OF DATA RELATIVE TO THE MODIFICATION OF DEVELOPER AND HARDENER SOLUTIONS FOR HIGH-TEMPERATURE PROCESSING

Temperature F.	*Regular x-ray developer*	*Hardener—Kodak SB-4*	*Fixer*
80°	Standard solution	Standard solution	Standard solution
90°	Modified solution (see below)	Standard solution	Standard solution
95°	Modified solution (see below)	Modified solution (see below)	Standard solution

	Developer			*Hardener*		
Temperature (degrees F.)	80°	90°	95°	80°	90°	95°
Ounces of sodium sulfate (desiccated) added per gallon of solution.	0	10 oz.	20 oz.	0	0	7 oz.

Chapter 26

Rapid Processing of Surgical Radiographs

As AN EXPEDIENT in the course of a surgical operation, it is occasionally necessary to inspect, at the earliest possible moment, radiographs that are made as a part of the surgical procedure. In such situations, the normal processing time can be reduced several minutes by the use of a developer solution prepared according to the following formula:

Kodak Developer D-8 (Stock Solution)

Water	96 ounces.
Sodium Sulfite, desiccated	12 ounces.
Hydroquinone	6 ounces.
Sodium Hydroxide (caustic soda)	5 ounces.
Potassium Bromide	4 ounces.
Water to make	1 gallon.

Note. Dissolve the chemicals in the order given.

PROCEDURE

For use, two parts of stock solution are mixed with one part of water. The x-ray film is developed in it for about 60 seconds at 68° F. The development time may be lowered to 45 seconds by decreasing to 1 ounce the amount of potassium bromide in the above formula. By so doing, however, appreciable fog may result. The employment of the tray method of processing rather than the tank method is advisable because the keeping quality of the developer is poor when diluted as recommended above. The solution should be discarded after use. The stock solution will retain its properties for about 2 months when kept in a well-stoppered brown bottle.

Since caustic soda is one of the components of the developer, it is recommended that rubber gloves be worn during development and dental x-ray film clips be employed to facilitate handling of films.

Following development, it is important that the film be rinsed thoroughly before it is immersed in the fixer. This step is necessary to preclude the formation of stains or dichroic fog. If fresh fixer solution is employed, the radiograph should be ready for viewing after having been immersed approximately 1 minute with frequent agitation. After inspection, it should be returned to the fixer solution for approximately 10 minutes to insure thorough hardening of the emulsion. It may then be washed in the usual manner.

Glossary

Absorption, x-ray: Absorption (x-ray) concerns the reduction in intensity of x-rays as they traverse body tissues and emerge to expose an x-ray film.

Accelerator, developer: An accelerator in a developer is an alkaline chemical (sodium carbonate, sodium hydroxide, or sodium metaborate) that makes possible the activity of the developing agents. It softens the gelatin to permit the reducing agents' easy access to the exposed silver bromide contained in the emulsion.

Acid: An acid is a solution containing less hydrogen ions than water. Its pH is *less* than 7. The H ions can be replaced by metals and can form salts. Test for acidity: blue litmus paper turns pink when immersed in the acid solution.

Acidifier: The acidifier in a fixer provides an acid medium for proper fixation of the radiograph. It also serves to neutralize carry-over of alkaline developer. The usual acids employed are acetic and citric.

Agent, clearing: The clearing agent in the fixing bath is a chemical (sodium, or ammonium thiosulfate) whose function is to remove unexposed and undeveloped silver halide crystals in the x-ray film emulsion.

Agents, developing: Developing or reducing agents in a developer are chemicals that change the exposed silver bromide crystals to black metallic silver. Substances commonly employed are elon and hydroquinone.

Agent, hardening: The fixing bath hardener is a chemical (potassium alum) used to harden and shrink an x-ray film emulsion after the unexposed and undeveloped silver bromide crystals have been removed.

Agent, wetting: A wetting agent is a solution used following the washing process to accelerate the flow of water from both film surfaces and to hasten the drying of radiographs.

Alkali: An alkali is a solution containing *more* hydrogen ions than water. Its pH is *greater* than 7. Alkalis can react with acids to form salts. It reacts with red litmus paper and turns it blue.

Ampere: The ampere is the unit of current that will flow through a conductor with a potential of 1 volt and 1 ohm of resistance.

Ångstrom: An ångstrom is a unit employed in expressing the length of light waves. It is equal to one ten-thousandth of a micron. Symbol: Å.

Anode, x-ray tube: An x-ray tube anode is a heavy copper bar containing a tungsten target (focal spot) at the end facing the cathode, that can be bombarded by an electron stream from the cathode resulting in x-ray production. The face of the target in stationary tubes is cut to an angle of 18-20°; in rotating anode tubes the face is 13-15°. It is the positive electrode in the x-ray tube.

Artifacts: Artifacts are those markings on a radiograph that are foreign to the image.

Attenuation, x-ray: X-ray attenuation is a situation in which the x-rays on passing through tissues are reduced in intensity or altered in direction (secondary radiation).

Atom: The atom is the smallest unit of matter (element) remaining unchanged in chemical reactions. It consists of a central positively charged nucleus surrounded by enough electrons to produce an equivalent negative charge to make the atom electrically neutral. The number of positive charges on the nucleus (atomic number) and thus the number of electrons around the nucleus determines the properties of the atom.

Beam, x-ray: The x-ray beam is the bundle of x-rays that emerges from the portal of an energized x-ray tube. For radiographic purposes, it comprises primary radiation and remnant radiation when an object is in its path. The center of the beam is known as the central ray (CR).

Capacity, tank: Tank capacity is the volume of solution held in an x-ray processing tank. It is computed by multiplying the width, depth (minus 1 inch), and length, in inches and dividing the product by 231. The answer is in gallons.

Cassette: A cassette is a book-like, light-tight box arrangement designed so as to enclose two x-ray intensifying screens between which is sandwiched an x-ray film. Its front is radiotransparent; the lid is backed with thin lead sheet or is made with heavy steel. The cassette is used for exposure of the x-ray film.

Cathode, x-ray tube: An x-ray tube cathode contains a spirally wound filament that can become incandescent and produce electrons when a low voltage electric current is passed through it. It is so designed that it can focus an electron beam on the focal spot of the anode. It is the negative electrode in the x-ray tube.

Central ray: The central ray is the center of the x-ray beam. The term is employed to designate the direction of the x-rays in a given projection. The central ray may be considered to extend from the focal spot of the x-ray tube to the x-ray film. The symbol is CR.

Compound, chemical: A compound is a substance each molecule of which contains at least one atom of each of at least two elements.

Compression (of tissues): Compression of body tissues serves to reduce the thickness of tissue being radiographed. It makes possible a reduction in MaS, the production of secondary radiation fog, and the depth of tissue to be penetrated.

Cone: A cone is an apparatus accessory that aids in controlling secondary radiation by limiting the volume of tissue exposed. By limiting the area exposed, secondary radiation which would normally be generated in adjacent areas is eliminated and greater contrast is obtained. It is made of radiopaque metal in various sizes and may be fitted to the x-ray tube portal.

Contrast, emulsion: Emulsion contrast refers to the ability of the emulsion to affect the contrast of the radiograph under specific conditions of exposure, development, and type of tissue being examined. Different emulsions can produce different contrasts despite the same exposure and development.

Contrast, long-scale: Long-scale contrast is recognized by the large number of translucent densities that makes possible the visualization of an abundance of image details. The transition between image densities is small. Silver deposits representative of both thick and thin parts are usually present. It is produced by relatively short wave length x-radiation.

Contrast, optimum: Optimum contrast in a radiograph makes possible the visualization of all image details within a given part with a full range of translucent densities or tones rendered throughout the image.

Contrast, radiographic: Radiographic contrast comprises the differences in radiographic density that enable image details to become visible. Whenever there is a visible difference in the light transmission between two or more densities on a radiograph, radiographic contrast is said to exist. Contrast is directly influenced by the applied kilovoltage, the proportion of secondary radiation and the character of the tissues being examined.

Contrast, scale. The scale of contrast in a radiograph constitutes the range of visible densities in an image and determines the number of details that can be visualized.

Contrast, short-scale: Short-scale contrast characterizes an image produced by long wave length x-radiation. The transition between densities as to silver content is large and exaggerated. The range of densities is small. Silver deposits (details) representative of *both* thick and thin parts are seldom shown. Detail visibility in these image areas is diminished and in most instances is diagnostically worthless. Opacities and absence of image silver denotes short-scale contrast.

Contrast, tissue: Tissue contrast refers to the relative differences in tissue density and thickness of the components of an anatomic part with respect to their x-ray absorbing properties. Radiographically, tissue contrast is evidenced by the variations in radiographic densities caused by the *differences* in absorbing power of the different kinds of tissue traversed by an x-ray beam resulting in reduced intensities that reach the film.

Current, alternating: Alternating electric current is a type that reverses its direction at regular intervals. Symbol: AC.

Current, direct: Direct current is electricity flowing in one direction only. Symbol: DC.

Current, electric: An electric current is a flow of electrons through a conductor.

Current, high tension: High tension current possesses high voltage and relatively low amperage.

Current, low tension: Low tension current possesses low voltage but relatively high amperage.

Current, unidirectional: Unidirectional, as applied to a current of electricity, is a current that flows only in one direction.

Definition: Definition is the degree of distinctness with which radiographic details are recorded on an x-ray film. It is dependent upon optimum image sharpness.

Density, radiographic: Radiographic density is the resultant deposit of black metallic silver in the x-ray film emulsion produced by x-ray exposure and subsequent processing. All usable densities transmit light from an x-ray illuminator and are translucent. Density is the radiographic measure of the quantity of radiation absorbed by the film.

Density, regulation of: When a fixed kilovoltage is employed, the radiographic density is regulated by increasing or decreasing the MaS to a correct value so that the remnant radiation will be sufficiently intense to produce a satisfactory image.

Density, tissue: Tissue density may be considered as the resistance of the tissues to the passage of x-rays.

Detail, radiographic: Radiographic detail comprises a multitude of deposits of black metallic silver of varying translucency to the light of an x-ray illuminator and represents the structural configuration of body tissues in the form of a radiographic image. Visibility of detail is dependent upon optimum image sharpness and radiographic contrast.

Developer, constituents: There are 6 chemicals found in an x-ray developer solution. These chemicals and their functions are as follows:

1. Water—solvent
2. Elon—reduces the exposed silver emulsion
3. Hydroquinone—reduces the exposed silver emulsion
4. Sodium carbonate—accelerates rate of development
5. Sodium sulfite—preserves developer, controls solution oxidation
6. Potassium bromide—restrains or controls rate of development

Developer, dilution: The effect of dilution of a developer beyond that recommended is to cause the film to be underdeveloped when a standard time-temperature development is employed. Frequently, the capacity of tanks is incorrectly estimated and insufficient developer chemicals are dissolved in the solution.

Developer, inactivity: Lack of developer activity may be the result of:

1. Incorrect solution mixing
2. An error in dilution
3. Inadequate replenishment
4. Excessive dilution with water
5. Aerial oxidation
6. Fixer or stop-bath contamination
7. Low solution temperature

Developer, rapid: A rapid developer is one in which a strong alkali such as Kodalk or potassium hydroxide is employed as the accelerator.

Developer, regular: A regular developer is one in which sodium carbonate is employed as the accelerator. It possesses less developing speed than rapid developer and tends to produce gas when neutralized by the fixing bath.

Developer, temperature of: The temperature of the developer solution influences the rate of development. The higher the temperature, the greater the rate and vice versa.

Development: Development is the chemical process of converting exposed silver bromide (latent image) to black metallic silver (silver image). The rate of development is influenced by the time and temperature of the developer and its chemical activity. The optimum temperature range of development is 60°-75° F.

Development, accelerated: Accelerated development may be caused by:

1. Errors in dilution when mixing solutions
2. Use of more replenisher than necessary
3. Excessively high temperatures

Development, degree of: The degree of development depends on development time, temperature, amount of agitation and activity of the developer.

Development, exhaustion system: In the exhaustion system of development, the activity of the developer diminishes slowly with use, and radiographic density is maintained by gradually increasing the development time and adding fresh developer to maintain solution volume. The system requires that the solution retained by the film be drained back to the tank.

Development, inspection: Development by inspection is poor practice. Errors in judgment occur as to when development is complete because of:

1. Failure in rapid eye accommodation from bright light to processing room light and vice versa.
2. Low level of illumination.
3. Opacity of uncleared film.
4. Differences in appearance of film made by direct x-ray or screen exposures.

Development, over-: The gain in density or contrast obtained with development of a correctly exposed radiograph beyond 5 minutes at 68°F. is relatively small. The slight density gain is largely due to development of unexposed silver bromide crystals that show as fog. There is little or no increase in film speed by such practice. Prolonged development of the properly exposed film may cause chemical fogging of the image. Overdevelopment cannot produce silver deposits (detail) on the radiograph if the x-rays employed do not reach the emulsion to expose it.

Development, replenishment system: In the replenishment system of development, a constant developing time can be maintained by frequent addition of small quantities of replenisher solution. A replenished developer should be discarded when 125, 14 to 17 inch films per gallon of solution have been passed through it —or, at the end of three months. The excess developer from the film must be drained to the waste.

Development, temperature compensation: As the temperature of a developing solution changes, the rate of development can be compensated by the development time.

Diaphragm, aperture: An aperture diaphragm is a radiographic device composed of a sheet of radiopaque lead or brass in which is cut an aperture of a size to permit x-ray coverage of a desired film area. Its function is comparable to that of a cone.

Diaphragm, grid: A grid diaphragm is a radiographic device employed to prevent or reduce the amount of secondary radiation generated by the tissues from reaching and fogging the x-ray film. Grids may be stationary or moving.

Dielectric: A dielectric is an insulator or material of low electrical conductivity or none at all. Examples: porcelain, rubber, air, etc.

Distance, focus-film: The focus-film distance is the distance from the focal spot of the x-ray tube to the x-ray film. It is used as a radiographic exposure factor and influences radiographic density and image sharpness. Symbol: FFD.

Distance, object-film: The object-film distance is the distance from the body part to the x-ray film. As a factor of projection, it influences the size and shape of the image (magnification and distortion) and image sharpness. Symbol: OFD.

Distortion, image: Distortion in the image is the perversion of the true size and shape of the body part being examined and caused by reason of the OFD and the angulation of the x-rays passing through the part.

Dose, permissible: The x-ray permissible dose is the total amount of radiation that a person may receive day after day without demonstrable damage to the tissues (including the blood and reproductive cells). The tolerances are established periodically by competent radiologic authority.

Drying, process: The drying process is the removal of water from the emulsion of an x-ray film so that it may be freely handled.

Effect, heel: The heel effect is the intensity variation within an x-ray beam that is materially influenced by the angle at which it is projected from the focal spot to either side (anode or cathode) of the central ray. The intensity is *greatest* on the cathode side of the x-ray beam and progressively diminishes on the anode side. The effect is materially influenced by the focus-film distance, kilovoltage, and range of tissue densities being examined. It diminishes as the FFD and KvP increases.

Electricity: As a source of power, electricity is a flow of electrons through a closed conducting circuit. The flow is governed by an excess of electrons at one point and a deficiency at another point. The flow is in the direction of least electron concentration (lower potential).

Electricity, static: Static electricity is stationary electricity as opposed to electricity in motion as an electric current.

Electrolyte: An electrolyte is a chemical compound that can be ionized.

Electron: An electron is the smallest atomic particle; an elementary particle of *negative* electricity.

Element: An element is a substance each molecule of which contains one or more like atoms.

Eliminator, hypo: A solution which chemically alters the fixing salts contained in the gelatin of the x-ray film and thus aids in shortening the washing time.

Elon, function: Elon is a reducing agent that starts action on the exposed emulsion within a few seconds and the entire image appears rapidly. Fine detail is produced but the contrast is low.

Exposure, MaS: When a fixed kilovoltage is employed, the radiographic density is regulated by increasing or decreasing the MaS to its correct value so that the remnant radiation will be sufficiently intense to produce a satisfactory image. The KvP and focus-film distance remain as constants.

Exposure, over-: An overexposure is evidenced in a radiograph after incorrect exposure and full development and the image contains excessive silver deposits, many of which are opaque to transmitted light.

Exposure, radiographic: A radiographic exposure is dependent upon the quantity of x-radiation of a given quality that emerges from the body part for a given period of time and absorbed by the x-ray film to expose it.

Exposure, under-: An underexposure is evidenced in a radiograph when the image displays insufficient silver deposits following full development.

Filament, x-ray tube: The x-ray tube filament is the spiral tungsten wire mounted in the cathode of the x-ray tube; when heated by a low voltage current, it emits electrons. The greater the flow of electrons, the greater the Ma.

Film, base: X-ray film base is the cellulose supporting medium for the radiographic emulsion. It is transparent, slightly blue in color, is slow-burning and approximately $^{8}/_{1000}$-inches thick. Its stiffness and flatness satisfies the purpose of handling.

Film, direct-exposure: Direct-exposure film is highly sensitive to the direct action of x-rays but has low sensitivity to screen fluorescence. It has a greater silver content. It should not be employed with screens.

Film, emulsion. An x-ray film emulsion is a light and x-ray sensitive coating on both sides of a transparent film base, consisting of crystals of silver bromide, chloride or iodide held in suspension and apart in gelatin. The emulsion $^{1}/_{1000}$-inch thick. X-ray film emulsions vary as to contrast, speed, fogging characteristics and rate of development. In these respects, films of different manufacture vary quite widely and from an exposure and processing standpoint cannot be considered interchangeable.

Film, screen-exposure: Screen-exposure film is sensitive to the fluorescent light of intensifying screens and not so sensitive to the direct action of x-rays. It may be employed with or without screens.

Film, substratum: A film substratum (subbing) is a very thin coating of a gelatin-like material on x-ray film base, glass, or paper that facilitates the adhesion of the silver emulsion.

Film, x-ray: X-ray film is the medium used to contain a radiographic image after it has been exposed and processed. It consists of a transparent, blue-tinted, cellulose plastic base upon both sides of which is coated a gelatin emulsion of silver salts.

Filter: A filter consists of any substance interposed in a beam of radiation for the purpose of changing the quality and intensity of the emitted x-rays.

Filtration: Filtration of the x-ray beam alters its intensity and quality. As filtration is increased, radiographic contrast decreases. In radiography, a 1 mm. minimum thickness of aluminum should always filter the x-ray beam.

Fixation: Fixation is the chemical removal of unexposed and undeveloped silver bromide crystals from an x-ray film after the exposed crystals have been reduced to silver by the development process. It occurs in an acid medium. This is the clearing function of the fixer. The second function of fixation is to harden and shrink the emulsion so that the film may be dried and handled safely.

Fixation, clearing time: The clearing time is the period begun by immersion of the film in the fixer and ending with the disappearance of all undeveloped and unexposed crystals (milkiness). It is during this interval that the fixer dissolves the unexposed silver salts and removes them from the emulsion.

Fixation, rate: The rate of fixation is determined by the:

1. Concentration and nature of the fixer chemicals
2. Temperature of the solution
3. Degree of agitation in the fixer
4. Tank volume in relation to size and number of films fixed

Fixation, time: The general rule for applying the fixation time is to leave the films in the fixing bath twice the length of time it takes to clear them.

Fixer, constituents: There are 5 chemicals usually found in an x-ray fixing bath. The chemicals and their functions are as follows:

1. Water—solvent
2. Sodium, or ammonium thiosulfate—removes unexposed and undeveloped silver bromide
3. Sodium sulfite—preservative
4. Potassium alum—hardener
5. Acetic acid—acidifier

Fluorescence: Fluorescence is a type of luminescence in a substance that is continued as long as radiation such as x-rays is absorbed.

Fluorescent Screen: A surface coated with zinc sulfide (formerly platinobarium cyanide) which fluoresces when irradiated by x-rays. Used for visual examination by x-rays, in a darkened room. To protect the operator from the effects of the x-rays during this process, the outer surface is covered with lead glass. For radiography, screens are composed of calcium tungstate crystals that fluoresce only as long as they absorb x-rays. These screens are known as intensifying screens because they augment the x-ray exposure effect 20-30 times.

Fluids, body: Body fluids constitute the liquid make-up of tissues and consist of water, lymph, blood, urine, etc.

Focal Spot: The focal spot (FS) of an x-ray tube is the area of x-ray generation located on the tungsten target of the anode. It may vary in size depending upon the focus desired.

Fog, secondary radiation: Secondary radiation fog is a *supplemental* density that veils the radiographic image produced by the remnant radiation. It is produced by exposure of the x-ray film by secondary radiation. Since it tends to degrade radiographic contrast, it adversely influences radiographic quality. Control can be exercised by the proper use of kilovoltage, cones, aperture diaphragms, or grids.

Gelatin: Gelatin is a jelly-like protein substance obtained from animal tissues by boiling. It is used in x-ray film manufacture as a means for suspension of the sensitive silver salts on the film base.

Grid: A grid is a device which consists of a series of alternate radiopaque and radioparent strips deeper than wide which when interposed between patient and film allows primary rays to pass through the radiopaque strips, but the secondary radiation is absorbed by the radiopaque strips. There are two general types of grids—stationary and moving. The efficiency of a grid ranges from 80-95 per cent in the elimination of secondary radiation thereby enhancing contrast and increasing detail visibility.

Grid, radius: The strips in a grid are angled so that their planes converge toward a point usually the tube focal spot. The grid is said to have a radius or focus equal to the distance from this point to the surface of the grid.

Grid, ratio: The ratio of a grid is expressed as the relation of the *depth* of the lead strips to the *width* of the radiolucent separators between lead strips. For example—if the depth of the lead strips of a grid is eight times greater than the width of the separating strips, the grid is said to have a ratio of 8:1.

Hanger, processing: A processing hanger is a stainless steel frame containing film clips at each corner that hold the x-ray film firmly during the processing procedure.

Hardener, fixing bath: The fixing bath hardener is a chemical (potassium alum) used to harden and shrink the x-ray film emulsion after development.

Holder, exposure: An exposure holder is a radioparent cardboard and envelope device used to hold an x-ray film for exposure purposes. The back of the holder is lined with a thin sheet of lead to protect the film from radiation back-scatter. The envelope mounted between the cardboard covers is to enclose the x-ray film.

Hydroquinone, function: The function of the chemical hydroquinone in a developer is to build up contrast in the image so that the detail becomes readily visible.

Hypo: Hypo is the common name for sodium or ammonium thiosulfate, the chemicals used in fixing baths.

Illuminator, x-ray: An x-ray illuminator is a device before which radiographs are viewed. It consists of a metal box containing two fluorescent tubes that emits light of standard color (daylight) and intensity. The face of the illuminator consists of a sheet of blue-tinted opal glass or plastic to diffuse the transmitted light.

Image, latent: The latent image refers to the atomic changes that occur in the silver bromide crystals in the emulsion of an x-ray film upon x-ray exposure which renders the crystals reducible to metallic silver upon development.

Image, radiographic: A radiographic image is a pictorial record of the internal structural elements of a part of the body as projected by x-rays on an x-ray film. It consists of deposits of black metallic silver of varying concentration on the radiograph.

Immobilization: Immobilization is the act of rendering a body part immobile during a radiographic exposure to secure sharp images or to compress the tissues and reduce their thickness.

Impulse: In AC current, there are 120 impulses. Each impulse has a time span of $1/120$ second. The number of impulses in a time span of $1/20$ second would be 6.

Intensity, x-ray: X-ray intensity refers to the rate (roentgens per second) at which x-radiation reaching the film directly influences the over-all density of the radiograph.

Ion: An ion is an electrically charged atom or group of atoms. The fundamental part of a negative ion is an electron; a positive ion is one from which an orbital electron has been removed.

Ionization: Ionization is a process whereby electrically neutral atoms become electrically charged because of the loss or gain of extranuclear electrons. If an electron attaches itself to a neutral atom, a negative ion results. If an electron is lost, a positive ion results. The ionization of a molecule of silver bromide is expressed by the following equation wherein the silver atom loses an electron and the bromine atom gains an electron.

$$AgBr \rightleftarrows Ag^{+} + Br^{-}$$

Ions, negative: Negative ions (anions) are those possessing an excess of electrons, as Cl^{-}.

Ions, positive: Postitive ions (cations) are atoms that lack a normal complement of electrons, as Na^{+}. They are atoms that have lost valence electrons.

Kilovoltage: Kilovoltage (1000 volts) as an exposure factor is used in radiography to influence radiographic density, contrast, production of secondary radiation fog, penetration of tissues and exposure latitude. Electrically, it is the potential applied to an x-ray tube to drive the electrons emitted by the cathode toward the tungsten target located on the face of the anode. It directly influences the qualitative characteristics of the x-ray beam (wave length). Symbol: KvP.

Kilovoltage, optimum: An optimum or fixed kilovoltage is one that, for a given projection, will always penetrate the body part irrespective of size and will produce an image of satisfactory contrast when the MaS employed is practical in value.

Latitude, exposure: Exposure latitude is the range (exposure spread) between the minimum and maximum exposure that will provide a scale of translucent densities of a body part acceptable for diagnostic purposes. It is influenced by the scale of contrast, hence by KvP. The lower the KvP, the less the exposure latitude, and vice versa. Exposure latitude improves as the kilovoltage is increased until a point is reached where the scale of contrast becomes too long.

Law, inverse square: The inverse square law is used in radiography and states that the intensity of x-radiation varies inversely as the square of the focus-film distance.

Magnification, image: Magnification is the degree of image enlargement of body tissues.

MaS, basic: A basic MaS is one employed to provide an optimum density for all tissue thicknesses in an average thickness range as established for a given projection and kilovoltage.

Media, contrast: Contrast media are employed to render high contrast in a viscus that normally has very low tissue contrast. Barium sulfate is a common contrast medium for visualization of the alimentary tract.

Milliampere: Milliampere (Ma) is a radiographic exposure factor that regulates the intensity of radiation emitted by the x-ray tube. It directly influences the radiographic density. Electrically, the milliampere is $1/1000$ of an ampere of electric current.

Milliampere Seconds: Milliampere seconds are the product of milliamperes and seconds of time. Its symbol is MaS and is an important exposure factor in the regulation of the amount of silver deposit in the radiographic image.

Molecule: A molecule is composed of one or more particles known as atoms. It is the smallest quantity of matter (compound) which can exist by itself and retain its chemical properties.

Neutron: A neutron is an electrically neutral particle having an atomic weight equal to one. Its mass is approximately equal to the hydrogen atom. Neutrons are constituents of atomic nuclei (except hydrogen). Being uncharged, neutrons are able to penetrate nuclei and are, therefore, used for bombardment in nuclear disintegration experiments.

Nucleus: The nucleus is the compact central portion of an atom. It is characterized by the number of its positive charges and its mass. The nucleus contains about 99.97 per cent of the mass of the atom.

Number, atomic: The atomic number is the number of protons or positive charges on the nucleus of an atom and serves to identify an element. It is also equal to the number of electrons surrounding the nucleus.

Osteoblasts: Osteoblasts are bone forming cells.

Osteoclasis: Osteoclasis is the process of breaking down bone structure.

Osteoclasts: Osteoclasts are cells that break down or erode bone.

Osteoporosis: Osteoporosis is a condition wherein a loss in bone substance occurs resulting in a decrease in tissue density.

Osteosclerosis: Osteosclerosis is a condition that occurs when there is an abnormal increase in the deposition of bone resulting in an increase in tissue density.

Opalescence, fixation: Opalescence in a radiograph sometimes occurs in a freshly made fixer but soon disappears after washing and drying. This transient condition is caused by the reaction of the gelatin to the high concentration of sodium thiosulfate in the fresh fixer. There is little tendency for opalescence to appear when ammonium thiosulfate is used as a clearing agent.

Oxidation: Oxidation occurs in a chemical reaction when an electron is *removed* from an atom of a substance. The development of an exposed x-ray film is basically a matter of oxidation of the silver bromide emulsion. Oxidation signifies a *loss* of electrons.

$$\text{Silver atom} - \text{electron}^- = \text{Silver ion}^+ + \text{electron}^-$$

It is any process which increases the proportion of oxygen or acid-forming element or radical in a compound.

Penetration, tissue: The penetration of tissue is a function of x-radiation wave length and is controlled by the applied kilovoltage.

Penumbra: A penumbra is the ill-defined margin of a shadow produced by light. In radiography, it is the blurred margin of an image detail.

pH: pH is a value that expresses the hydrogen ion concentration of a solution—degree of acidity or alkalinity. Pure water is neutral and its pH is 7. Solutions with pH values *less* than 7 are acid in reaction; those above 7 are alkaline. A rapid developer is strongly alkaline and might have a pH of 14. A strong fixer is exceedingly acid in reaction and might have a pH value of about 3.

Photoelectron: A photoelectron is an electron emitted from a substance under the stimulus of light or other radiation of appropriate wave length.

Photography: Photography is the art or process of obtaining images on sensitized surfaces by the action of light or other radiant energy.

Photon: A "particle" of electromagnetic radiation. The energy of the photon (quantum) determines the type of radiation that it is. Thus, a red light photon has a small amount of energy, a violet light photon more, and an x-ray photon still more. A beam of light or x-rays may be considered as a stream of photons.

Photoradiography: Photoradiography is the technic of photographing the x-ray fluorescent screen image on 35 or 70 mm roll film or 4 x 10″ cut film.

Preservative: A preservative is a chemical placed in an x-ray developer and employed to reduce the amount of oxidation of the reducing agents by air. Sodium sulfite is the chemical usually employed. Due to its slight alkalinity, it contributes to the alkalinity of the developer. Sodium sulfite is also used in the fixer to prevent decomposition of the sodium thiosulfate by acid.

Processing: Processing is the chemical treatment of an exposed x-ray film that results in the production of a radiographic image. It involves the processes of development, rinsing, fixation, washing, and drying.

Proton: Protons are basic constituent particles of atomic nuclei. They have a positive charge numerically equal to that of the negative electron but have a mass 1840 times the mass of an electron.

Quality, radiographic: A radiograph may be said to possess radiographic quality when by reason of existing contrast and definition all required anatomical details within the body part being examined become visible in the image.

Quality, x-ray: X-ray quality is a property determined by the distribution of intensity among the various wave lengths.

Quantum: A quantum is the amount of energy associated with a photon; the x-ray energy reacting with or affecting a single atom or ion. A quantum is an elemental unit of radiant energy (x-rays). The term is almost synonymous with the term of photon.

Radiation, heterogeneous: Heterogeneous radiation contains a mixture of many different x-ray wave lengths as it leaves the portal of the x-ray tube.

Radiation, homogeneous: Homogeneous radiation is one consisting of x-rays of the same wave length; that is, monochromatic.

Radiation, primary: Primary radiation (PR) comprises the x-rays that emerge from the portal of an x-ray tube. The quality and quantity are influenced by the exposure factors KvP and MaS.

Radiation, remnant: Remnant radiation (RR) is the emergent radiation from a body part which has been selectively diminished in intensity by the various tissues traversed by the primary radiation. It is the radiation that produces the radiographic image and is influenced largely by the absorption characteristics of the tissues examined.

Radioactivity: The property possessed by certain elements of spontaneously emitting x-rays or gamma rays.

Radiograph: A radiograph contains the image of the internal structures of an object produced by the passage of x-rays and recorded by an x-ray film.

Radiography: Radiography is that procedure which depends on the differential absorption of x-rays traversing an object to emerge to expose an x-ray film and produce a radiographic image.

Radiolucent: Radiolucent (radiotransparent, radioparent) indicates the property of a structure to be partly or wholly permeable to the passage of x-rays to some degree.

Radiopaque: Radiopaque indicates the property of a structure to be impenetrable to the passage of x-rays.

Ratio, grid: The ratio of a grid is expressed as the relation of the *depth* of the lead strips to the width of the radiolucent separators between lead strips. For example—if the depth of the lead strips of a grid is eight times greater than the width of the separating strips, the grid is said to have a ratio of 8:1.

Ray, central: The central ray is the center of the x-ray beam. The term is employed to designate the direction of the x-rays in a given projection. The central ray may be considered to extend from the focal spot of the x-ray tube to the x-ray film. The symbol is CR.

Rays, gamma: Gamma rays are similar to x-rays though shorter in wave length. They are not affected by electric or magnetic fields. They ionize gases. They are detectable after passage through steel plate many inches thick and are electromagnetic photons, or quanta. They travel with the velocity of light. Their wave lengths are in general shorter than ordinary x-rays.

Reaction, chemical: A chemical reaction is an exchange of atoms between molecules to form molecules of a different kind. The result of a chemical reaction is illustrated by an equation.

$$NaCl + AgNO_3 \rightarrow NaNO_3 + AgCl \downarrow$$

Reciprocity: The reciprocity law is an important law formulated by Bunsen and Roscoe. It states that the reaction of a photographic emulsion to light is equal to the product of the intensity of the light and the duration of the exposure. The law is valid for direct x-ray exposures but fails for exposures with intensifying screens.

Reduction: Reduction occurs in a chemical reaction when an electron is *added* to an ion of a chemical to form an atom. Reduction signifies a *gain* in electrons.

$$\text{Silver ion}^{+} + \text{electron}^{-} = \text{Silver atom.}$$

Reduction is any process which increases the proportion of hydrogen or base-forming elements or radicals in a compound.

Replenishment System: The replenishment system of development or fixation makes possible the use of a constant development or fixing time by constant chemical replenishment of the solutions to maintain a standard strength.

Restrainer, developer: A restrainer is a chemical (potassium bromide) used in a developer to check development of the unexposed silver bromide and to control the working speed of the developer with respect to the exposed silver bromide.

Rinsing: After development the film is saturated with alkali. When the film is placed in the fixer, development continues until the alkali is neutralized by the acid fixer. This causes artifacts on the film and hastens exhaustion of the fixer and destroys its hardening properties. To maintain the correct chemical balance in the fixer, all films after removal from the developer should be thoroughly rinsed in flowing water or an acid rinse bath for at least 30 seconds.

Roentgen: The *roentgen* is the international unit of quantity of both x-rays and gamma rays. It is designated by the symbol *r*. It is the physical unit of quantity of radiation based on the amount of ionization produced by its absorption in air.

Rule, heel effect: Align the long axis of the tube with the long center axis of the part and film, and direct the cathode portion of the x-ray beam toward the anatomic area of greatest tissue density or thickness.

Rule-of Thumb: A photographic rule-of-thumb to change radiographic density by workable amounts may be employed by either halving or doubling the MaS, provided the kilovoltage employed is optimum for the part being examined.

Safelight: A safelight consists of a sheet of dyed gelatin sandwiched between glass, which when put in the window of a safelight lamp containing the correct wattage bulb, will transmit illumination in which x-ray film may safely be handled for a limited period of time. Safelights currently in use employ the amber series 6B type.

Screens, x-ray intensifying: X-ray intensifying screens consist of a finely powdered fluorescent material (usually calcium tungstate) mixed with a binder and coated on a cardboard or plastic support. When excited by x-rays, the fluorescent salt emits visible light. They are a means for reducing exposure in radiography.

Secondary Radiation: Secondary radiation (SR) is x-radiation that is generated by body tissues or other objects when exposed to a beam of x-rays. It is dependent upon the quality and quantity of the primary radiation and the atomic number of its tissue source. Light elements such as water, tissue, and wood generate large quantities of secondary radiation. The primary exposure factor influencing the production of secondary radiation is KvP.

Speed, emulsion: Emulsion speed is a measure of the minimum exposure required to produce a predetermined density. The speed, therefore, depends upon the nature of the emulsion and activity of developer.

Spot, focal: The focal spot (FS) of an x-ray tube is the area of x-ray generation located on the tungsten target of the anode.

Technic, optimum KvP: The optimum kilovoltage technic is based upon standardization of the processing procedure and the reduction of all exposure factors to constants for a given projection with the exception of one variable—MaS. The kilovoltage is fixed for a given projection and the MaS is the variable.

Thickness, average range: Average thickness ranges are employed for radiographic projections as a guide to exposure. They are based on the frequency with which certain groups of thicknesses occur as measured for a given projection.

Tissues, body: Body tissues are construed as the solid portions of the body structures and comprise muscle, bone, fat, skin, etc. These tissues are classified as organic, and inorganic in composition.

Tone: A tone (or brightness) value represents the amount of light transmitted through a radiographic density from a conventional x-ray illuminator; all tones are translucent. The x-ray absorption differences of tissues are rendered as differences in density or tones. The light transmission is dependent upon the silver concentration in the image.

Transparent: A material is transparent when it has the property of transmitting rays of light so that objects can be seen through it.

Translucent: A material that is translucent admits the passage of light, but does not permit objects to be distinctly seen through it.

Tube, x-ray: An x-ray tube is a highly evacuated glass container in which two electrodes—cathode and anode—are mounted and designed to produce x-rays.

Umbra: An umbra is a complete shadow produced by light, with sharply demarcated margins. In radiography, it is a sharply delineated image detail.

Underexposure: An underexposure is evidenced in a radiograph when the image displays insufficient silver deposits.

Valence: The valence of an element (or radical) is measured by the number of atoms of hydrogen with which it can combine, or by the number of atoms of hydrogen that it can replace by reaction with an acid.

Volt: A volt is the electrical unit of pressure that moves or tends to move electrons.

Washing: Washing is the terminal part of the processing procedure. The film saturated with fixing bath and soluble silver salts is washed until these salts are removed. The rate of washing is dependent upon the temperature of the water and the rate and volume of the water flow.

Wave Length, x-ray: The wave length of x-rays is confined to a useful band for medical radiography of 0.50 to 0.100 *ångstrom* units.

Weight, atomic: The number of protons and neutrons found in the nucleus of the atom is known as the atomic weight.

X-rays: X-rays consist of electromagnetic radiation of very short wave length possessing the properties of (1) penetration of matter, (2) exposure of photographic materials, (3) excitation of fluorescence; and, (4) ionization of matter. The useful band of wave lengths employed for medical radiography is 0.50 to 0.100 *ångstrom* units.

X-rays, generation of: X-rays are generated in an x-ray tube when a high speed beam of electrons is bombarded against a tungsten target.

Reference Reading

BODY TISSUES

Living Bone in Health and Disease. Stein, I., Stein, R. O., and Beller, M. L. Philadelphia and Montreal, Lippincott, 1955.

Factors Determining the Deposition and Demineralization of Bone. Haldeman, K. O. *J. Bone & Joint Surg., 32A*:596-600, 1950.

Influence of Mechanical Factors on the Development and Structure of Bone. Townsley, W. *Am. J. Phys. Anthropol., 6*:25-45, 1948.

An Electron-Microscopic Study of the Crystalline Inorganic Component of Bone and Its Relationship to the Organic Matrix. Robinson, R. A. *J. Bone & Joint Surg., 34A*:389-435 and 476, 1952.

Roentgenographic Estimation of the Mineral Content of Bone. Henny, G. C. *Radiology, 54*:202-210, 1950.

Defective Skeletal Mineralization. Swenson, P. C., and Jeffrey, R. B. *G. P., 7*:34-45, 1953.

The Quantitative Evaluation of Bone Density. Mack, P. B., Brown, W. N., Jr., and Trapp, H. D. *Am. J. Roentgenol., 61*:808-825, 1949.

Problems in the Measurement of Bone Density. Jackson, H. *Brit. J. Radiol., 24*:613-616, 1951.

The Record of Metabolism Imprinted on the Skeleton. Todd, T. W. *Am. J. Orthodontics, 24*:811-825, 1938.

Fundamentals of Tissue Differentiation. Gould, D. R. *Radiography, 6*:83-92, 1940.

The Biology of Human Starvation. Keys, A., *et al. Am. J. Phys. Anthropol., 10*:229-233, 1952.

Further Observations on Total Body Water, I. Normal Values Throughout the Life Span. Edelman, I. S., *et al. Surg., Gynec. & Obst., 95*:1-12, 1952.

Further Observations on Total Body Water, II. Changes of Body Composition in Disease. Moore, F. D., *et al. Surg., Gynec. & Obst., 95*:155-180, 1952.

The Relation of Body Fluid Compartments to Body Fat. Hardy, J. D., Sen, P. K., and Drabkin, D. L. *Surg., Gynec. & Obst., 93*:103-106, 1951.

Fat-Bone Index as a Sex-Differentiating Character in Man. Reynolds, E. L. *Human Biol., 21*:199-204, 1949.

Evaluation of Leanness-Fatness in Man: Survey of Methods. Brozek, J. and Kays, A. *Nutrition Abstr. & Rev., 20*:247-256, 1950-51.

Differences in the Distribution of Subcutaneous Fat with Sex and Maturity. Edwards, D. A. W. *Clin. Sc., 10*:305-315, 1951.

Physical Diagnosis. Walker, H. St. Louis, Mosby, 1952.

Das Verhältnis Der Belichtungszeit Zur Spannung Und Objektdicke In Der Röntgenphotographie. Francis, T. *Acta radiol., 21*:510-517, 1940.

EXPOSURE

Rationale of Radiographic Exposure. Fuchs, A. W. *X-ray Tech., 22*:62-68, 1950.

Control of Radiographic Density. Fuchs, A. W. *X-ray Tech., 20*:271-273, 1949.

Relationship of Tissue Thickness to Kilovoltage. Fuchs, A. W. *X-ray Tech., 19*:287-293, 1948.

Relation Between Tension and Exposure Times in Radiography. Bierman, A. and Boldingh, W. H. *Acta radiol., 35*:22-25, 1951.

Exposure Latitude, Range of Depth (Permissible Variation of Depth) and Field of Applicability in Roentgenography. Francis, T. *Acta med. scandinav., Suppl. 131*, pp. 146-153, 1948.

Story of Contrast and Definition. Spiegler, G. *Radiography, 16*:177-182, 1950.

Analysis of Physical Factors Controlling Diagnostic Quality of Roentgen Images; Contrast and Intensity Distribution Function of Roentgen Image. Morgan, R. H. *Am. J. Roentgenol., 55*:67-89, 1946.

Analysis of Physical Factors Controlling Diagnostic Quality of Roentgen Images; Contrast and Film Contrast Factor. Morgan, R. H. *Am. J. Roentgenol., 55*:627-633, 1946.

Factors Determining Detection of Shadows in Radiographs. Barclay, A. E. and Franklin, K. J. *Brit. J. Radiol., 10*:689-692, 1937.

Aids to Radiographic Definition. Watson, W. *Radiography, 17*:67-78, 1951.

Demonstration of the Geometrical Principles Underlying Radiography. Greening, J. R. *Radiography, 15*:268-269, 1949.

Respiratory Blurring in Routine Roentgenography. Kraft, E. *Quart. Bull. Sea View Hosp., 5*:167-174, 1940.

Determination of Physical Factors Influencing Quality of Radiographic Image (Reproduction Number Method and Its Application). Nelson, A. *Acta radiol., Suppl. 76*, pp. 1-87, 1949.

Anode "Heel" Effect in Radiography. Fuchs, A. W. *X-ray Tech., 18*:158-163, 1947.

FILM

X-ray Films, Their Manufacture and Their Characteristics. Longmore, T. A. *Radiography, 16*:200-207, 1950.

Production of Photographic Gelatin. Cohen, J. H. *J.P.S.A. 19B*:105-108, 1953.

Fluorescence in the Photographic Emulsion. Friedman, J. S. and Horowitz, L. *Photo. Sc. and Tech., 2*:42-47, 1955.

Sensitometry of Roentgenographic Films and Screens. Morgan, R. H. and Van Allen, W. W. *Radiology, 52*:832-845, 1949.

Sensitometry of Roentgen Films and Interpretation of Sensitometric Data. Henny, G. C. *Am. J. Roentgenol., 45*:895-908, 1941.

Historical Evolution of Roentgen-Ray Plates and Films. Martin, F. C. and Fuchs, A. W. *Am. J. Roentgenol., 26*:540-548, 1931.

Radiographic Recording Media and Screens, in The Science of Radiology. Glasser, Otto, editor. Springfield, Thomas, 1933.

Evolution of Roentgen Film. Fuchs, A. W. *Am. J. Roentgenol., 75*:30-48, 1956.

HISTORY

On a New Kind of Rays. Sitzungsberichte der Wurzburger Physikalischen-Medicinischen gesellschaft. Röntgen, W. C. 1895 and 1896.

The Rontgen Rays. Houston, E. J. and Kennelly, A. E. *J. Franklin Inst. 141*:241-278, 1896.

From Immigrant to Inventor. Pupin, M. New York, Scribner, 1930.

History of Photography. Newhall, B. New York, Simon & Schuster, Inc., 1949.

Technical Highlights of the Past Fifty Years. Matthews, G. E. *Am. Photo., 45*:93-100, 1951.

Edison and Roentgenology. Fuchs, A. W. *Am. J. Roentgenol., 57*:145-156, 1947.

PROCESSING

Some Fundamentals in the Processing of X-ray Films. Herz, R. H. *Photo. J., 83*:343, 1943.

Photographic Development. James, T. H. *Scient. Am., 187*:30-33, 1952.

Developer Solutions for X-ray Films. Crabtree, J. I and Henn, R. W. *M. Radiog. & Photog., Part 1, 23:*2-12; *Part 2, 23:*38-46, *Part 3, 24:*10-14, 1947.

New Stop Bath and Fixing Bath Formulas. Crabtree, J. I., Muehler, L. E. and Russell, H. D. *J. Soc. Mot. Pict. Engineers*, pp. 353-372, 1942.

Some Properties of Fixing Baths. Crabtree, J. I., and Hartt, H. A. *Tr. Soc. Mot. Pict. Engineers, 13:*364-405, 1929.

The Removal of Hypo and Silver Salts from Photographic Materials as Affected by the Composition of the Processing Solutions. Crabtree, J. I. Eaton, G. T. and Muehler, L. E. *J. Soc. Mot. Pict. Engineers*, pp. 39-68, 1943.

Fixer Solutions for X-ray Films. Crabtree, J. I. and Russell, H. D. *Radiog. and Clin. Photog., 21:*26-33, 1945.

How to Save Water in Photographic Processing. Crabtree, J. I. *J.P.S.A. 16B:*70-74, 1950.

Scums, Sludges, and Stains. Crabtree, J. I. and Henn, R. W. *J.P.S.A. 14:*201-209, 1948.

Artifacts in Roentgen Films. Henny, G. C. *Radiology 24:*350-356, 1935.

Study of the Static Electricity Problem in the X-ray Darkroom. Roderick, J. F. and Sutherland, B. *X-ray Tech. 23:*343-366, 1952.

Reduction of Static Disturbances in Dark Rooms. Mattsson, O. *Acta radiol. 45:*383-388, 1956.

Photographic Chemicals and Solutions. Crabtree, J. I. and Matthews, G. E. Boston, Am. Photo. Pub. Co.

Processing Chemicals and Formulas for Black-and-White Photography. Kodak Data Book, 1954.

THEORY

The Theory of the Photographic Process. Mees, C. E. K. New York, Macmillan, 1942.

Fundamentals of Photographic Theory. James, T. H. and Higgins, G. C. New York, Wiley, 1948.

Recent Advances in Our Knowledge of the Photographic Process. Mees, C. E. K. *Scient. Month. 55:*293-300, 1942.

The Latent Image. Webb, J. H. *Physics Today, 3:*8-15, 1950.

The Latent Image in Photography. Friedman, J. S. *Am. Photo. 45:*484-487, 1951.

Formation of the Photographic Latent Image. Webb, J. H. *J.P.S.A. 7:*136-143, 1941.

Formation of the Latent Image by X-rays. Larson, E. T. *J.P.S.A. 17B:*19-24, 1951.

Photographic Photometry of Roentgen Rays. Wilsey, R. B. *Am. J. Roentgenol. 32:*789-804, 1935.

The Sensitometry of Roentgenographic Materials. Hodgson, M. B. *Am. J. Roentgenol., 4:*610-617, 1917.

A Discussion on Radiographic Sensitivity. Hastings, C. H. *Am. Soc. Test. Materials, 96:*60-69, 1949.

Physical Foundations of Chest Roentgenography. Wilsey, R. B. *Am. J. Roentgenol. 30:* 234-241, 388-400, 523-528, 1933.

Recent Hypotheses Concerning the Mechanism of Photographic Development. James, T. H. *J.P.S.A. 13:*608-614, 1947.

The Photographic Function. Levenson, G. I. P. *Functional Photo., 1:*10-11, 1950.

Atoms in Action. Poultney, L. *Radiographer, 5:*7-10, 1954.

Meet the Electron. Levenson, G.I.P. *Functional Photo., 1:*15-17, 1950.

Reduction and Oxidation. Levenson, G. I. P. *Functional Photo., 1:*19-22, 1950.

Practical Roentgenographic Importance of Reciprocity Law Failure. Frantzell, A. *Acta Radiol. 34:*6-15, 1950.

SCREENS

Sensitometry of Roentgenographic Films and Screens. Morgan, R. H. and Van Allen, W. W. *Radiology, 52:*832-845, 1949.

Screen Intensification Systems and Their Limitations. Sturm, R. E., and Morgan, R. H. *Am. J. Roentgenol. 62:*617-634, 1949.

Edison and Roentgenology. Fuchs, A. W. *Am. J. Roentgenol. 57:*145-156, 1947.

Radiographic Recording Media and Screens. Fuchs, A. W. In the Science of Radiology, Otto Glasser, editor. Springfield, Thomas, 1933.

SECONDARY RADIATION

Remarks on the Measurements of Scattered Radiation. Hodgson, M. B. *Am. J. Roentgenol. 8:*338-339, 1921.

Intensity of Scattered X-rays in Radiography. Wilsey, R. B. *Am. J. Roentgenol. 8:*328-338, 1921.

The Effects of Scattered X-rays in Radiography. Wilsey, R. B. *Am. J. Roentgenol. 8:* 589-598, 1921.

The Efficiency of the Bucky-Diaphragm Principle. Wilsey, R. B. *Am. J. Roentgenol. 9:* 58-66, 1922.

The Reduction of Secondary Radiation and of Excessive Radiographic Contrast by Filtration. Seeman, H. E. *Am. Soc. Test. Materials, 40:*1289-1296, 1940.

TECHNIC

The Optimum Kilovoltage Technique in Military Roentgenography. Fuchs, A. W. *Am. J. Roentgenol. 50:*358-365, 1943.

Selection of Optimum Kilovoltage for Dental Radiography. Wuehrmann, A. H. and Monacelli, C. J. *Radiology, 57:*240-246, 1951.

Military Photoroentgen Technique Employing Optimum Kilvolt (Peak) Principles. Fuchs, A. W. *Am. J. Roentgenol. 53:*587-596, 1945.

Suggestions for Simplifying Technique in Diagnostic Roentgenology. Huyler, W. C. *Am. J. Roentgenol. 39:*967-971, 1938.

Roentgenographic Soft Tissue Study in an Orthopedic Hospital. Lewis, R. W. *Am. J. Roentgenol. 48:*634-642, 1942.

The Contrast Problem in High Kilovoltage Medical Radiography. Nemet, A., Cox, W. F., and Hills, T. H. *Brit. J. Radiol. 26:*185-192, 1953.

The Miniature X-ray Chest Film. Potter, H. E., *et al. Radiology, 34:*283-291, 1940.

A Thickness Technique for Radiography of the Chest. Steven, G. D. *Radiography, 22:* 220-222, 1956.

Simplification of Roentgenography by High Kilovoltage Technique. Teplick, J. G. *Am. J. Roentgenol. 56:*660-667, 1946.

High Voltage Radiography. Trout, E. D., Graves, D. E., and Slauson, D. B. *Radiology, 52:*669-683, 1949.

Trend for Higher Kilovoltage for Adequate Penetration. Yurcessen, E. H. *X-ray Tech. 25:*96-99, 1954.

Soft Tissue Radiography. Frantzell, A. *Acta Radiol., Suppl. 85,* 1951.

Radiology of Soft Tissue. Drey, L. *Brit. J. Radiol. 26:*619-627, 1953.

Radiography of Air and Fluids. Jaundrell-Thompson, F. *Radiography, 19:*233-245, 1953.

Use of Additional Filtration in Medical Radiography. Gifford, D. and Truscott, D. E. *Brit. J. Radiol. 27:*113-116, 1954.

Compensating Filters in Medical Radiography. Funke, T. *X-ray Tech. 27:*12-27, 1955.

MISCELLANEOUS

Medical Photography, Radiographic and Clinical. Longmore, T. A. London and New York, Focal Press, 1955.

Practical Photographic Problems in Radiography. Mattson, O. *Acta Radiol., Suppl. 120,* 1955.

Fundamentals of Radiography, 7th Ed. Rochester, New York, Eastman Kodak Company, 1951.

Index

Clarence W. Donnelly, R.T. (ARRT)